50% OFF

Online CMA Prep Course!

By Mometrix

Dear Customer,

We consider it an honor and a privilege that you chose our Certified Medical Assistant Study Guide. As a way of showing our appreciation and to help us better serve you, we are offering **50% off our online CMA Prep Course**. Many Certified Medical Assistant courses are needlessly expensive and don't deliver enough value. With our course, you get access to the best CMA prep material, and **you only pay half price**.

We have structured our online course to perfectly complement your printed study guide. The CMA Prep Course contains **in-depth lessons** that cover all the most important topics, **30+ video reviews** that explain difficult concepts, over **750+ practice questions** to ensure you feel prepared, and more than **300+ digital flashcards**, so you can study while you're on the go.

Online Certified Medical Assistant Prep Course

Topics Included:

- Clinical Competency
  - Medical Terminology
  - First Aid, CPR, and Emergency Response
  - The Systems of the Body
- General
  - Therapeutic Communication
  - Grief and Loss
- Administrative
  - Financial Bookkeeping
  - Medical Transcription
  - Business Practices

Course Features:

- CMA Study Guide
  - Get content that complements our best-selling study guide.
- 4 Full-Length Practice Tests
  - With over 750+ practice questions, you can test yourself again and again.
- Mobile Friendly
  - If you need to study on the go, the course is easily accessible from your mobile device.
- CMA Flashcards
  - Our course includes a flashcard mode with 300+ content cards to help you study.

To receive this discount, visit us at mometrix.com/university/cma/ or simply scan this QR code with your smartphone. At the checkout page, enter the discount code: **cma50off**

If you have any questions or concerns, please contact us at support@mometrix.com.

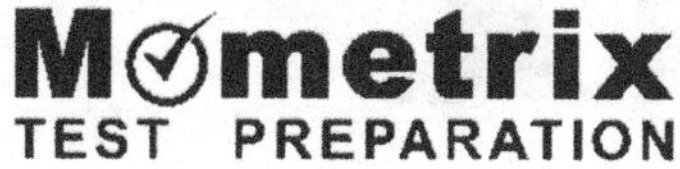

FREE Study Skills Videos/DVD Offer

Dear Customer,

Thank you for your purchase from Mometrix! We consider it an honor and a privilege that you have purchased our product and we want to ensure your satisfaction.

As part of our ongoing effort to meet the needs of test takers, we have developed a set of Study Skills Videos that we would like to give you for FREE. These videos cover our *best practices* for getting ready for your exam, from how to use our study materials to how to best prepare for the day of the test.

All that we ask is that you email us with feedback that would describe your experience so far with our product. Good, bad, or indifferent, we want to know what you think!

To get your FREE Study Skills Videos, you can use the **QR code** below, or send us an **email** at studyvideos@mometrix.com with *FREE VIDEOS* in the subject line and the following information in the body of the email:

- The name of the product you purchased.
- Your product rating on a scale of 1-5, with 5 being the highest rating.
- Your feedback. It can be long, short, or anything in between. We just want to know your impressions and experience so far with our product. (Good feedback might include how our study material met your needs and ways we might be able to make it even better. You could highlight features that you found helpful or features that you think we should add.)

If you have any questions or concerns, please don't hesitate to contact me directly.

Thanks again!

Sincerely,

Jay Willis
Vice President
jay.willis@mometrix.com
1-800-673-8175

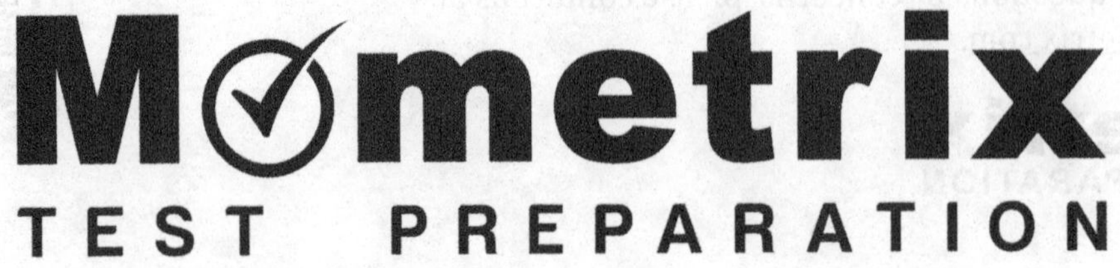

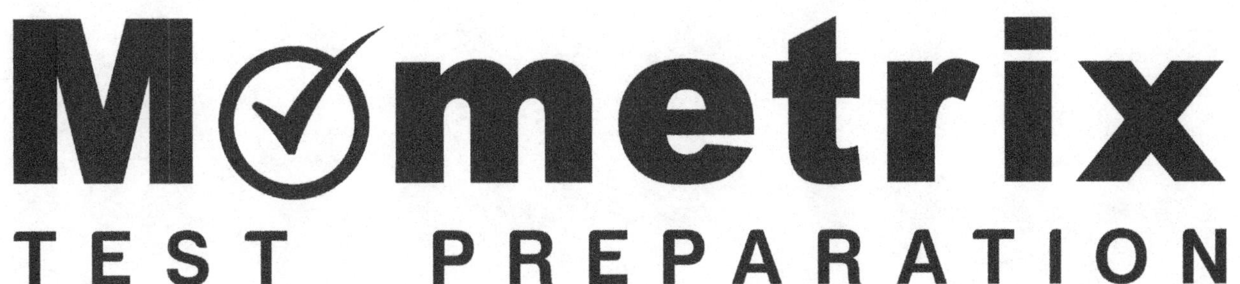

Certified Medical Assistant Exam Prep Book 2023-2024

750+ Practice Test Questions

CMA Secrets Study Guide with Detailed Answer Explanations

4th Edition

Written and edited by Mometrix Test Prep

Printed in the United States of America

This paper meets the requirements of ANSI/NISO Z39.48-1992 (Permanence of Paper).

Paperback
ISBN 13: 978-1-5167-2193-1
ISBN 10: 1-5167-2193-4

Dear Future Exam Success Story

First of all, **THANK YOU** for purchasing Mometrix study materials!

Second, congratulations! You are one of the few determined test-takers who are committed to doing whatever it takes to excel on your exam. **You have come to the right place.** We developed these study materials with one goal in mind: to deliver you the information you need in a format that's concise and easy to use.

In addition to optimizing your guide for the content of the test, we've outlined our recommended steps for breaking down the preparation process into small, attainable goals so you can make sure you stay on track.

We've also analyzed the entire test-taking process, identifying the most common pitfalls and showing how you can overcome them and be ready for any curveball the test throws you.

Standardized testing is one of the biggest obstacles on your road to success, which only increases the importance of doing well in the high-pressure, high-stakes environment of test day. Your results on this test could have a significant impact on your future, and this guide provides the information and practical advice to help you achieve your full potential on test day.

Your success is our success

We would love to hear from you! If you would like to share the story of your exam success or if you have any questions or comments in regard to our products, please contact us at **800-673-8175** or **support@mometrix.com**.

Thanks again for your business and we wish you continued success!

Sincerely,
The Mometrix Test Preparation Team

Need more help? Check out our flashcards at:
http://MometrixFlashcards.com/MedicalAssistant

TABLE OF CONTENTS

Introduction

Thank you for purchasing this resource! You have made the choice to prepare yourself for a test that could have a huge impact on your future, and this guide is designed to help you be fully ready for test day. Obviously, it's important to have a solid understanding of the test material, but you also need to be prepared for the unique environment and stressors of the test, so that you can perform to the best of your abilities.

For this purpose, the first section that appears in this guide is the **Secret Keys**. We've devoted countless hours to meticulously researching what works and what doesn't, and we've boiled down our findings to the five most impactful steps you can take to improve your performance on the test. We start at the beginning with study planning and move through the preparation process, all the way to the testing strategies that will help you get the most out of what you know when you're finally sitting in front of the test.

We recommend that you start preparing for your test as far in advance as possible. However, if you've bought this guide as a last-minute study resource and only have a few days before your test, we recommend that you skip over the first two Secret Keys since they address a long-term study plan.

If you struggle with **test anxiety**, we strongly encourage you to check out our recommendations for how you can overcome it. Test anxiety is a formidable foe, but it can be beaten, and we want to make sure you have the tools you need to defeat it.

Secret Key #1 – Plan Big, Study Small

There's a lot riding on your performance. If you want to ace this test, you're going to need to keep your skills sharp and the material fresh in your mind. You need a plan that lets you review everything you need to know while still fitting in your schedule. We'll break this strategy down into three categories.

Information Organization

Start with the information you already have: the official test outline. From this, you can make a complete list of all the concepts you need to cover before the test. Organize these concepts into groups that can be studied together, and create a list of any related vocabulary you need to learn so you can brush up on any difficult terms. You'll want to keep this vocabulary list handy once you actually start studying since you may need to add to it along the way.

Time Management

Once you have your set of study concepts, decide how to spread them out over the time you have left before the test. Break your study plan into small, clear goals so you have a manageable task for each day and know exactly what you're doing. Then just focus on one small step at a time. When you manage your time this way, you don't need to spend hours at a time studying. Studying a small block of content for a short period each day helps you retain information better and avoid stressing over how much you have left to do. You can relax knowing that you have a plan to cover everything in time. In order for this strategy to be effective though, you have to start studying early and stick to your schedule. Avoid the exhaustion and futility that comes from last-minute cramming!

Study Environment

The environment you study in has a big impact on your learning. Studying in a coffee shop, while probably more enjoyable, is not likely to be as fruitful as studying in a quiet room. It's important to keep distractions to a minimum. You're only planning to study for a short block of time, so make the most of it. Don't pause to check your phone or get up to find a snack. It's also important to **avoid multitasking**. Research has consistently shown that multitasking will make your studying dramatically less effective. Your study area should also be comfortable and well-lit so you don't have the distraction of straining your eyes or sitting on an uncomfortable chair.

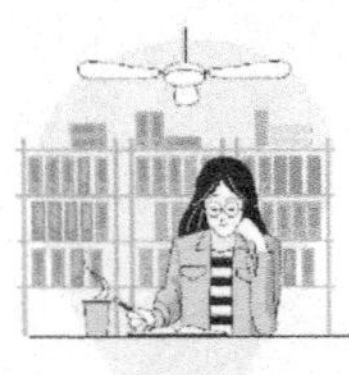

The time of day you study is also important. You want to be rested and alert. Don't wait until just before bedtime. Study when you'll be most likely to comprehend and remember. Even better, if you know what time of day your test will be, set that time aside for study. That way your brain will be used to working on that subject at that specific time and you'll have a better chance of recalling information.

Finally, it can be helpful to team up with others who are studying for the same test. Your actual studying should be done in as isolated an environment as possible, but the work of organizing the information and setting up the study plan can be divided up. In between study sessions, you can discuss with your teammates the concepts that you're all studying and quiz each other on the details. Just be sure that your teammates are as serious about the test as you are. If you find that your study time is being replaced with social time, you might need to find a new team.

Secret Key #2 – Make Your Studying Count

You're devoting a lot of time and effort to preparing for this test, so you want to be absolutely certain it will pay off. This means doing more than just reading the content and hoping you can remember it on test day. It's important to make every minute of study count. There are two main areas you can focus on to make your studying count.

Retention

It doesn't matter how much time you study if you can't remember the material. You need to make sure you are retaining the concepts. To check your retention of the information you're learning, try recalling it at later times with minimal prompting. Try carrying around flashcards and glance at one or two from time to time or ask a friend who's also studying for the test to quiz you.

To enhance your retention, look for ways to put the information into practice so that you can apply it rather than simply recalling it. If you're using the information in practical ways, it will be much easier to remember. Similarly, it helps to solidify a concept in your mind if you're not only reading it to yourself but also explaining it to someone else. Ask a friend to let you teach them about a concept you're a little shaky on (or speak aloud to an imaginary audience if necessary). As you try to summarize, define, give examples, and answer your friend's questions, you'll understand the concepts better and they will stay with you longer. Finally, step back for a big picture view and ask yourself how each piece of information fits with the whole subject. When you link the different concepts together and see them working together as a whole, it's easier to remember the individual components.

Finally, practice showing your work on any multi-step problems, even if you're just studying. Writing out each step you take to solve a problem will help solidify the process in your mind, and you'll be more likely to remember it during the test.

Modality

Modality simply refers to the means or method by which you study. Choosing a study modality that fits your own individual learning style is crucial. No two people learn best in exactly the same way, so it's important to know your strengths and use them to your advantage.

For example, if you learn best by visualization, focus on visualizing a concept in your mind and draw an image or a diagram. Try color-coding your notes, illustrating them, or creating symbols that will trigger your mind to recall a learned concept. If you learn best by hearing or discussing information, find a study partner who learns the same way or read aloud to yourself. Think about how to put the information in your own words. Imagine that you are giving a lecture on the topic and record yourself so you can listen to it later.

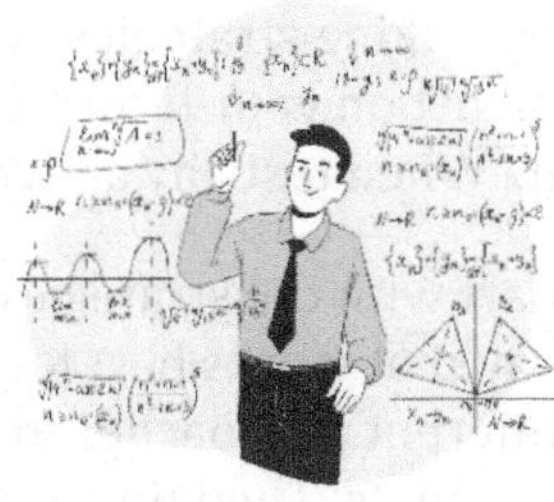

For any learning style, flashcards can be helpful. Organize the information so you can take advantage of spare moments to review. Underline key words or phrases. Use different colors for different categories. Mnemonic devices (such as creating a short list in which every item starts with the same letter) can also help with retention. Find what works best for you and use it to store the information in your mind most effectively and easily.

Secret Key #3 – Practice the Right Way

Your success on test day depends not only on how many hours you put into preparing, but also on whether you prepared the right way. It's good to check along the way to see if your studying is paying off. One of the most effective ways to do this is by taking practice tests to evaluate your progress. Practice tests are useful because they show exactly where you need to improve. Every time you take a practice test, pay special attention to these three groups of questions:

- The questions you got wrong
- The questions you had to guess on, even if you guessed right
- The questions you found difficult or slow to work through

This will show you exactly what your weak areas are, and where you need to devote more study time. Ask yourself why each of these questions gave you trouble. Was it because you didn't understand the material? Was it because you didn't remember the vocabulary? Do you need more repetitions on this type of question to build speed and confidence? Dig into those questions and figure out how you can strengthen your weak areas as you go back to review the material.

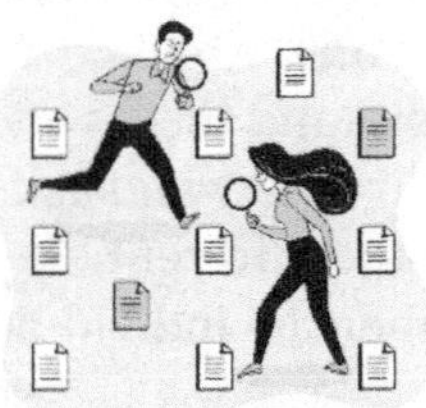

Additionally, many practice tests have a section explaining the answer choices. It can be tempting to read the explanation and think that you now have a good understanding of the concept. However, an explanation likely only covers part of the question's broader context. Even if the explanation makes perfect sense, **go back and investigate** every concept related to the question until you're positive you have a thorough understanding.

As you go along, keep in mind that the practice test is just that: practice. Memorizing these questions and answers will not be very helpful on the actual test because it is unlikely to have any of the same exact questions. If you only know the right answers to the sample questions, you won't be prepared for the real thing. **Study the concepts** until you understand them fully, and then you'll be able to answer any question that shows up on the test.

It's important to wait on the practice tests until you're ready. If you take a test on your first day of study, you may be overwhelmed by the amount of material covered and how much you need to learn. Work up to it gradually.

On test day, you'll need to be prepared for answering questions, managing your time, and using the test-taking strategies you've learned. It's a lot to balance, like a mental marathon that will have a big impact on your future. Like training for a marathon, you'll need to start slowly and work your way up. When test day arrives, you'll be ready.

Start with the strategies you've read in the first two Secret Keys—plan your course and study in the way that works best for you. If you have time, consider using multiple study resources to get different approaches to the same concepts. It can be helpful to see difficult concepts from more than one angle. Then find a good source for practice tests. Many times, the test website will suggest potential study resources or provide sample tests.

Practice Test Strategy

If you're able to find at least three practice tests, we recommend this strategy:

Untimed and Open-Book Practice

Take the first test with no time constraints and with your notes and study guide handy. Take your time and focus on applying the strategies you've learned.

Timed and Open-Book Practice

Take the second practice test open-book as well, but set a timer and practice pacing yourself to finish in time.

Timed and Closed-Book Practice

Take any other practice tests as if it were test day. Set a timer and put away your study materials. Sit at a table or desk in a quiet room, imagine yourself at the testing center, and answer questions as quickly and accurately as possible.

Keep repeating timed and closed-book tests on a regular basis until you run out of practice tests or it's time for the actual test. Your mind will be ready for the schedule and stress of test day, and you'll be able to focus on recalling the material you've learned.

Secret Key #4 – Pace Yourself

Once you're fully prepared for the material on the test, your biggest challenge on test day will be managing your time. Just knowing that the clock is ticking can make you panic even if you have plenty of time left. Work on pacing yourself so you can build confidence against the time constraints of the exam. Pacing is a difficult skill to master, especially in a high-pressure environment, so **practice is vital.**

Set time expectations for your pace based on how much time is available. For example, if a section has 60 questions and the time limit is 30 minutes, you know you have to average 30 seconds or less per question in order to answer them all. Although 30 seconds is the hard limit, set 25 seconds per question as your goal, so you reserve extra time to spend on harder questions. When you budget extra time for the harder questions, you no longer have any reason to stress when those questions take longer to answer.

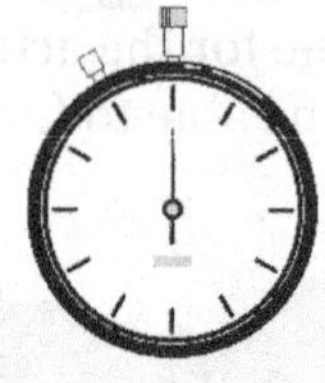

Don't let this time expectation distract you from working through the test at a calm, steady pace, but keep it in mind so you don't spend too much time on any one question. Recognize that taking extra time on one question you don't understand may keep you from answering two that you do understand later in the test. If your time limit for a question is up and you're still not sure of the answer, mark it and move on, and come back to it later if the time and the test format allow. If the testing format doesn't allow you to return to earlier questions, just make an educated guess; then put it out of your mind and move on.

On the easier questions, be careful not to rush. It may seem wise to hurry through them so you have more time for the challenging ones, but it's not worth missing one if you know the concept and just didn't take the time to read the question fully. Work efficiently but make sure you understand the question and have looked at all of the answer choices, since more than one may seem right at first.

Even if you're paying attention to the time, you may find yourself a little behind at some point. You should speed up to get back on track, but do so wisely. Don't panic; just take a few seconds less on each question until you're caught up. Don't guess without thinking, but do look through the answer choices and eliminate any you know are wrong. If you can get down to two choices, it is often worthwhile to guess from those. Once you've chosen an answer, move on and don't dwell on any that you skipped or had to hurry through. If a question was taking too long, chances are it was one of the harder ones, so you weren't as likely to get it right anyway.

On the other hand, if you find yourself getting ahead of schedule, it may be beneficial to slow down a little. The more quickly you work, the more likely you are to make a careless mistake that will affect your score. You've budgeted time for each question, so don't be afraid to spend that time. Practice an efficient but careful pace to get the most out of the time you have.

Secret Key #5 – Have a Plan for Guessing

When you're taking the test, you may find yourself stuck on a question. Some of the answer choices seem better than others, but you don't see the one answer choice that is obviously correct. What do you do?

The scenario described above is very common, yet most test takers have not effectively prepared for it. Developing and practicing a plan for guessing may be one of the single most effective uses of your time as you get ready for the exam.

In developing your plan for guessing, there are three questions to address:

- When should you start the guessing process?
- How should you narrow down the choices?
- Which answer should you choose?

When to Start the Guessing Process

Unless your plan for guessing is to select C every time (which, despite its merits, is not what we recommend), you need to leave yourself enough time to apply your answer elimination strategies. Since you have a limited amount of time for each question, that means that if you're going to give yourself the best shot at guessing correctly, you have to decide quickly whether or not you will guess.

Of course, the best-case scenario is that you don't have to guess at all, so first, see if you can answer the question based on your knowledge of the subject and basic reasoning skills. Focus on the key words in the question and try to jog your memory of related topics. Give yourself a chance to bring the knowledge to mind, but once you realize that you don't have (or you can't access) the knowledge you need to answer the question, it's time to start the guessing process.

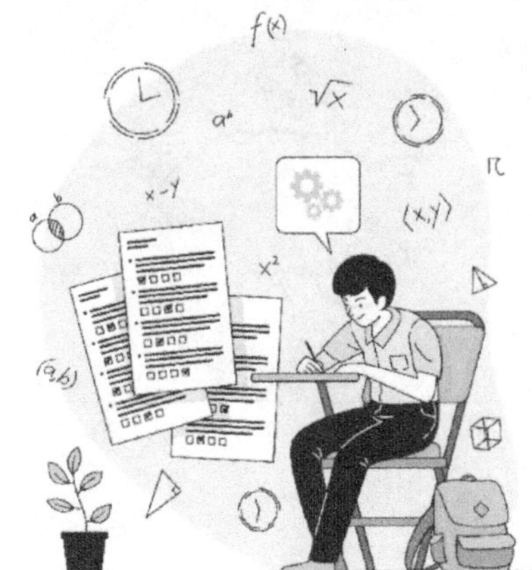

It's almost always better to start the guessing process too early than too late. It only takes a few seconds to remember something and answer the question from knowledge. Carefully eliminating wrong answer choices takes longer. Plus, going through the process of eliminating answer choices can actually help jog your memory.

Summary: Start the guessing process as soon as you decide that you can't answer the question based on your knowledge.

How to Narrow Down the Choices

The next chapter in this book (**Test-Taking Strategies**) includes a wide range of strategies for how to approach questions and how to look for answer choices to eliminate. You will definitely want to read those carefully, practice them, and figure out which ones work best for you. Here though, we're going to address a mindset rather than a particular strategy.

Your odds of guessing an answer correctly depend on how many options you are choosing from.

Number of options left	5	4	3	2	1
Odds of guessing correctly	20%	25%	33%	50%	100%

You can see from this chart just how valuable it is to be able to eliminate incorrect answers and make an educated guess, but there are two things that many test takers do that cause them to miss out on the benefits of guessing:

- Accidentally eliminating the correct answer
- Selecting an answer based on an impression

We'll look at the first one here, and the second one in the next section.

To avoid accidentally eliminating the correct answer, we recommend a thought exercise called **the $5 challenge**. In this challenge, you only eliminate an answer choice from contention if you are willing to bet $5 on it being wrong. Why $5? Five dollars is a small but not insignificant amount of money. It's an amount you could afford to lose but wouldn't want to throw away. And while losing $5 once might not hurt too much, doing it twenty times will set you back $100. In the same way, each small decision you make—eliminating a choice here, guessing on a question there—won't by itself impact your score very much, but when you put them all together, they can make a big difference. By holding each answer choice elimination decision to a higher standard, you can reduce the risk of accidentally eliminating the correct answer.

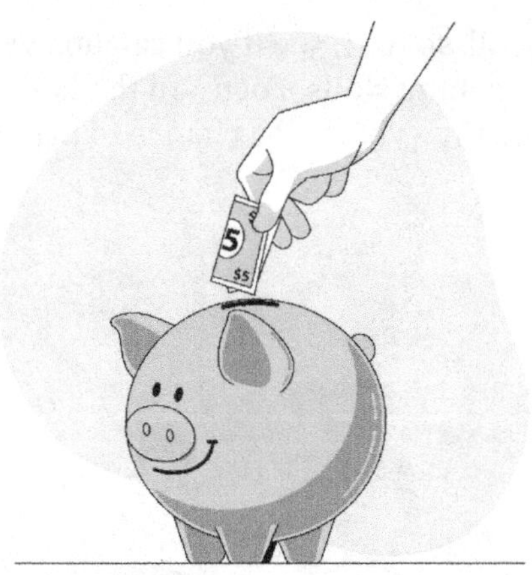

The $5 challenge can also be applied in a positive sense: If you are willing to bet $5 that an answer choice *is* correct, go ahead and mark it as correct.

Summary: Only eliminate an answer choice if you are willing to bet $5 that it is wrong.

Which Answer to Choose

You're taking the test. You've run into a hard question and decided you'll have to guess. You've eliminated all the answer choices you're willing to bet $5 on. Now you have to pick an answer. Why do we even need to talk about this? Why can't you just pick whichever one you feel like when the time comes?

The answer to these questions is that if you don't come into the test with a plan, you'll rely on your impression to select an answer choice, and if you do that, you risk falling into a trap. The test writers know that everyone who takes their test will be guessing on some of the questions, so they intentionally write wrong answer choices to seem plausible. You still have to pick an answer though, and if the wrong answer choices are designed to look right, how can you ever be sure that you're not falling for their trap? The best solution we've found to this dilemma is to take the decision out of your hands entirely. Here is the process we recommend:

Once you've eliminated any choices that you are confident (willing to bet $5) are wrong, select the first remaining choice as your answer.

Whether you choose to select the first remaining choice, the second, or the last, the important thing is that you use some preselected standard. Using this approach guarantees that you will not be enticed into selecting an answer choice that looks right, because you are not basing your decision on how the answer choices look.

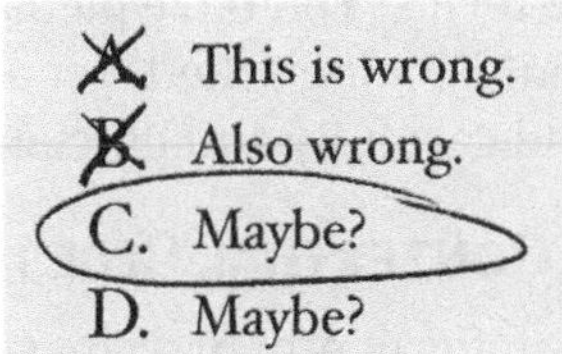

This is not meant to make you question your knowledge. Instead, it is to help you recognize the difference between your knowledge and your impressions. There's a huge difference between thinking an answer is right because of what you know, and thinking an answer is right because it looks or sounds like it should be right.

Summary: To ensure that your selection is appropriately random, make a predetermined selection from among all answer choices you have not eliminated.

Test-Taking Strategies

This section contains a list of test-taking strategies that you may find helpful as you work through the test. By taking what you know and applying logical thought, you can maximize your chances of answering any question correctly!

It is very important to realize that every question is different and every person is different: no single strategy will work on every question, and no single strategy will work for every person. That's why we've included all of them here, so you can try them out and determine which ones work best for different types of questions and which ones work best for you.

Question Strategies

☑ Read Carefully

Read the question and the answer choices carefully. Don't miss the question because you misread the terms. You have plenty of time to read each question thoroughly and make sure you understand what is being asked. Yet a happy medium must be attained, so don't waste too much time. You must read carefully and efficiently.

☑ Contextual Clues

Look for contextual clues. If the question includes a word you are not familiar with, look at the immediate context for some indication of what the word might mean. Contextual clues can often give you all the information you need to decipher the meaning of an unfamiliar word. Even if you can't determine the meaning, you may be able to narrow down the possibilities enough to make a solid guess at the answer to the question.

☑ Prefixes

If you're having trouble with a word in the question or answer choices, try dissecting it. Take advantage of every clue that the word might include. Prefixes can be a huge help. Usually, they allow you to determine a basic meaning. *Pre-* means before, *post-* means after, *pro-* is positive, *de-* is negative. From prefixes, you can get an idea of the general meaning of the word and try to put it into context.

☑ Hedge Words

Watch out for critical hedge words, such as *likely, may, can, sometimes, often, almost, mostly, usually, generally, rarely,* and *sometimes.* Question writers insert these hedge phrases to cover every possibility. Often an answer choice will be wrong simply because it leaves no room for exception. Be on guard for answer choices that have definitive words such as *exactly* and *always.*

☑ Switchback Words

Stay alert for *switchbacks.* These are the words and phrases frequently used to alert you to shifts in thought. The most common switchback words are *but, although,* and *however.* Others include *nevertheless, on the other hand, even though, while, in spite of, despite,* and *regardless of.* Switchback words are important to catch because they can change the direction of the question or an answer choice.

✓ Face Value

When in doubt, use common sense. Accept the situation in the problem at face value. Don't read too much into it. These problems will not require you to make wild assumptions. If you have to go beyond creativity and warp time or space in order to have an answer choice fit the question, then you should move on and consider the other answer choices. These are normal problems rooted in reality. The applicable relationship or explanation may not be readily apparent, but it is there for you to figure out. Use your common sense to interpret anything that isn't clear.

Answer Choice Strategies

✓ Answer Selection

The most thorough way to pick an answer choice is to identify and eliminate wrong answers until only one is left, then confirm it is the correct answer. Sometimes an answer choice may immediately seem right, but be careful. The test writers will usually put more than one reasonable answer choice on each question, so take a second to read all of them and make sure that the other choices are not equally obvious. As long as you have time left, it is better to read every answer choice than to pick the first one that looks right without checking the others.

✓ Answer Choice Families

An answer choice family consists of two (in rare cases, three) answer choices that are very similar in construction and cannot all be true at the same time. If you see two answer choices that are direct opposites or parallels, one of them is usually the correct answer. For instance, if one answer choice says that quantity x increases and another either says that quantity x decreases (opposite) or says that quantity y increases (parallel), then those answer choices would fall into the same family. An answer choice that doesn't match the construction of the answer choice family is more likely to be incorrect. Most questions will not have answer choice families, but when they do appear, you should be prepared to recognize them.

✓ Eliminate Answers

Eliminate answer choices as soon as you realize they are wrong, but make sure you consider all possibilities. If you are eliminating answer choices and realize that the last one you are left with is also wrong, don't panic. Start over and consider each choice again. There may be something you missed the first time that you will realize on the second pass.

✓ Avoid Fact Traps

Don't be distracted by an answer choice that is factually true but doesn't answer the question. You are looking for the choice that answers the question. Stay focused on what the question is asking for so you don't accidentally pick an answer that is true but incorrect. Always go back to the question and make sure the answer choice you've selected actually answers the question and is not merely a true statement.

✓ Extreme Statements

In general, you should avoid answers that put forth extreme actions as standard practice or proclaim controversial ideas as established fact. An answer choice that states the "process should be used in certain situations, if..." is much more likely to be correct than one that states the "process should be discontinued completely." The first is a calm rational statement and doesn't even make a definitive, uncompromising stance, using a hedge word *if* to provide wiggle room, whereas the second choice is far more extreme.

⊘ Benchmark

As you read through the answer choices and you come across one that seems to answer the question well, mentally select that answer choice. This is not your final answer, but it's the one that will help you evaluate the other answer choices. The one that you selected is your benchmark or standard for judging each of the other answer choices. Every other answer choice must be compared to your benchmark. That choice is correct until proven otherwise by another answer choice beating it. If you find a better answer, then that one becomes your new benchmark. Once you've decided that no other choice answers the question as well as your benchmark, you have your final answer.

⊘ Predict the Answer

Before you even start looking at the answer choices, it is often best to try to predict the answer. When you come up with the answer on your own, it is easier to avoid distractions and traps because you will know exactly what to look for. The right answer choice is unlikely to be word-for-word what you came up with, but it should be a close match. Even if you are confident that you have the right answer, you should still take the time to read each option before moving on.

General Strategies

⊘ Tough Questions

If you are stumped on a problem or it appears too hard or too difficult, don't waste time. Move on! Remember though, if you can quickly check for obviously incorrect answer choices, your chances of guessing correctly are greatly improved. Before you completely give up, at least try to knock out a couple of possible answers. Eliminate what you can and then guess at the remaining answer choices before moving on.

⊘ Check Your Work

Since you will probably not know every term listed and the answer to every question, it is important that you get credit for the ones that you do know. Don't miss any questions through careless mistakes. If at all possible, try to take a second to look back over your answer selection and make sure you've selected the correct answer choice and haven't made a costly careless mistake (such as marking an answer choice that you didn't mean to mark). This quick double check should more than pay for itself in caught mistakes for the time it costs.

⊘ Pace Yourself

It's easy to be overwhelmed when you're looking at a page full of questions; your mind is confused and full of random thoughts, and the clock is ticking down faster than you would like. Calm down and maintain the pace that you have set for yourself. Especially as you get down to the last few minutes of the test, don't let the small numbers on the clock make you panic. As long as you are on track by monitoring your pace, you are guaranteed to have time for each question.

⊘ Don't Rush

It is very easy to make errors when you are in a hurry. Maintaining a fast pace in answering questions is pointless if it makes you miss questions that you would have gotten right otherwise. Test writers like to include distracting information and wrong answers that seem right. Taking a little extra time to avoid careless mistakes can make all the difference in your test score. Find a pace that allows you to be confident in the answers that you select.

⊘ Keep Moving

Panicking will not help you pass the test, so do your best to stay calm and keep moving. Taking deep breaths and going through the answer elimination steps you practiced can help to break through a stress barrier and keep your pace.

Final Notes

The combination of a solid foundation of content knowledge and the confidence that comes from practicing your plan for applying that knowledge is the key to maximizing your performance on test day. As your foundation of content knowledge is built up and strengthened, you'll find that the strategies included in this chapter become more and more effective in helping you quickly sift through the distractions and traps of the test to isolate the correct answer.

Now that you're preparing to move forward into the test content chapters of this book, be sure to keep your goal in mind. As you read, think about how you will be able to apply this information on the test. If you've already seen sample questions for the test and you have an idea of the question format and style, try to come up with questions of your own that you can answer based on what you're reading. This will give you valuable practice applying your knowledge in the same ways you can expect to on test day.

Good luck and good studying!

Clinical Competency

Transform passive reading into active learning! After immersing yourself in this chapter, put your comprehension to the test by taking a quiz. The insights you gained will stay with you longer this way. Scan the QR code to go directly to the chapter quiz interface for this study guide. If you're using a computer, simply visit the bonus page at **mometrix.com/bonus948/certmedasst** and click the Chapter Quizzes link.

Vital Signs

Stable Vital Signs

Stable vital signs (those maintained within the normal range for the individual's age) indicate good health (homeostasis). Ill or injured patients have vital signs outside the normal range. The severity of the illness or injury is often indicated by the variability of vital sign measurements. Wide variations mean the patient is unstable. Their vital signs should be checked every five minutes. For stable patients, vital signs can be checked less frequently, depending on the circumstance. The following parameters are considered vital signs:

- Pulse
- Respiration rate
- Blood pressure
- Oxygen saturation
- Temperature

Pulse

The pulse is a surge of blood through an artery that occurs when the heart contracts (during systole). The key **pulse points** are:

- **Apical**: Over the heart
- **Brachial**: In the elbow bend (most common site for palpation in children under 1 year)
- **Carotid**: In the neck (for pulse checks in unconscious patients; be sure to only palpate one side at a time to maintain perfusion to the brain)
- **Dorsalis pedis**: On top of the foot
- **Facial**: On the jaw under the mouth
- **Femoral**: In the groin (for pulse checks in unconscious patients)
- **Popliteal**: On the back of the knee
- **Posterior tibial**: On the back of the ankle
- **Radial**: On the anterior wrist below the thumb (most common site for palpation in patients older than 1 year)
- **Temporal**: On the temple
- **Ulnar**: On the anterior wrist below the little finger

Pulse **rate** varies by age:

Normal Resting Pulse Rate	Age
60-100 beats per minute	Adult
80-100 beats per minute	Child

Normal Resting Pulse Rate	Age
100 beats per minute	Toddler
100-140 beats per minute	Infant under one year
up to 150 beats per minute	Newborn (neonate)

Distal Pulse and Pulse Deficit

If a **distal pulse** cannot be felt in the patient's limbs, first utilize a doppler machine to find the pulse. If it still cannot be found, find the apical pulse in the chest. Count to the 5th rib space in the middle of the left side of the chest or midclavicular line. If the apical pulse is regular, count for 30 seconds and record the reading. If the apical pulse is irregular, count for a full minute and record the reading. Report an irregular pulse to the doctor to evaluate for possible pulse deficit. A **pulse deficit** occurs when the radial pulse in the wrist is slower than the apical pulse in the chest. A pulse deficit can indicate that the patient has weak heart contractions, which fail to transmit beats to the peripheral arterial system.

Tachycardia and Bradycardia

Tachycardia is a pulse rate over 100 beats per minute, which may be caused by anxiety, fear, stress, pneumonia, anemia, low blood pressure, dehydration, fever, infection, hyperthyroidism, and heart conditions.

Bradycardia is a resting heart rate less than 60 beats per minute, which may be caused by a heart attack (MI), hypothermia, heat exhaustion, obstructive jaundice, skull fracture, malnutrition, hypothyroidism, and many adverse drug reactions. Olympic athletes may have bradycardia because their hearts are extremely efficient.

Measuring Respirations

Measuring respirations is done to assess the number of times per minute the patient breathes. Typically, when a person is made aware of his breathing, he does not breathe deeply or regularly. Do not tell the patient when measuring the respiration rate, as it may make them aware of their breathing and produce an inaccurate result. The ideal time to measure the patient's respiration rate is after checking the patient's pulse. Count the number of times the patient breathes, counting one rise and fall of the chest wall as one respiration. Count the number of breaths for one minute, noting the depth of the breath and any use of accessory muscles. Record the respiratory rate on the patient's chart.

Indications of Abnormal Respirations

The normal range for respiratory rate for adults is 12-20 breaths per minute. A number of factors may affect the rate of the patient's breathing. The patient may breathe more slowly if resting or if he is positioned on his back. Certain narcotics may also depress the respiratory drive, resulting in fewer breaths per minute. A rapid respiration rate may be caused by increased activity, pain, or stress. An elevated temperature or an infection may cause the patient's respiratory rate to be quicker. Other conditions, such as respiratory distress, fluid overload, or a heart attack, may also cause an elevated respiratory rate.

Blood Pressure

Increased blood pressure contributes to stroke and heart disease. Low blood pressure is associated with shock, trauma, bleeding, or severe infection. Blood pressure is defined by the following parameters:

- Normal adult blood pressure: Systole <120 mmHg, diastole <80 mmHg
- Prehypertension: Systole 120-129, diastole <80
- Hypertension stage 1: Systole 130-139, diastole 80-89
- Hypertension stage 2: Systole ≥140, diastole ≥90
- Hypotension (low blood pressure): 90/50 or less

False BP reading can occur from the following:

- **Incorrect cuff size**: If the patient is obese, use a thigh cuff on the upper arm. Bariatric blood pressure cuffs also exist. If the patient is a child, use a pediatric cuff.
- **Deflating the cuff more rapidly** than 2–3 mmHg per second can inhibit the ability to accurately record both systole and diastole.
- **Venous congestion** makes it difficult to hear the blood pressure sounds. Elevating the patient's arm after positioning the cuff but before inflating it can decrease venous congestion.
- Loud **environmental noises**
- **Operator error**

Aneroid Sphygmomanometer

Blood pressure is measured as systolic and diastolic pressure by means of a stethoscope and an **aneroid sphygmomanometer** (portable blood pressure cuff). For example, if the reading is 120/80 mmHg, 120 is the systole, and 80 is the diastole. The first Korotkoff sound the medical assistant hears is the systole; the last Korotkoff sound is the diastole. Position the blood pressure cuff so it is 1-2 cm from the antecubital fossa and two fingers can slide between the cuff and the arm. The width of the cuff bladder should exceed the diameter of the patient's arm by 20% or more. Place the stethoscope's diaphragm over the patient's brachial artery of the same arm, and insert the earpieces into one's ears. Inflate the cuff quickly, in 7 seconds or less. Deflate the blood pressure cuff slowly, at a rate of 2-3 mmHg per second. Listen for the "lub" and "dub," while mentally noting the mmHg when each sound was made. Remove the cuff and stethoscope. Record the measurement in the patient's chart immediately.

Oxygen Saturation

Pulse oximetry non-invasively measures a patient's oxyhemoglobin (oxygen saturation) level using a small clip-like device with a light that measures the oxygen saturation of the site it is attached to. This is a painless method of monitoring an individual's respiratory status and perfusion over a period of time when attached continuously, or in a single moment as part of a physical assessment. Attach the oximeter sensor to one of the patient's first three fingers (index, middle or ring). If the patient's hands are damaged, use a toe or earlobe. Consider using the forehead, nose, or other parts of the foot only as a last resort. Normal range should fall between 95% and 100%, although patients with certain conditions, such as COPD, may have a chronically lower saturation. If a patient's oxygen saturation falls below normal range persistently, the medical assistant must inform the doctor that the patient is hypoxic. Many pulse oximeters also measure the patient's heart rate at the same time. A pulse oximeter is not accurate if the patient is very anemic, has poor circulation (due to being cold or having vascular abnormalities), is edematous, moves a lot, or wears artificial nails or very dark nail polish. Adjust the room temperature, lighting, and move electronic equipment to get a good reading.

Body Temperature

A live patient's body temperature is measured to determine if he or she is storing and releasing heat properly, to detect abnormally high or low body temperatures, and to assess the effectiveness of some types of medications. The coroner measures temperature to determine time of death. Adult normal temperature ranges are as follows:

- Normal range: 97-99 °F (36.1-37.2 °C)
- Hypothermia (too cold): <95°F (<35 °C)
- Pyrexia (fever): >100.4 °F (>38 °C)
- Hyperpyrexia (lethal fever): >106.7 °F (>41.5 °C)

Temperature is at its lowest around 4:00 a.m. and highest around 6:00 p.m. Temperature spikes often occur after meals. Ovulation in women creates a temperature rise of 0.5-1.0 °F when measured before arising from bed in the morning (basal body temperature). Individual temperature differences in healthy people are due to the rate of metabolism. Patients with hypothyroidism tend to be cold. Body temperature differs at different sites. Normal oral temperature is 98.6 °F, while rectal temperature is 0.5-1.0 °F higher than oral temperature, and axillary temperature is usually 0.5-1.0 °F lower than oral temperature. Do not take the patient's oral temperature for 30 minutes after eating or drinking, as it will be raised with hot food, and lowered with cold drinks.

Medical Terminology

Reference Sources for Medical Terminology

Reliable sources to check spelling, selection, and use of medical terminology include the following:

- **Abbreviations**: Use safe terms and definitions from The American Society for Testing and Materials' (ASTM). Obtain a list of dangerous abbreviations to be avoided from the Institute for Safe Medication Practices.
- **Style guides**: Provide guidelines for format and presentation in documents. Use the *American Medical Association Manual of Style: A Guide for Authors and Editors* for an overview.
- **Anatomy and physiology texts**: Contain essential information regarding body structure, function of body parts, disease processes, and common health disorders. *Grey's Anatomy* is one classic example.
- **Specialty texts**: Assist with specialty transcriptions. Try Sloan's *Medical Word Book*, Tessier's *Surgical Word Book*, and Pagana's *Laboratory and Diagnostic Tests*.
- **English dictionary**: Helps with spelling, definitions, and pronunciation. *Cambridge Dictionary of American English* is one example.

Origin of Medical Terminology Used in the U.S.

Most medical terms are derived from Greek or Latin. If the Greek or Latin word is broken into its root, prefix and suffix, unfamiliar terminology can be understood. To avoid awkward pronunciation when there is no vowel between the root word and suffix, add an "o" to the combining form. For instance, adding the suffix "metry" (meaning the measure of) to the root word for eye, "opt," creates the word "optometry".

There also are a few English-, French-, and German-originating medical terms:

- Examples of **English terminology** include: Epstein-Barr virus, HIV-positive, 100-mL sample, oxygen-dependent, or self-image. English words use a dash instead of a joining vowel.
- An example of **French terminology** is *grand mal* (the big sickness) for epileptic seizures (although they are now referred to as a generalized or tonic-clonic seizures).
- An example of **German terminology** is *mittelschmerz* (middle pain) for the discomfort of ovulation. French and German do not have convenient combining forms, so they must be memorized.

Prefix, Root, and Suffix

Medical terms have three parts:

- **Root** containing the basic meaning
- **Prefix** before the root that modifies the meaning
- **Suffix** after the root that modifies the meaning

Examples:

- Menorrhagia is excessive bleeding during menstruation and at irregular intervals. The prefix is meno-, meaning menstruation and the suffix is -rrhagia, meaning a flow that bursts forth.
- Rhinoplasty is a "nose job." The root is rhino, meaning nose. The suffix is -plasty, meaning reconstructive surgery.
- Antecubitum is the bend of the arm where blood is often drawn. The root is cubitum, meaning elbow. The prefix is ante-, meaning forward or before.

When confronted with an unfamiliar term, break it into its root, prefix, and suffix to understand its meaning.

Common Prefixes

Common prefixes that the medical assistant must be familiar with include the following:

Prefix	Meaning	Example
Ab-	from, not here, off the norm	Abnormal
Ad-	toward, in the direction of	Adduct
Ante-	prior to, in front of, previously	Antecedent
Anti-	hostile to, against, contradictory	Antisocial
Be-	make, aligned with, greatly	Benign
Bi-	two, occurring twice	Bipolar
De-	away, versus, reduce	Deduct
Dia-	transverse, across	Diameter
Dis-	contradictory, disparate, away	Disjointed
En-	create, put in or on, surround	Engulf
Syn-	by means of, together, same	Synthesis
Trans-	across, far away, go through	Transvaginal
Ultra-	extreme, beyond in space	Ultrasound
Un-	opposing, antithetical, not	Uncooperative

Common Suffixes

Common suffixes that the medical assistant must be familiar with include the following:

Suffix	Meaning	Example
-fication/-ation	manner or process	classification
-gram	written down or illustrated	cardiogram
-graph	a machine or instrument that records data	cardiograph
-graphy	the process of recording of data	cardiography
-ics	science or skill of	synthetics
-itis	red, inflamed, swollen	bursitis
-meter	means of measure	thermometer
-metry	action of measuring	telemetry
-ology/-ogy	the study of	biology
-phore	bearer or maker	semaphore
-phobia	intense, irrational fear	arachnophobia
-scope	instrument used for visualizing data	microscope
-scopy	visualize or examine	bronchoscopy

Pluralizing Medical Terms

Most medical laboratory terms derive from Latin and Greek. Most Latinate terms originated from the Greek. The basic **rules for pluralizing medical terms** are as follows:

Rule	Examples
-a changes to -ata	Stigm*a* to stigm*ata* Condylom*a* to condylom*ata*
-on changes to -a	Criteri*on* to criteri*a* Phenomen*on* to phenomen*a*
-s changes to -des	Iri*s* to iri*des* Arthriti*s* to arthriti*des*
Feminine -a ending changes to -ae	Uln*a* to uln*ae* Conch*a* to conch*ae*
Masculine ending -us changes to -i	Radi*us* to radi*i* Muscul*us* to muscul*i*
Neutral ending -um changes to -a	Bacteri*um* to bacteri*a* Trepone*um* to Trepone*a*
-osis changes to -oses	Diagn*osis* to diagn*oses* Anastom*osis* to anastom*oses*
-x changes to -ces or -ges	Phalan*x* to phalan*ges* Vari*x* to vari*ces*

Standardized Terminology and Abbreviations

Standardized terminology and abbreviations are vital for patient safety. Use abbreviations to save time and space only when there is no potential for confusion over the meaning of the message. Avoid Latin if there is an accepted English equivalency. The Medical Records manager decides acceptable terminology and forbidden abbreviations. If working in a small office and the medical assistant is in charge of Medical Records, use the list of safe terms from The American Society for Testing and Materials' (ASTM) and the list of dangerous abbreviations from the Institute for Safe Medication Practices (ISMP). The Joint Commission also has a "Do Not Use" List for medical abbreviations and symbols that are included on the ISMP's more comprehensive list. Post them throughout the office. Use one type of units only. For example, do not use SI units (International System of Measurement) for Lab and Imperial units for Pharmacy without listing equivalencies. Adopt the U.S. Postal Service database's two-letter abbreviations for states.

Forms of Abbreviations

Health professionals use abbreviations to save time when charting or to be discreet when speaking around a patient. Abbreviations take these forms:

- **Brief form** means shortening a common term or difficult to pronounce term (e.g., *telephone* into *phone* and *Papanicolaou smear* into *Pap smear*).
- **Acronym** means making a new word from the first letter of each word in a phrase, pronounced as a word (e.g., laser for **l**ight **a**mplification by **s**timulated **e**mission of **r**adiation).
- **Initialism** means referring to a phrase by its initials, pronounced as a series of letters (e.g., MRI for **m**agnetic **r**esonance **i**maging or HIV for **h**uman **i**mmunodeficiency **v**irus).
- **Eponym** means naming a test or sign for its discoverer (e.g., Coombs' test and McBurney's sign).

COMMON ABBREVIATIONS FOUND IN DOCTOR'S NOTES

Common abbreviations found in doctor's notes include the following:

Term	Meaning
a.d.	right ear, auris dextra*
a.s.	left ear, auris sinistra*
a.u.	both ears, auris utraque*
o.d.	right eye, oculus dexter* [NOTE: Do not confuse with OD (once daily)]
o.s.	left eye, oculus sinister*
o.u.	both eyes, oculus uterque*
a.c.	before meals
p.c.	after meals
h.s.	hour of sleep, bedtime
ad lib	freely or whenever desired
p.r.n.	as needed
q.4h.	every four hours
q.d. or OD	once daily* [NOTE: Do not confuse with o.d. (right eye)]
b.i.d.	twice a day
t.i.d	three times a day
q.i.d.	four times a day*

*These terms are on ISMP's list of error prone abbreviations.

USE OF MEDICAL SLANG

Medical staff should not write slang terms in written reports because they may:

- Be vague and not give the precise meaning required in a subpoenable medical document
- Make the report seem condescending or disparaging to the patient, portraying the author as prejudiced, offensive, or unprofessional
- Leave the report open to interpretation, which could be used against the author in a court of law

Brief forms are contractions of words that can be found in a medical dictionary, which have been accepted and recognized as suitable for court documents through common usage. They include exam, lab, Pap smear, and prepped. The following jargon can be safely used when talking privately with medical colleagues:

- Appy: Appendectomy
- BP: Blood pressure
- Cath: Catheter (generally referring to urinary catheters)
- Chem: Blood test (CBC)
- Coag: Blood test (coagulation profile)
- D/C: Dilation and curettage
- Dig: Digoxin
- Echo: Echocardiogram
- Lytes: Electrolytes
- Meds: Medications
- Nitro: Nitroglycerin
- Peds: Pediatrics
- ROMI: Rule-out myocardial infarction
- Script: Prescription
- Temp: Temperature
- tib-fib: Tibia fibula (generally relating to a fracture)
- Trach: Tracheostomy
- URI: Upper respiratory infection
- UTI: Urinary tract infection
- V-tach or V-fib: Ventricular tachycardia or ventricular fibrillation

The rule for charting is: "When in doubt, write it out."

Naming of Common Medical and Surgical Specialties

The suffix -ology means "the study of" and the suffix –iatrics means "medical treatment." Add the body system root to obtain the name of the **specialty**:

- Anesthesiology: Study of pain relief
- Bariatrics: Treatment of obesity
- Cardiology: Study of the heart
- Dermatology: Study of the skin
- Endocrinology: Study of the hormone system
- Gastroenterology: Study of the digestive system
- Geriatrics: Treatment of the elderly
- Hematology: Study of the blood
- Neurology: Study of the nervous system
- Obstetrics: Treatment of pregnant women
- Pediatrics: Treatment of children
- Psychiatry: Treatment of the mind
- Radiology: Study of radiation (for medical imaging)
- Rheumatology: Study of rheumatoid diseases, like arthritis
- Toxicology: Study of poisons
- Urology: Study of the urinary system

Common Surgical Procedures

Common surgical procedures that the medical assistant should be familiar with include the following:

Appendectomy	Removal of the vermiform appendix
Breast Biopsy	Removal of suspicious tissue to detect cancer
Cesarean Section	Birth through the mother's abdomen
Cholecystectomy	Gall bladder removal
Coronary Artery Bypass Graft	CABG grafts a vessel from the aorta to the coronary artery to relieve angina or blockage
Debridement	Removal of foreign matter and dead or damaged skin from a wound
Free Skin Graft	Detach skin from one body part to repair another
Hemorrhoidectomy	Removal of swollen veins in the anus
Hysterectomy	Removal of the uterus
Inguinal Hernia Repair	Pulling a loop of bowel that protrudes through the groin back into place
Mastectomy	Removal of the breast
Partial Colectomy	Removal of part of the large intestine
Prostatectomy	Removal of the prostate gland
Release of Peritoneal Adhesions	Removal of the peritoneum membrane from abdominal organs to which it is sticking
Tonsillectomy	Removal of lymphatic tissue at the back of the throat

Anatomical Position

The anatomical position is the medical standard used when describing the orientation and location of the parts of the human body. A patient in the anatomical position stands with the feet facing to the front. The hips and shoulders are square and level. The feet are placed slightly apart. The arms are held straight at the sides of the body with the palms of the hands facing forward. The little fingers are therefore nearest the body, and the thumbs point away from the body. The arms do not touch the trunk but are held close to it. The head faces forward, as do the eyes.

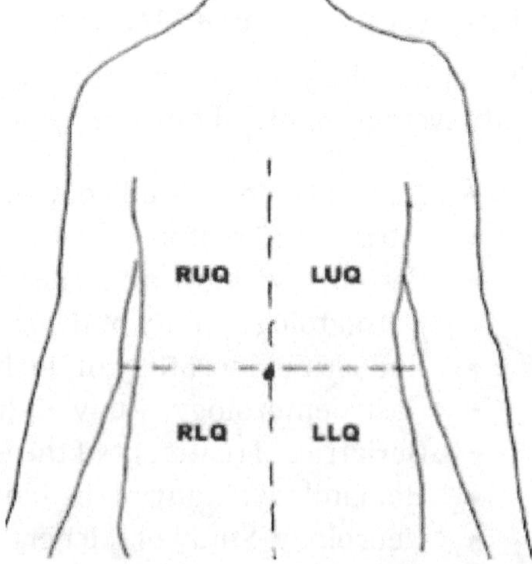

Abdominal Quadrants

The four abdominal quadrants are:

- Right Upper Quadrant (**RUQ**)
- Left Upper Quadrant (**LUQ**)
- Right Lower Quadrant (**RLQ**)
- Left Lower Quadrant (**LLQ**)

Body Planes

The six body planes are:

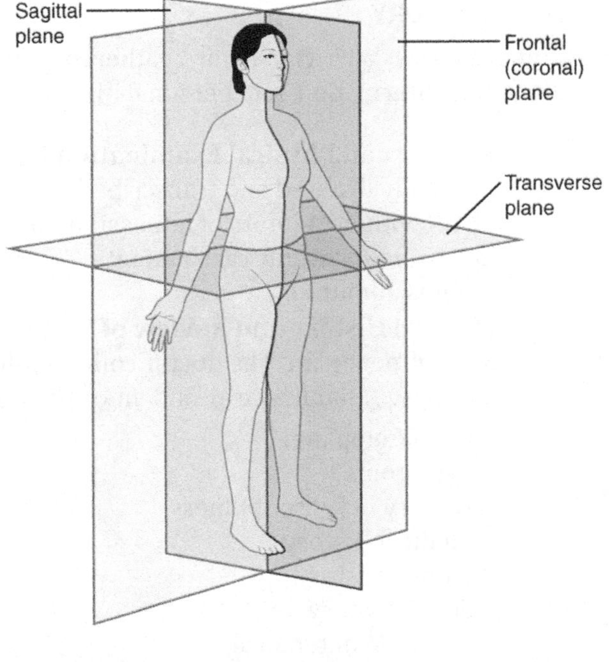

- **Transverse plane** divides the patient's body into imaginary upper (superior) and lower (inferior or caudal) halves.
- **Sagittal plane** divides the body, or any body part, vertically into right and left sections. The sagittal plane runs parallel to the midline of the body.
- Equal halves are the **midsagittal plane.**
- **Median plane** divides the body into right and left halves. The median plane runs vertically through the midline of the body, or any body structure. The median plane is a type of sagittal plane.
- **Coronal plane** divides the body, or any body structure, into front and back (anterior and posterior sections). The coronal plane runs vertically through the body at right angles to the midline. The coronal plane is also called anterior or frontal plane.
- **Posterior plane** is the back, also called the **dorsal plane.**

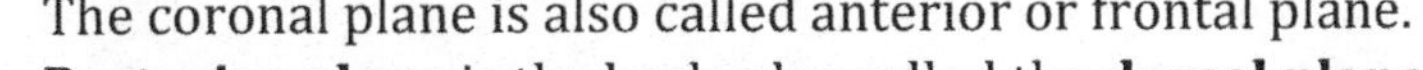

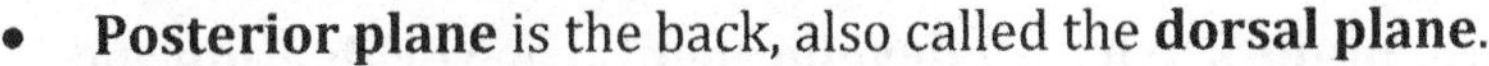

Body Tissue

The four major types of body tissue are:

- **Connective tissue** (e.g., bones, tendons, and ligaments) joins and protects the organs and keeps them in their proper position.
- **Muscle tissue** contracts and expands to allow movement and pump blood, lymph, and other fluids.
- **Nerve tissue** transmits messages from the brain and spinal cord to all of the peripheral parts of the body.
- **Epithelial tissue**, the most common type of tissue, is the skin (integument) covering the body and the lining inside organs and tracts.

Body tissue is 55-78% water, depending on the patient's age and sex. Infants contain the most water. Adult women contain the least. If tissue has too little water, the patient is dehydrated. If tissue is oversaturated with water, the patient has edema (swelling).

Patient Interview and Documentation

Patient History

A patient history is a written record gathered from a patient interview, listing past and present health, family information, and personal information pertinent to health, such as occupation.

- A **History and Physical Examination Report (H&P)** is a single report with two segments. It is usually dictated and transcribed, but can also be a form. The Joint Commission requires an H&P within 24 hours of admission for acute care patients and within 30 days prior to admission for chronic care patients. This must then be updated within 24 hours after the patient is admitted.
- A **Medical History and Review of Systems** forms the basis for the provisional diagnosis and treatment plan. The doctor collects information from the patient, guardian, or a reliable source (e.g., ambulance attendant or personal support worker). The headings are as follows:
    - Chief Complaint
    - Symptoms
    - History of Present Illness
    - Medical History
    - Family History
    - Social History
    - Health Maintenance
    - Review of Systems
- The Joint Commission requires **minors** to have a **developmental age evaluation** and educational needs assessment, also.

Data Collected in Patient Admission/Assessment

Objective data is that which can be directly measured or observed. Objective data may include blood pressure, pulse rate, respiratory rate, height, weight, size of wound, ECG tracings, gender, oxygen saturation, and description (brown hair, blue eyes, ambulatory). Objective data should be easily verified by other observers.

Subjective data, on the other hand, is not measurable or observable but is reported or assumed. Subjective data includes almost anything that the patient reports, including reports of symptoms (headache, diarrhea, pain, dizziness) or anything associated with feelings or assumptions (patient appears tired, angry, upset, anxious). For example, if a patient reports he had been coughing up thick yellow sputum the day prior, this information is subjective. If, however, the patient is observed coughing up thick yellow sputum into a sputum cup, this information is objective.

Charting Techniques

FACT System

All entries in a patient's chart must follow the FACT system and be:

- **Factual**: Patient complaints should be clearly described; for instance, a report of pain should include its specific location, quality (sharp and stabbing or dull ache), duration, and medications taken to relieve it.
- **Accurate**: Information reflects the patient's condition and is not assumed. Information is documented and signed off by the individual who conducted the assessment. In paper charts, entries are legible and in ink. Never use correction fluid or an eraser. Draw a single line through mistakes. The provider should write "error" beside mistakes along with his or her name and title or initials, according to unit policy.
- **Complete**: All fields should be completed to the best of the health care provider's ability. If unable to assess, the field should be marked as such. In paper charting, never leave lines completely or partially blank. Place a single line through the space to prevent someone else from adding to the line.
- **Timely**: Include a time stamp on all entries. This is automatic in electronic charting, but should be written out in paper charting.

HIPAA requires healthcare providers to maintain confidentially of all patient records. Release information on a need-to-know basis only. Never leave a paper chart or computer screen open to prying eyes. Report to the head nurse, IT, and security if approached by the press, an insurance company, or suspicious persons. Keep passwords secure and log off all sessions.

SOAP Note

The SOAP note format for composing chart notes is a reliable method of organizing and documenting information from the patient assessment. Do not transcribe in the chronological order in which the doctor dictates, but put the applicable parts of his or her dictation under these headings in this order:

- S: The **subjective** portion of the report is the chief complaint the patient or guardian makes.
- O: The **objective** portion includes all of the definite findings and observations dictated by the physician or nurse practitioner.
- A: The **assessment** portion of the report is where the physician reports the diagnosis.
- P: The **plan** section is where the physician prescribes the treatment program.

Review Video: SOAP
Visit mometrix.com/academy and enter code: 543158

Roles of the Patient Chart

The patient's chart is a legal document of the events and procedures carried out during a treatment. It can be subpoenaed in court as a way to explain what care the patient did or did not receive. Charting is a method of communication between staff members about the patient, and it provides continuity of care from shift to shift. The chart is a diagnostic aid and the foundation upon which decisions are made concerning changes in medical therapy. The patient's chart also provides data for infection control, risk management, and quality control purposes and is subject to inspection by various regulating bodies, such as Medicare.

Health and Wellness

Lifestyle Choices That Influence Wellness

Lifestyle choices that influence wellness include:

- **Exercise**: Children should exercise at least 3 times weekly for 30 minutes and adults at least 30 minutes daily or 150 minutes per week. Daily exercise is an important component of health but should be age- and condition-appropriate.
- **Smoking**: All those smoking should be encouraged to begin smoking cessation as smoking increases risks of cardiopulmonary disease, bladder cancer, and other disorders.
- **Substance abuse**: Users need to stop use or participate in rehabilitation programs. Substance abuse may lead to serious health problems, such as heart attack, overdose, stroke, and death.
- **Nutrition**: Diet must provide adequate nutrients to promote growth and development.
- **Weight control**: Obesity is a risk factor for cardiac disease, diabetes, hypertension, and hypercholesteremia, so dietary management and strategies to reduce weight are especially important.

Nutritional Elements That Influence Wellness

The nutritional elements that influence wellness include:

- **Fats**: 9 calories per gram. Fat provides the slowest but most efficient form of energy (taking 5 hours to metabolize). Fat should comprise 30% of the diet (with saturated fats no more than 10% of the diet).
- **Carbohydrates**: 4 calories per gram. Simple carbohydrates (sugars, fruits, dairy products) are the fastest source of energy (30 minutes). Complex carbohydrates (whole grains, vegetables) convert more slowly to energy (2 hours). Should comprise about 55% of the diet.
- **Proteins**: 4 calories per gram. Protein (meat, fish, dairy products, eggs, tofu), metabolizes more slowly (3 hours) and provides a long-lasting source of energy. Protein should provide about 15% of the diet.
- **Vitamins**: Organic compounds comprised of carbon, oxygen, hydrogen, nitrogen, and other elements. Vitamins are utilized for cellular biochemical reactions and include both fat soluble (A, D, E, and K) and water-soluble forms (thiamine [B_1], riboflavin [B_2], Niacin [B_3], pyridoxine [B_6], folate [B_{12}], pantothenic acid, biotin, and vitamin C).
- **Minerals**: Include calcium, phosphorus, potassium sulfur, sodium, chloride, iron, copper, zinc, magnesium, fluoride, selenium, chromium, and molybdenum. Minerals are needed for many bodily functions, including fluid balance, nerve transmission, muscle contraction, blood clotting, and BP regulation.

Common Screening Measures and Preventive Care

Common screening measures performed in the comprehensive assessment of an adult include the following:

Breast cancer	Manual exam, mammogram, ultrasound, MRI
Cervical cancer	Pap smear, pelvic exam
Skin cancer	Skin evaluation, encourage use of sunscreen
Lung cancer	Assess history of smoking (pack years), chest x-ray, encourage smoking cessation
Colorectal cancer	Fecal occult blood test, stool DNA test (Cologuard), sigmoidoscopy, double-contrast barium enema, standard colonoscopy, or virtual colonoscopy
Testicular cancer	Manual exam, ultrasound
Prostate cancer	Manual exam, PSA
Osteoporosis	History, physical exam, and bone density scan, encourage exercise and adequate calcium and vitamin D in diet.
Sexually transmitted infections	History, testing for those having unprotected sex, campaign to encourage the use of condoms and safe sex practices
Domestic violence	Ask all patients in privacy (not with a partner or other person present) if they are victims of abuse in non-judgmental manner, discussing confidentiality and mandatory reporting requirements.

Smoking Risks and Cessation Methods

Smoking damages the lining of the respiratory tract and the blood vessels, resulting in risk of respiratory disease (COPD, asthma attack) and heart disease (hypertension, heart attack). Smoking causes 90% of lung cancers and increases risk of coronary heart disease and stroke by 2-4 times, and is a factor in developing rheumatoid arthritis. Chemicals from smoking are filtered into the urine and increase risk of bladder cancer. Smoking increases the risk of preterm delivery and stillbirth and impairs male fertility. **Cessation methods** include:

- **Planned cessation**: Set a date, tell friends and family, remove smoking paraphernalia, list reasons, identify triggers, develop strategies for coping, establish a support system, and provide incentive rewards for compliance.
- **Support groups**: Online and in person support groups may help the patient cope with withdrawal and cravings.
- **Cold-turkey**: This approach is only successful if the patient is very motivated.
- **Medication-assisted**: Nicotine gum, nicotine patches, oral medications (varenicline) can help to control and manage cravings if taken in reduced doses.

Alternative Therapeutic Modalities

Complementary and Alternative Medicine

Complementary medicine is a group of diagnostic and therapeutic disciplines that is used in conjunction with conventional Western medicine. Examples of **complementary medicine** include acupuncture, aromatherapy, biofeedback, chiropractic, hypnosis, massage, naturopathy, nutrition therapy, osteopathic manipulation, qi gong, reflexology, Reiki, traditional Chinese medicine, and yoga. Complementary medicine is often useful to relieve pain after surgery when conventional Western methods are not sufficient. The complementary method acts to complement conventional medicine.

Alternative medicine is used instead of conventional Western medicine. Examples of alternative medicine include dietary supplements, herbs, magnet therapy, vitamin megadoses, and spiritual healing.

Complementary and alternative medicine (CAM) often lacks the support of scientific research studies, instead relying on anecdotal evidence. Patients should be encouraged to discuss their use of complementary and alternative treatments during the collection of their history due to the possible interactions that alternative methods (specifically herbal and dietary supplements) have with standard medications.

Heat Treatments

Externally applied **heat sources** penetrate only the superficial layers of the skin (1-2 cm after about 30 minutes) but are believed to relax deeper muscles by reflex, decrease pain, and increase metabolism (there has been evidence suggesting a 10% increase in oxygen consumption for every 1 °C increase in skin temperature). Therapeutic temperature range for heat therapy is 40-45 °C (104-113 °F). Various methods of heat therapy exist:

- **Hot packs** utilize dry heat (hot water bottles, microwaved heat packs, and heating pads). Hot packs are applied for 15-20 minutes at a time.
- **Moist heat packs**, such as cloth moistened with warm water, are placed on the skin and secured by several layers of towels to provide insulation, applied for 15-30 minutes at a time.
- **Paraffin (wax) baths** (at temperatures of 52-54 °C or 126-130 °F) involve the hand, foot, or elbow being dipped 7 times, cooling between dippings, and then wrapped with plastic and towels for 20 minutes.
- **Whirlpool baths** are used to increase circulation and promote healing. Water temperature is 35-40 °C (95-104 °F, adjusted for the individual) and should be deep enough to completely submerge the affected part. The body part should be cleaned with soap and water before immersion for about 20 minutes.
- **Heat lamps** provide deep heat that differs from superficial heat in that the heat penetrates 3-5 cm deep and is generated internally using ultrasound, short wave, and microwave diathermy rather than applied to the surface of the skin.

Cold Treatments

Therapeutic cold treatment is used to cool the surface of the skin and underlying subcutaneous tissues in order to decrease blood flow, pain, swelling and metabolism. Initial response to cold therapy causes vasoconstriction to occur within the first 15 minutes, but if the tissues are cooled to -10 °C (14 °F), then the body responds with vasodilation. Cryotherapy affects sensory response so the person will at first feel cold, which progresses to burning, aching, and finally to numbness and tingling. Treatment is usually given for 15-30 minutes. Treatment options include:

- **Ice packs** such as refrigerated gel packs (-5 °C or 23 °F) or plastic bags filled with water and ice chips are applied directly to the skin for 10-15 minutes for superficial cooling and 15-20 minutes for greater penetration.
- **Cold compress**: A towel or heavy gauze compress is dipped in an ice and water slurry and then applied to the affected area to provide cold therapy, but this is best used only for emergency situations when ice packs are unavailable, as the compress must be changed frequently as the skin warms the towel rapidly.

Range-of-Motion Exercises

Range-of motion exercises are active or passive exercises intended to maintain mobility of joint, muscles, and tendons by moving the joints through all of their normal ranges:

- **Neck (pivot joint)**: Flexion, extension, lateral flexion, and rotation
- **Shoulder (ball and socket joint)**: Flexion, extension, abduction, adduction, circumduction, and external and internal rotation
- **Elbow (hinge joint)**: Flexion, extension, supination, and pronation
- **Wrist (condyloid joint)**: Flexion, extension, abduction, and adduction
- **Hands and fingers (condyloid and hinge joints)**: Flexion, extension, abduction, and adduction
- **Thumb (saddle joint)**: Flexion, extension, abduction, adduction, and opposition (touching finger tips)
- **Hip (ball and socket joint)**: Flexion, extension, abduction, adduction, circumduction, and internal and external rotation
- **Knee (hinge joint)**: Flexion and extension
- **Ankle (hinge joint)**: Flexion and extension
- **Foot (gliding joint)**: Eversion and inversion
- **Toes (hinge, gliding)**: Flexion and extension
- **Trunk (gliding)**: Extension, lateral flexion, and rotation

Nutrition

Fat-Soluble Vitamins

Fat-soluble vitamins that are integral in the body's growth, development, and immunity include the following:

- **Vitamin A (retinol)** aids growth, development, immune function, and maintains night vision. Sources include butter, egg yolks, cod liver oil, yellow and green leafy vegetables, and prunes. Deficiency causes night blindness, poor visual acuity, skin disorders, and bronchopulmonary dysplasia in low-birth-weight newborns.
- **Vitamin D (calciferol)** aids calcium and phosphorus absorption for bone and teeth formation and is necessary for normal growth and development. Sources include milk, cod liver oil, butter, and egg yolks. Sunlight activates Vitamin D. Deficiency causes rickets, osteomalacia (soft bones, bowed legs) and dental caries.
- **Vitamin E (tocopherols)** is an antioxidant found in sunflower seeds, wheat germ, egg yolks, vegetable oils, almonds, olives, and papaya. Deficiency causes hemolytic anemia of premature newborns.
- **Vitamin K (quinones)** is a necessary for normal clotting of the blood and is found in green leafy vegetables, meat, dairy products, alfalfa, fishmeal, oats, wheat, and rye. Deficiency causes hemorrhagic disease of the newborn. Caution must be taken if anticoagulants are being used as this may affect the clotting of the blood.

The small intestine absorbs fat-soluble vitamins, so patients who have had bowel resections, cystic fibrosis or malabsorption may have deficiencies. Excessive intake of fat-soluble vitamins may cause them to accumulate in fat and in the liver, which can be toxic.

Water-Soluble Vitamins

Water-soluble vitamins that are integral in the body's growth, development, and immunity include the following:

- **Thiamin (B_1)** is found in whole grains, egg yolk, legumes, nuts, pork, and brewer's yeast. Deficiency causes beriberi, confusion, muscle weakness, and poor growth.
- **Riboflavin (B_2)** is in meat, whole grains, brewer's yeast, green vegetables, milk, and eggs. Deficiency causes growth retardation, cracked mouth, and light sensitivity.
- **Niacin (B_3)** is found in meat, fish and poultry, whole grains, dairy products, brewer's yeast, and legumes. Deficiency causes pellagra, dermatitis, and malabsorption.
- **Pantothenate (B_5)** is found in cheese and dairy products, eggs, peanuts, beef, fish, legumes, and soy. Deficiency causes dermatitis and depression.
- **Pyridoxine (B_6)** is in whole grains, nuts, legumes, eggs, meat, fish, bran, and yeast. Deficiency causes dermatitis, cracked mouth, insomnia, weakness, irritability, a strange gait, and seizures.
- **Biotin (B_7)** is in egg yolks, liver, brewer's yeast, and royal jelly. Deficiency is rare.
- **Folic acid (B_9)** is in green, leafy vegetables, organ meat, beef, whole grains and cereals, and legumes. Deficiency causes anemia, neural tube defects.
- **Cobalamin (B_{12})** is in liver, milk, and eggs. Deficiency causes pernicious anemia. Loss of balance and nerve damage.
- **Ascorbic acid (C)** is found in citrus fruits, strawberries, melons, and vegetables such as broccoli, peppers, tomatoes, potatoes, and green leafy vegetables. Deficiency causes scurvy, pyorrhea, bleeding gums, tooth and bone defects, and poor wound healing.

Macrominerals and Trace Minerals

The body requires seven macrominerals in large quantities, and some trace minerals are necessary for good health. The seven **macrominerals** are:

- **Calcium** for muscle contraction, conduction of nerve impulses, bone and tooth maintenance, and blood clotting
- **Phosphorous** for energy transfer, pH balance, and bone and tooth maintenance
- **Sodium** for fluid balance, function of nerves and muscles
- **Potassium** for fluid balance in the blood, acid-base balance, muscle building, and protein synthesis
- **Chloride** for pH balance and needed for digestive juices
- **Sulfur**, an essential component of protein that helps energy metabolism
- **Magnesium** for energy metabolism, muscle function, enzymes, and protein synthesis

Important **trace minerals** include:

- **Chromium** for metabolism of fats and carbohydrate
- **Cobalt** for red blood cell maintenance
- **Copper** for blood, nerves, bones, and immune function
- **Fluoride** to strengthen bones and teeth
- **Iodine** for thyroid function and metabolism
- **Iron** to make red blood cells and protein
- **Manganese** for formation of connective and skeletal tissue, reproduction, growth, and metabolism
- **Molybdenum** helps breakdown sulfites, nitrogen metabolism, enzyme function
- **Selenium** to protect against free radicals
- **Zinc** for immune response, tissue growth, and wound healing

Condition-Specific Dietary Guidelines

Various diets exist to address the needs and deficiencies of specific conditions, including the following:

Weight loss	Diets vary: low carbohydrate, low fat, and/or low calorie. Most include more whole grains, vegetables, and fruit and less refined sugar and flour.
Diabetes mellitus	Patients eat 3 meals daily and sometimes two small snacks, but calories and portion size are usually limited. Patients avoid sugar and high carbohydrate foods and eat food high in fiber, lean meats/fish, vegetables, and limited amounts of fruit.
Hypertension	DASH diet (2,000 calories/day) is plant-focused and high in vegetables, fruits, and nuts and with limited fat, lean meats, and sweets/sugar.
Lactose intolerance	Diet is free of milk products (cheese, milk) because the patient lacks the enzyme necessary to metabolize milk. Some patients may take lactase tablets in order to tolerate milk products.
Gluten intolerance/ Celiac disease	Gluten is a protein found in wheat, rye, and barley, so patients must avoid all products containing these grains, including pastas, breads, and pastries. Gluten is commonly found in many prepared foods and seasonings (chicken broth, salad dressings, soy sauce, frozen foods), which must also be avoided.

Meal Modifications

When the doctor admits a patient to a hospital, rehab, or hospice, check the chart for known allergies, religion, and other conditions that may affect eating. For example, patients with alcoholism and liver disease or who are nursing mothers may need extra calories and supplements, whereas patients with diabetes and PKU have dietary restrictions. Flag this information to alert the dietitian and nurse at the receiving facility by checking off the appropriate boxes on the meal card and admitting forms.

Dysphagia

Esophageal **dysphagia** is difficulty swallowing. It is distinct from odynophagia, which is painful swallowing. Dysphagia can result from:

- Strictures, tumors, or foreign bodies
- Motility disorders, including achalasia
- Spasms of the esophagus

Patients present with difficulty swallowing, choking, or coughing during eating, chronic weight loss and aspiration pneumonia. The doctor diagnoses the cause of dysphagia with endoscopy, barium swallow, and manometric studies of the esophagus. Patients with stroke, Parkinson's disease, multiple sclerosis, Lou Gehrig's disease, myasthenia gravis, muscular dystrophy, and various palsies are prone to dysphagia in their end stages. The treatment approach depends on the underlying cause of the dysphagia, and may include physiotherapy to retrain swallowing muscles, acid blocking medications, surgery to remove obstructions, or placement of a gastrostomy tube.

Eating Disorders

Eating disorders are a health risk for young adult females (from puberty to age 40, most commonly) although males sometimes also have eating disorders, often presenting as excessive exercise. The most common eating disorders include:

- **Anorexia nervosa** is a profound fear of weight gain and severe restriction of food intake, often accompanied by abuse of diuretics and laxatives, which can cause electrolyte imbalances as well as kidney and bowel disorders and delay or cessation of menses. Anorexics may become emaciated and risk death. Self-image is severely impaired, and patients are often in denial.
- **Bulimia nervosa** includes binge eating followed by vomiting often along with use of diuretics, enemas, and laxatives. Gastric acids can damage the throat and teeth. While bulimics may maintain a normal weight, they are at risk for severe electrolyte imbalances that can be life threatening.

Treatment for both eating disorders may include psychotherapy, cognitive behavioral therapy, family therapy, nutritional counseling, and nutritional monitoring.

Anemia

Anemia is lack of blood or a deficiency in red blood cells. It occurs from increased red blood cell destruction from sickle-cell anemia, thalassemia, G6PD deficiency, autoimmune reaction, inherited disorders, hemolytic poison, or an enlarged spleen. Signs and symptoms of anemia are fatigue, thirst, rapid pulse, pallor, dizziness, sweating, shortness of breath, abdominal or chest pain, leg cramps, and syncope. Aplastic anemia results from suppressed bone marrow due to leukemia, radiation, or poisoning. Protein deficiency causes kwashiorkor anemia. Strict vegetarianism and chronic bleeding (e.g., heavy menstruation) deplete iron stores (ferritin), thereby causing iron deficiency anemia. Vitamin B_{12} deficiency causes pernicious anemia.

Humans need iron, folate, Vitamin B_6, Vitamin B_{12}, Vitamin C, Vitamin E, Vitamin K, riboflavin, copper, zinc, and protein to **manufacture blood in the bone marrow**. Even if these nutrients are adequate, the patient cannot produce sufficient blood without the hormone erythropoietin from the kidneys. Therefore, patients with end-stage renal failure who are on dialysis become anemic.

TPN

Many end-stage patients report anorexia (lack of appetite) and changes in the taste of food from medications, disease, or treatments. Anorexia means decreased food consumption, problems meeting the patient's nutritional needs, and distress for the patient's family. **Total parenteral nutrition (TPN)** replaces all or some of the patient's food with liquid nutrients delivered through a surgically implanted central line catheter in the subclavian vein under the collarbone, the jugular vein of the neck, the umbilical vein in the abdomen, or a PICC line in the arm. TPN can be given over the course of the day or overnight depending upon the patient's condition. A TPN bag will range in size from 500-3,000 mL and requires an infusion pump and IV pole to administer. TPN must be provided under the most sterile of conditions to reduce the risk for infection. There are many complications that can be associated with TPN including clotting issues, infection, and liver disease. Close monitoring by the healthcare team is essential. TPN can cause discord in the family and ethical issues for caregivers because it prolongs life artificially. TPN removes the patient's pleasure and sense of normalcy from eating.

Infectious Diseases

Viral Infections

Herpes Simplex Virus Infections

There are 2 types of the herpes simplex virus (HSV), human herpesvirus 1 and 2. **HSV-1** usually causes a **gingivostomatitis** (often referred to as "cold sores" or "fever blisters") and is transmitted through **close contact. HSV-2** usually causes painful **genital lesions** through **sexual contact**. Either may be found in other areas of the body.

- **Incubation** period is around 2-12 days.
- The primary infection is usually more severe (causes systemic **symptoms**) than the reactivated infection, but it may be asymptomatic. After the primary infection, the virus remains dormant in the nerve ganglia, and can be reactivated especially during times of stress, illness, immunosuppression, or sun exposure. While patients are most contagious during times of active lesions, the disease may be spread while asymptomatic. The frequency of the outbreaks usually decreases over time.
- HSV **lesions** are grouped vesicles with an erythematous base. They are usually painful, and a prodrome of tingling, pain, or burning sensations may be felt hours to a couple days before the eruption. Lesions last for approximately 2-3 weeks in primary infection (up to 4 weeks with genital HSV), and 1-2 weeks in recurrent infections.
- HSV is **diagnosed** clinically and confirmed with a + culture, PCR test, or HSV antibody tests (HSV-1 or HSV-2: IgM= active or recent infection; IgG= previous infection).
- Symptomatic **treatment**, proper wound care, and antivirals (acyclovir, valacyclovir, or famciclovir) may be given.
- **Complications** include perinatal infection, keratitis, herpetic whitlow, herpes gladiatorum, secondary infections, and encephalitis.

Epstein-Barr Infection

Epstein-Barr virus (EBV) is a **herpesvirus** (human herpesvirus 4) and is responsible for causing **infectious mononucleosis**. After the initial infection, it remains latent in B cells and epithelial cells. It has been linked to certain epithelial and lymphatic neoplasms (e.g., nasopharyngeal carcinoma, Burkitt lymphoma, Hodgkin lymphoma).

- EBV is **transmitted** through **body fluids** like saliva, so it is sometimes referred to as the kissing disease. It is most common in teenagers and college-age young adults
- **Incubation** period is typically 30-50 days.
- **Symptoms** of EBV infection range from being asymptomatic to swollen painful lymph nodes, pharyngitis (can mimic strep pharyngitis), extreme fatigue, fever, and possibly hepatosplenomegaly. The WBC count is elevated (~10,000-20,000 cells/mL) with 10-30% atypical lymphocytes in the differential.
- Confirm **diagnosis** with a Mono Spot test or EBV antibody serology tests.
- **Treatment** is supportive, and antibiotics are not helpful in treating this viral infection. Therefore, avoid unnecessary antibiotics in those with EBV, especially since administration of ampicillin or amoxicillin is often associated with a pruritic, maculopapular rash. Analgesics, warm salt water gargles, increased fluid intake, and rest will help to relieve some of the symptoms. Symptoms may last for several weeks and fatigue may last even longer. Patients should avoid contact sports for up to 2 months.
- **Complications** include hepatitis, cytopenias (e.g., thrombocytopenia), Guillain Barré syndrome, and splenic rupture.

Measles, Mumps, and Rubella

Measles (rubeola) virus is highly contagious, is spread through **respiratory secretions** (incubation is 7-14 days), and peaks in late winter to spring. It causes a prodrome of high fever (4-7 days), cough, congestion, conjunctivitis; then Koplik spots (pathognomonic), and finally a maculopapular rash (spreads cephalocaudally). Report suspected cases immediately to the health dept. **Diagnose** with a + IgM antibody test (collected after 3 days of rash), viral culture, or PCR. **Treatment** is supportive.

Mumps (parotitis) is a viral infection that is spread via **saliva** (incubation is 12-24 days), and often occurs during winter and spring. It causes painful swelling of the salivary glands (parotid). Report to health dept. Supportive **treatment**. Complications include orchitis (infertility), pancreatitis, and meningitis.

Rubella (German measles) is a virus that spreads via **respiratory droplets** (incubation is 2-3 weeks), and peaks in the spring. There is a mild prodrome (fever, aches, sore throat, conjunctivitis, swollen nodes [esp. suboccipital, postauricular, & posterior cervical]), then a maculopapular rash (face first, then down). Report to health dept. Confirm with rubella antibodies IgM or IgG. Symptomatic care.

Influenza

Influenza is a highly contagious viral infection that affects the entire **respiratory system** from the nose to the lungs. There are 3 types of **influenza virus**: **A** (causes epidemics), **B** (only in humans), and **C**. Types A and B are seen most often and are the strains that the annual flu vaccine is most effective against; and type C is not as common and much less severe.

- Prevention is key and annual, age-appropriate influenza **vaccines** should be given to those ≥6 months; 2 vaccines are required in first-time vaccine patients if 6 mo. through 8-year-olds (separated by 28 days).
- **Incubation** period is 1-4 days and it is spread via respiratory droplets.
- Though **symptoms** can be very similar, the flu and the common cold differ in that the flu has a very sudden onset. Symptoms of influenza include a high fever (may last up to 5 days), headache, myalgias, dry cough, rhinorrhea, and fatigue. There may also be vomiting and diarrhea, although children are more prone to this.
- Clinical judgement, community patterns, and rapid influenza tests (high specificity, but lower sensitivity) aid in **diagnosis**, but RT-PCR or viral culture definitively confirm the diagnosis; pulse oximetry and CXR as needed for pulmonary issues.
- Antibiotic **treatment** is not effective unless there is a secondary bacterial infection (e.g., pneumonia). Look for signs of secondary infections (e.g., dyspnea, cyanosis, fever that goes away and returns, confusion/lethargy). Supportive treatment with rest, fluids, and analgesics. Antivirals should be considered in those who are at high risk (<5 years old, elderly, pregnant, chronic conditions). These are most effective if initiated within 24-48 hours of symptom onset. The neuraminidase inhibitors (oseltamivir, zanamivir) treat type A, type B, and avian H5N1. There is extensive resistance to the adamantanes (amantadine, rimantadine) so they are rarely used.
- **Complications** include pneumonia, ARDS, and death.

Coronavirus

A coronavirus is a common virus that causes cold-like symptoms, including a cough, runny nose, sore throat, and congestion. Most cases of coronavirus are not dangerous and are often given little attention or go entirely unnoticed. However, specific coronavirus strains have led to two worldwide pandemics. The first, **severe acute respiratory syndrome (SARS)**, appeared in China in 2002 and quickly spread worldwide. Presenting symptoms of SARS were fever, cough, dyspnea, and general malaise. It was extremely virulent, spreading easily from person to person through close contact by way of contaminated droplets produced by coughing or sneezing. SARS was also very deadly, with a case fatality rate of nearly 10%. High rates of infection occurred in health care workers and others in contact with infected patients, so prompt diagnosis and proper isolation were essential. By 2004, there were no longer any documented active cases of SARS.

The most recent coronavirus outbreak was the **COVID-19** strain, which first appeared in December of 2019, in the Chinese city of Wuhan, and quickly became a global pandemic. Presentation of COVID-19 was similar to that of SARS, with the notable additional symptom of acute loss of taste/smell as a unique identifier. Much is still unknown about this strain, including exact transmission methods (though droplet transmission is suspected), effective treatment protocols, and long-term effects.

Precautions to take when treating patients with pandemic coronavirus include the following:

- Contact and droplet precautions, including eye protection and appropriate personal protection equipment.
- Airborne precautions (recommended by the CDC), especially with aerosol-producing procedures (ventilators, nebulizers, intubation).
- Immediate notification of public health authorities and institution of contact tracing.
- Activity restrictions of exposed health care workers planned in coordination with public health officials.

Cytomegalovirus

Cytomegalovirus (CMV) is a herpes virus, occurring in most people by the time they are adults.

- **Transmission** can occur through secretions during personal contact and from mother to baby before, during or after birth.
- Most cases have no **symptoms**, although a few infants will have fetal damage, such as jaundice, hepatitis, brain damage, or growth retardation.
- **Treatment** for those with severe infections is with ganciclovir, an antiviral drug.

Respiratory Syncytial Virus

Respiratory syncytial virus (RSV) is a virus that infects the respiratory tract, causing symptoms of nasal congestion, cough, sore throat, and headache. Severe cases can lead to high fever, breathing difficulties, severe cough, and cyanosis.

- Respiratory syncytial virus may **manifest** as a cold in adults and older children; however, there are some children who are more at risk of developing complications.
- **Transmission** is through contact with droplets from an infected person's nose or throat, generally through coughing and sneezing.
- Infants born prematurely, children with chronic lung disease, children with cystic fibrosis, and children who are in an immunocompromised state because of surgery or illness are at **high risk** of breathing difficulties, poor oxygenation, and even death from RSV.

FIFTH DISEASE

Fifth disease, or **erythema infectiosum**, is a viral illness caused by parvovirus B19. It is most prevalent in the spring, with outbreaks in preschools, daycares, and elementary schools.

- The **incubation** period is 4-20 days, and it may be communicable for several days before the rash appears.
- **Transmission** occurs through oral and nasal secretions and possibly blood.
- **Symptoms** are possible fever, headache, nasal congestion, general unwell feeling, and rash starting on the cheeks (slapped cheek appearance). The rash typically spreads to the rest of the body as a lacy red rash that may come and go for up to a month.
- Use over-the-counter fever medications as needed and provide **supportive care**.
- The virus can cause fetal death if contracted during pregnancy. There is no vaccine for fifth disease, and because it is a viral infection, it is not treated with antibiotics.

CHICKENPOX

Chickenpox (Varicella) is a viral infection, most prevalent in the late winter and early spring in children under 10 years of age.

- It has an **incubation** period of 10-21 days and is communicable from 1-2 days before the rash appears to after all lesions have dried up.
- **Transmission** is through direct contact and contact with respiratory droplets.
- **Symptoms** are low fever and feeling unwell, followed by the itchy rash (raised red bumps that develop vesicles which then ooze and crust over).
- The patient should be isolated until all lesions are dry. Aveeno baths and Benadryl help with the itching. Ibuprofen or acetaminophen can be used for the fever, and acyclovir is indicated in some cases. Encourage the patient not to scratch the lesions to prevent secondary infections. Provide supportive care as indicated.

ROSEOLA

Roseola is a viral illness, most prevalent in children 6-24 months of age.

- The **incubation** period is about 9 days.
- **Transmission** may be through oral and nasal.
- The illness begins with a high fever for 3-5 days; the patient appears well otherwise. The fever drops and then the rash appears. The rash is a light pink maculopapular rash which lasts 1-2 days.
- Parents should **treat the fever** as needed with anti-inflammatory medications.

POLIOMYELITIS

Poliomyelitis (commonly referred to as **polio**) is caused by an enterovirus and occurs most often in babies and young children.

- The **incubation** period is 3-14 days, and transmission occurs through direct contact with respiratory secretions and the oral-fecal route.
- The **symptoms** are slight fever, sore throat, general malaise, nausea and vomiting, headache, stomach ache, and constipation, but there can be severe pain, muscular weakness, and then paralysis.
- There are no drug therapies for polio. Observe for respiratory distress, provide general support measures, and provide for physical therapy.

ROTAVIRUS

Rotavirus is a viral illness that causes diarrhea, fever, and vomiting in children.

- It can be extremely **contagious** within groups where large numbers of children are present, such as in daycare centers, preschools, pediatric offices, clinics, and children's units in hospitals.
- Rotavirus can be prevented through **immunization** with a vaccine, as recommended by the American Academy of Pediatrics. Immunization can prevent up to 98% of severe cases of the illness.
- Children should wash their hands before eating and after using the bathroom to avoid spreading the disease. Caregivers should wash their hands before preparing food, after changing diapers, and after using the bathroom; they should avoid letting small children place toys or other items in their mouths and should disinfect surfaces after use.

BACTERIAL INFECTIONS

DIPHTHERIA

Diphtheria, caused by ***Corynebacterium diphtheriae***, is most prevalent in fall and winter.

- The **incubation** period is 2-7 days, possibly longer, and transmission is through direct contact with nasal, eye, and oral secretions.
- The **symptoms** are slight fever, nasal discharge, sore throat, feeling unwell, poor appetite, and swelling of the airway.
- If the disease is severe, death can result. The patient requires isolation, bed rest, fluids, antibiotics, medication for fever, and an antitoxin. The patient may also require oxygen therapy and tracheostomy if the airway is obstructed.

TETANUS

Tetanus, caused by ***Clostridium tetani***, occurs all over the world. The spores formed by the bacillus are present in soil, dust, and the GI tracts of animals and humans.

- The **incubation** period is 3-21 days.
- **Symptoms** start with headache, irritability, jaw muscle spasms, and inability to open the mouth. This is followed by severe back muscle spasms, seizures, incontinence, and fever.
- **Treatment** requires human tetanus immune globulin, penicillin G, Valium, and placement on a ventilator. The environment should be kept quiet because the spasms are initiated by stimuli.

SCARLET FEVER

Scarlet fever, caused by **group A beta-hemolytic streptococci**, is most prevalent in school-age children during the fall, winter, and spring.

- The **incubation** period is 1-7 days, and transmission occurs through direct or indirect contact with oral and nasal secretions.
- The illness begins with a high fever, very sore throat, headache, malaise, chills and possibly vomiting and stomach pain. A rash appears in about 12 hours as sandpapery red pinpoints in creases of the skin, flushed face and then a strawberry tongue.
- Antibiotics will be prescribed, but patients should be isolated until taking the antibiotic for 24 hours. Analgesics are needed to bring down the fever and the patient should be encouraged to drink plenty of fluids.

Whooping Cough

Whooping cough, caused by ***Bordetella pertussis*** **bacillus**, is most prevalent in infants and children who were not immunized.

- The **incubation** period is 6-20 days, and transmission occurs through direct contact with oral and nasal secretions.
- The **symptoms** are cold symptoms for 1-2 weeks, when the cough will worsen and progress to a whoop sound, usually occurring at night. Vomiting will usually follow an episode of intense coughing. As the patient recovers, the coughing will subside. In babies, a mucus plug or apnea can result in death by respiratory arrest. Hospitalization is usually required for infants less than 6 months of age and those with a severe case of pertussis.
- The patient needs isolation and bed rest, with a calm, quiet environment to limit coughing spells. Fluid intake needs to be monitored and humidified air will help.
- Watch for signs of respiratory distress and give antibiotic and pertussis immune globulin as prescribed.

Impetigo

Impetigo is a skin infection that is most commonly seen in preschool children or those in young childhood.

- Impetigo causes blister-like sores on skin areas that may already be compromised, such as under the nose, on the hands or neck, or in the diaper area. It is caused by a bacterial infection, most commonly *Staphylococcus aureus* or group A *Streptococcus*. The sores may itch or the patient may already have irritation at the site, such as a diaper rash.
- To **prevent the spread of infection**, children and caregivers should wash their hands frequently and avoid scratching the sores and then touching items. Isolation by staying home from school or daycare may be necessary until the sores have crusted over. Treating skin irritations, such as poison ivy or eczema, can also prevent infection from spreading to impetigo.

Fungal Infections

Cryptococcosis

Cryptococcosis is an infection resulting from inhaling the **fungus** *Cryptococcus neoformans,* which is found worldwide in soil (can be associated with bird droppings), or *Cryptococcus gattii,* which is associated with certain trees in the Northwest.

- Cryptococcosis is most often due to *C. neoformans*. It is often found among those with compromised immune systems and is an **AIDS-defining opportunistic infection**.
- Healthy patients may be asymptomatic and the only finding may be pulmonary lesions on CXR that resolve spontaneously. The fungus can disseminate and cause meningitis, encephalitis, cutaneous lesions, and affect long bones and other tissues. **Symptoms** are based on the area of involvement. Patients may experience cough, pleuritic chest pain, weight loss, and fever if there is pulmonary involvement; headache, double vision, light sensitivity, N/V, and confusion if CNS involvement; cutaneous lesions (papules, pustules, nodules, ulcers) if the skin is involved.
- **Diagnosis** includes microscopic analysis, culture (gold standard), or an antigen test (highly sensitive; good for detecting early infection) for *Cryptococcus* using CSF, tissue, sputum, blood, or urine. Check CSF by India ink (limited sensitivity) or culture so meningitis can be ruled out. Confirm that no mass lesion is present by CT or MRI before LP is performed.

- Mild cases may only require monitoring to ensure that the infection does not spread. In more advanced cases, the infection is treated with different antifungal medications (e.g., fluconazole for pulmonary infections, amphotericin B ± flucytosine for meningitis). The patient should also be monitored for CNS infection and medication side effects. AIDS patients may need lifelong antifungals.
- **Complications** include cryptococcal meningitis, neural deficits, optic nerve damage, and hydrocephalus.

HISTOPLASMOSIS

Histoplasmosis is an infection caused by inhalation of **spores** from the fungus *Histoplasma capsulatum* that is found in soil and is associated with bird and bat droppings (e.g., chicken coops, caves).

- Healthy patients are usually asymptomatic and those with symptoms are typically immunocompromised or those who've had a heavy exposure to spores. The primary **pulmonary infection** occurs 3-17 days after exposure and can present with flu-like symptoms. It is typically self-limited but may become chronic. Histoplasmosis can also spread through the **blood** and can cause progressive disseminated disease in the immunocompromised (high mortality rate); this is an **AIDS-defining illness**.
- **Diagnose** through antigen tests (urine, serum), histopathology, or cultures; order a CXR. Mild and even moderate acute pulmonary histoplasmosis may resolve on its own.
- If needed, **treat** mild to moderate infections with itraconazole and severe illness with amphotericin B.

PNEUMOCYSTIS

Pneumocystis jiroveci is a **fungus** (previously known as *Pneumocystis* carinii) that causes **pneumonia** (PJP, previously PCP) in the immunocompromised. Most people have been exposed to this by the age of 3 or 4.

- **Symptoms** of PJP include a dry nonproductive cough, fever, dyspnea, and weight loss.
- CXR may show diffuse bilateral infiltrates or it may be normal; and pulse oximetry may be low, especially on exertion. **Diagnosis** is confirmed with sputum histopathology using sputum induction or bronchoalveolar lavage.
- **Treat** immediately with TMP-SMX (trimethoprim/sulfamethoxazole) for 21 days if HIV + and for 14 days in other cases. Steroids may be added for HIV patients with severe PJP. HIV/AIDS patients with CD4 counts <200/μL should receive PJP prophylaxis with TMP-SMX. Dapsone and pentamidine are alternatives.
- **Complications** include ARDS and death.

Candidal Infections

Candida is a type of yeast that may cause a variety of infections:

- **Oral thrush** is commonly seen in diabetic patients and those who are immunosuppressed (HIV or underlying neoplasm). Patients often complain of burning on the tongue or in the mouth, associated with "curd-like" white patches that can be scraped away leaving reddish tissue underneath. Diagnosis is with KOH prep. Treatment is with oral or topical antifungals, including nystatin (swish and swallow or troches).
- **Candida esophagitis** also occurs in the immunosuppressed population, and patients may complain of dysphasia, odynophagia, and chest pain. This is diagnosed on EGD and may be treated with oral or IV antifungals (ketoconazole).
- **Candidal intertrigo**, or diaper rash, presents with beefy-red lesions at skin fold areas as well as satellite lesions. Treatment is with topical antifungals.
- **Candidemia** is diagnosed with fungal blood cultures and may lead to osteomyelitis, endocarditis, and other complications. Treatment is with IV antifungals.

Ringworm

Ringworm is caused by an infection from the ***Tinea* fungus**, which produces patches on the skin that have normal centers, giving the appearance of a ring.

- The fungus can cause hair loss and patches of scaly skin that may develop blisters that ooze or crust.
- It is **transmitted** by touching the affected skin or through objects that have touched the affected skin.
- Ringworm may be **diagnosed** by viewing the skin section under a Wood's lamp. Skin cultures may also be taken for examination to identify the fungus. A potassium hydroxide (KOH) exam involves scraping the affected skin and placing the skin sample in KOH to test for the presence of the fungus.

Vector-Borne and Parasitic Infections

Malaria

Malaria is a **blood-borne disease** caused by a **parasite** from the genus *Plasmodium and* found in tropical areas. There are 4 known to cause disease in humans (*P. malariae, P. vivax, P. ovale*, and *P. falciparum*). These protozoa are transmitted by the **female *Anopheles* mosquito**. They travel to the **liver** where they multiply, are released, and then infect the RBCs, where they continue to multiply. Incubation time can be as little as 9 days or as much as multiple years depending on the species of the infecting parasite.

- **Signs and symptoms** include headache, high fever with shaking chills and sweating (rigors; occurs when merozoites, an immature form of the parasite, are released from RBCs), jaundice, anemia, and hepatosplenomegaly. Take a thorough history including recent travel.
- **Diagnose** with 3 thin and thick blood smears (gold standard) stained with Giemsa (preferred) and obtained 12-24 hours apart. Labs typically show elevated LDH, thrombocytopenia, and atypical lymphocytes. Rapid antigen tests are also available as well as PCR.
- **Treat** with chloroquine. If travelling, chemoprophylaxis depends on the area of travel due to species and resistance patterns, and may include chloroquine, primaquine, mefloquine, Malarone, or doxycycline. Report infections to your local or state health department.
- **Complications** include severe anemia and hemolysis, organ failure (liver, spleen, kidneys), cerebral malaria, ARDS, and death.

LYME DISEASE

Lyme disease occurs from a bite from a **deer tick** (blacklegged tick) infected with the **spirochete bacterium** *Borrelia burgdorferi*. It is the most common tick-borne disease in the U.S. and is more prevalent in heavily wooded areas. Adult ticks are more active during colder times whereas the nymphs (<2 mm in size) are more active in the warm, spring or summer months. Once the tick bites, it stays attached; however, it takes about 36-48 hours for nymphs and about 48-72 hours for adult ticks before the spirochete is transmitted to the person. **Incubation** period is 3-30 days. There are 3 stages to this disease: early localized, early disseminated, and chronic disseminated.

- At **Stage 1**, 75% have the characteristic expanding red rash (erythema migrans; can be large, ~30cm) which can progress to have central clearing (bull's eye), headache, fever, chills, myalgias, and fatigue.
- **Stage 2** occurs weeks to months after initial infection and involves systemic symptoms (flu-like), neck stiffness, headaches, migrating pain in muscles and joints, rashes, paresthesias, Bell's palsy, confusion, fatigue, myocarditis, and heart palpitations.
- **Stage 3** occurs months to years after initial infection and involves neurologic (e.g., encephalitis) and rheumatologic issues, especially arthritis of large joints (e.g., knee).

DIAGNOSIS AND TREATMENT OF LYME DISEASE

Diagnose Lyme disease using 2-tiered testing: antibodies (IgM, IgG), then Western blot. Antibiotic treatment for localized Lyme disease involves 2-3 weeks of doxycycline, amoxicillin, or cefuroxime axetil is started immediately after diagnosis. IV antibiotics may be needed for severe disease (e.g., IV ceftriaxone). Prevention is key by wearing clothes covering the skin, using tick repellents, showering soon after being outdoors in tick-prone areas, and thoroughly checking for ticks (especially in hard to see areas by using a mirror). The Lyme vaccine is no longer available and previous vaccine recipients are still at risk of contracting the disease as protection decreases over time. Complications are prevalent with untreated Lyme disease and include chronic arthritis, fatigue, chronic musculoskeletal issues, acrodermatitis chronica atrophicans, and memory and concentration issues. Report cases to the local health dept.

ROCKY MOUNTAIN SPOTTED FEVER

Rocky Mountain spotted fever is a tick-borne illness caused by **Rickettsia rickettsii**. It tends to occur in spring and summer throughout the United States.

- **Incubation** period is about one week.
- **Symptoms** include headache, fever, nausea, vomiting, loss of appetite, muscle pain, and rash on the ankles and wrists.
- **Treatment** requires an antibiotic, usually Vibramycin.

Zika Virus in Pregnant Women

Zika virus is a **flavivirus** that is transmitted by the *Aedes* mosquito and through sexual contact. This virus can be passed on to an unborn baby causing severe congenital defects while causing mild or no disease in the mother. It is advised that all pregnant women avoid traveling to areas with the Zika virus (e.g., Central and South America, Mexico, Caribbean, Africa).

- **Incubation** period is 3-14 days and symptoms may last 4-7 days. The virus has been found to remain longer in semen than in other body fluids.
- If **symptoms** are present, they may include fever, headache, myalgias, arthralgias, a maculopapular rash, and conjunctivitis. Congenital defects include severe microcephaly, severe brain abnormalities, macular scarring, hearing loss, motor disabilities (e.g., hypertonia), and contractures. Women should be screened for Zika exposure at each prenatal visit.
- **Diagnostic** testing is recommended for all asymptomatic pregnant women who have continued exposure to Zika and for all symptomatic pregnant women who have possibly been exposed to the Zika virus. Testing includes RNA NAT testing on serum and urine, and serum IgM Zika antibody testing. Prenatal ultrasound helps determine if the effects of Zika are present. Report cases to the state health department; and the CDC can be consulted.
- There is **no treatment** or cure for the Zika virus.

Helminth Infestations

Helminth infestations (worms) include **roundworms** [nematodes: *Ascaris*, hookworms (cause anemia), **filariae** (cause elephantiasis)] and **flatworms** [tapeworms (cause weight loss); **flukes** (intestinal or liver)]. **Pinworms** are a type of roundworm that cause enterobiasis and is the most common helminth infestation. Pinworms are more prevalent in warmer areas of the country and infestations occur more frequently in children. The worms lay eggs within the digestive tract and then travel to the anal area where they are usually found. Pinworms are highly contagious. As a patient itches the anal area where the eggs are located, the eggs cling to the fingers and can easily be transmitted to other people either directly or through food or surfaces. The eggs can survive for 2-3 weeks on inanimate objects.

- Patients may be asymptomatic or have intense anal itching that is usually worse at night and can cause insomnia. Abdominal pain, nausea, and vomiting can also occur.
- **Diagnose** with the "tape test" which involves pressing cellophane tape over the perianal area to pick up eggs or worms and examine under the microscope. Most other helminth infestations can be diagnosed with a stool sample for ova and parasites; filariasis requires a blood smear or antigen test.
- Anthelmintic medications are given in a single dose and repeated in 2 weeks to kill the pinworms and their larvae (mebendazole, albendazole, or pyrantel pamoate). The entire family and close contacts should be treated simultaneously since pinworms are so contagious.

Giardia Lamblia

Giardia lamblia is a **protozoan** that infects water supplies and spreads to children through the fecal-oral route. It is the most common cause of non-bacterial diarrhea in the United States, causing about 20,000 cases of infection each year in all ages.

- Children often become infected after swallowing recreational waters (pools, lakes) while swimming or putting contaminated items into the mouth. *Giardia* live and multiply within the small intestine where cysts develop.
- **Symptoms** occur 7-14 days after ingestion of 1 or more cysts and include diarrhea with greasy floating stools (rarely bloody), stomach cramps, nausea, and flatulence, lasting 2-6 weeks. A chronic infection may develop that can last for months or years.
- **Treatment** includes Furazolidone 5-8 mg/kg/day in 4 doses for 7-10 days or Metronidazole 40 mg/kg/day in 3 doses for 7-10 days. Chronic infections are often very resistant to treatment.

Toxoplasmosis

Toxoplasmosis is an infection caused by the **parasite *Toxoplasma gondii***, which is commonly found in soil. It is widespread and transmitted through cat feces; however, it also may be contracted by eating undercooked meat (especially pork, lamb, or venison) or poorly washed vegetables. Toxoplasmosis can cause serious disease and can affect various organs; and immunocompromised and pregnant women and their unborn babies are especially likely to have side effects of the disease (the "T" in congenital TORCH infections).

- Healthy patients are usually asymptomatic; however, once infected the parasite can remain latent until the patient becomes immunocompromised and the parasite is reactivated causing **symptoms**. The disease can cause a flu-like illness with fever, myalgias, and lymphadenopathy. More serious effects include retinochoroiditis, brain lesions, and encephalitis. Congenital toxoplasmosis may cause retinochoroiditis, microcephaly, hydrocephalus, intellectual disability, and possibly miscarriage or stillbirth.
- **Diagnose** with serology for *Toxoplasma* antibodies IgM and IgG. Also, PCR may be used to test amniotic fluid, CSF, or tissue.
- **Treat** with pyrimethamine (preferred) plus folinic acid or sulfadiazine plus folinic acid. Pregnant women should avoid high-risk practices like changing the cat litter and should avoid sand boxes.

Asepsis

Modes of Infection Transmission

Modes of infection transmission include the following (with possible infectious diseases in parenthesis):

- **Direct contact**: Direct touching, kissing (mononucleosis) and sexual intercourse (gonorrhea, syphilis, chlamydia, HIV). Vertical transmission involves mother to infant during pregnancy, delivery, or breastfeeding (HIV, hepatitis B, gonorrhea, herpes).
- **Indirect contact**: A contaminated fomite (inanimate object), such as a doorknob, syringe, or catheter, spreads infection (*Clostridium difficile*).
- **Airborne**: Particles less than 5 μm in size inhaled from cough, sneeze, or exhalation. Particles stay suspended in the air and travel large distances (tuberculosis, measles, COVID-19).
- **Droplet**: Particles greater than 5 μm in size are inhaled from a cough, sneeze, or exhalation (influenza, mumps, meningitis, pertussis, pneumonia, rubella). Droplets travel less than 3 feet and do not stay suspended, therefore are less contagious than airborne particles.
- **Vehicle**: Contact with contaminated water, air, or food (*E. coli* diarrhea, Cryptosporidiosis, hepatitis A).
- **Vector (mechanical)**: Contact with an animal, insect, or device that carries infection from one host to another (such as a fly carrying bacteria from feces of an infected host to food [dysentery]).
- **Vector (biological)**: Infected biological vector (such as a tick or flea) transmits infection directly to another host (Chagas disease, malaria, West Nile virus, Lyme disease).

Chain of Infection and Natural Barriers to Infection

There are six components to the chain of infection:

- **Infectious microorganisms**: Bacteria, viruses, fungi, parasites
- **Reservoir**: The place the microorganism lives and reproduces (water, feces, body fluids, toilet seats, door knobs, blood)
- **Portal of exit**: The place where the microorganism leaves the reservoir (nose, mouth, rectum, blood, sputum)
- **Transmission mode**: The method (direct or indirect) by which a microorganism travels from one host to another
- **Portal of entry**: The site at which a microorganism enters a host (wounds, mucous membranes, feeding tubes, urinary catheter, ventilation tube, IV)
- **Susceptible host**: The host at risk of developing the infection

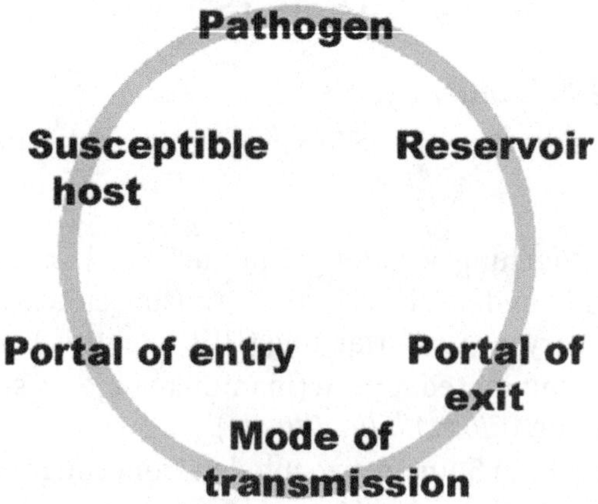

Pathogen

Reservoir

Portal of exit

Mode of transmission

Portal of entry

Susceptible host

Natural barriers to infection include an effective immune system, intact skin, adequate cough reflex and air filtering (nose and lungs), digestive acids and enzymes (destroy some pathogens), healthy mucous membranes (prevent infections), blood components (white blood cells), inflammation response (walls off infection), urethra (provides protection of urinary system), and fever (increases body defense system).

Infection Control Precautions

Various levels of infection control precautions exist to aid in the prevention of the spread of infection amongst health care workers and facilities:

- **Standard or universal precautions** are means through which healthcare workers control the spread of disease by assuming every patient's samples are infectious, and following the OSHA standards for proper hand washing, wearing gloves and other personal protective equipment (PPE), bagging specimens in biohazard bags, and disposing of needles and lancets in a sharps container.
- **Contact precautions** prevent direct and indirect contact transmission of infectious pathogens such as those found with herpes simplex, infected wounds, and infectious diarrhea. PPE includes wearing gloves and gown upon room entry and properly discarding before exiting the patient room.
- **Droplet precautions** are used to prevent the transmission of pathogens transmitted by respiratory droplets from coughing, sneezing, or talking. PPE includes a mask for the patient when being transported outside patient room, and a mask for medical personnel when entering the patient room.
- **Airborne precautions** are used for airborne transmission microbes such as tuberculosis, which require a negative pressure private room and a HEPA or fit-tested N95 mask.

Isolating infectious patients is essential to reduce the risk of infection.

- **Strict isolation** segregates infectious patients to one room, and visitors are restricted.
- **Modified isolation** attempts to limit infection with protective techniques, like donning gloves, gowns, and masks when handling the patient's body fluids.
- **Reverse isolation** protects a patient from others in a clean room, as after kidney transplant.

Antisepsis is reducing the flora and transient microorganisms on the skin for minor procedures like venipuncture. Clean gloves are worn. It requires a short-acting antiseptic like 70% isopropyl alcohol that can denature proteins.

Asepsis prevents the spread of infection by reducing pathogens. There are two types of asepsis: medical asepsis and surgical asepsis. Some procedures require surgical asepsis while others only require medical asepsis.

Medical Asepsis

Medical asepsis is defined as the absence of disease-causing microorganisms and is often referred to as **clean**. Medical asepsis is used to prevent the spread of hospital-acquired (nosocomial) disease and cross-infections (different pathogens passed between two patients):

- Wash hands using proper hand hygiene whenever visibly soiled, before and after any contact with patients, and after gloves are removed.
- Disinfect patient care materials before use with the proper chemical agent, according to the manufacturer's specifications.
- Maintain a clean patient care environment, with adequate space, ventilation, sunlight, and cool temperature.
- Dispose of infectious material as soon as soiling is discovered in the proper bin (concurrent cleaning).
- Disinfect patient care materials after a patient leaves the office, dies, or is transferred to another floor or facility (terminal cleaning).
- Use clean and dirty utility rooms to separate unused equipment from used equipment and prevent contamination.
- Store clean linen separate from used linen, and limit access to the clean linen room to authorized personnel only.

Surgical Asepsis

Surgical asepsis is defined as the absence of all microorganisms and is often referred to as **sterile**. Surgical asepsis is used in the sterilization of instruments, sutures, drapes, sponges, and other surgical equipment and storing them safely, so they do not become reinfected. The principles of surgical asepsis are used when the skin is not intact and when internal areas of the body are being entered, cared for, or treated. This includes wound care, surgical procedures, invasive procedures such as endoscopy, and insertion of internally placed tubes such as an indwelling urinary catheter or central IV line. Sterility is not required for instruments introduced into the vagina, ear canal, or mouth; a vaginal speculum, otoscope, or tongue depressor can be clean (disinfected), rather than sterile.

Appropriate technique for setting up sterile field and maintaining asepsis:

- Sterile gowns, gloves, and masks are worn by staff setting up or working with a sterile field.
- Only sterile items are placed on the sterile field.
- NEVER lean over a sterile field or turn your back to a sterile field.
- NEVER have the sterile field below waist level.
- Maintain a one-inch border around the sterile field that is not sterile. Sterile items are put inside of this one-inch border.
- Sterile field must remain dry. Coughing or sneezing over the sterile field contaminates the sterile field.
- Sterile liquids must be poured carefully into sterile containers on the sterile field without the solution running over.

If the sterile field is not maintained continuously throughout the procedure, the entire sterile field and its contents are discarded and the entire setup must be redone.

Hand-Washing Technique

Handwashing is the most effective way to prevent the spread of infection when done properly. To **wash hands correctly**, wet the hands with clean running water and apply soap. Lather hands by rubbing them together with soap, scrubbing the backs of hands, between fingers, and under nails for at least 20 seconds. Note any cuts, rashes, broken or long nails that need treatment before resuming work. Rinse well under clean running water and dry hands with paper towels, not a blow dryer. Use a clean paper towel to turn off the taps and to open the exit door.

If there is no sink nearby, a 60% alcohol-based hand sanitizer can be used. Rub gel over all the surfaces of hands and fingers until hands are dry, about 20 seconds. Although hand sanitizers are effective against most pathogenic microorganisms, they are not effective against Clostridium difficile.

Hands should be washed before and after each client contact, anytime they are visibly soiled, and before and after donning and removing gloves. Change gloves frequently by turning them inside out from the wrists.

Hazard Management

Safety Data Sheets (SDSs)

Safety Data Sheets (SDSs), formerly known as Material Safety Data Sheets (MSDSs), explain how to handle caustic substances in the event of an accident or injury and provide pertinent information on the composition and toxic effects of the chemicals in the lab. SDSs outline proper storage of chemicals, procedures for cleanup, and dumping of caustic substances as well as procedures in the event of a chemical spill or injury and proper locations in the facility for clean-up. The SDSs should also contain information indicating which substances may cause allergic effects or asthma from contact or inhalation. The medical assistant should obtain SDSs for common chemicals and products being used as a safety measure so that the information is readily available. Manufacturers and suppliers should have SDSs on file and can be contacted for copies. OSHA/EPA Occupational Chemical Database provides links for SDSs for some products. SDSs are available from various other sources, including Toxicology Data Network (TOXNET), Pathogen Safety Data Sheets (biological hazards), and Poison Control centers.

OSHA's Requirement to Glove for Specimen Collection

OSHA recommends all health care workers wear gloves during specimen collection due to the heightened risk of contact with the patient's blood during this procedure. Gloves should be changed between each patient. If the medical assistant does not change gloves between each patient, he or she runs the risk of contaminating patients with infectious body fluids. Remove the gloves after collection by turning them inside out from the wrist, not by pulling on the fingers. Wash hands after removing gloves. Hand hygiene should also be performed on the following occasions, at the very least:

- Before donning gloves
- Before and after washroom breaks and meals
- Before leaving the collection area
- Whenever gloves are punctured or torn
- Whenever gloves are soiled
- At the end of a shift

Disposal of Biohazardous Material

Biohazardous material must be appropriately disposed of to protect staff and patients from possible infectious diseases. Wear a gown, gloves, and mask when handling all tissue. Post biohazard signs on walls and containers. Properly label all containers. Ventilate biohazardous areas very well and consult the Safety Officer regarding fume hoods and filters. Avoid using aerosols, especially for quick freezing tissue, because they increase the risk of exposure to infectious material. Dispose of all soft waste material in red or yellow biohazard bags, and disposable blades in red or yellow sharps containers. Disinfect non-disposable objects, such as tables. The CDC and EPA recommend steam sterilization and incineration for all waste except pathological waste, which only needs incineration. Dispose of blood in the sink with adequately running water. If the medical assistant or a co-worker is exposed to hazardous materials, start decontamination procedures immediately. Familiarize oneself with the written procedures in the policy and procedures manual (P&P). By law, P&Ps must be readily available to all staff, and the employer must train staff fully to use them.

Protocols for Exposure/Contamination Via Eye Splash

Protocols for exposure/contamination from an eye splash should be made known to all staff. If any body fluids are sprayed or accidentally splashed into the eyes, the medical assistant must immediately flush the eyes with water for at least 20 minutes at an eye station if one is available or under a faucet. If possible, water should be lukewarm for comfort. It's important to leave contact lenses in for the initial flushing as they may provide some protection, but they should be removed at the end if they have not washed out. Avoid rubbing or bandaging the eyes. Report the splash and seek medical attention.

Emergency Preparedness and Management

TRIAGE

Triage refers to the dividing of casualties/emergencies into one of three groups: immediate, delayed, or non-transport. The triage officer commands, and should be the most qualified individual, regardless of rank and seniority.

Primary triage is conducted at the scene of the incident. The triage group sorts patients according to the severity of their injuries with a color-coding system:

- Red tag: first priority patient
- Yellow tag: second priority patient
- Green tag: delayed priority patient
- Black tag: the patient is deceased

Colored ribbon, tape, or labels are also appropriate.

Secondary triage is conducted in the treatment area to prioritize medical care and transportation to hospital. The treatment group arranges the medical care for patients after they have been triaged. The supply group obtains necessary resources and distributes these as needed. The transportation officer contacts the receiving hospital about the incoming casualties. The staging group directs incoming ambulances. The extrication group frees trapped patients. Minimal documentation is required for triage because treatment is top priority. Complete documentation after attending to the casualties.

START SYSTEM OF TRIAGING CASUALTIES

START is a triage system used at multi-casualty incidents. The acronym stands for **S**imple **T**riage **A**nd **R**apid **T**reatment. START assesses patients using three parameters: Respiration, perfusion, and mentation **(RPM)**. The assessment of a patient using START takes no more than 30 seconds. Patients are triaged using START according to:

- The patient's ability to walk away from the incident site
- Whether respiratory rate is under or over 30 respirations per minute
- Whether capillary refill is over or under 2 seconds and whether the patient has a radial pulse
- Whether the patient is able to follow basic commands

The medical assistant should ensure the safety of oneself, the safety of the general public, and the safety of the patient, in that order. Don appropriate personal protective equipment (PPE) before approaching a contaminated patient. Identifying a hazardous substance should not take precedence over the health and safety of the patient. Fire department officials or a Haz-Mat team are better able to identify the hazard. Medical assistants are not generally responsible for securing or controlling the scene of the emergency; that is a police function.

Being Seconded During a Natural Disaster

When a natural disaster strikes a community, the **Multi-Agency Coordination System (MACS)** responds. EMS (police, fire department, and ambulance), Red Cross, and military search and rescue teams conduct rescue efforts. Healthcare facilities and community agencies, such as public health agencies, the CDC, and community care nurses, are second-line responders. Mass casualties require the assistance of private doctors and allied health personnel, so the medical assistant may be **seconded** to help away from their usual post. Public buildings such as schools, sports arenas, and churches are used as shelters. Extra medical supplies, food, clean water, and morgues are secured by deputies in case of looting. U.S. states and Canadian provinces follow the **Standardized Emergency Management System (SEMS)** for natural disaster preparedness, mitigation, response, and recovery. The facility's manager helps to set up the **Incident Command System (ICS)** for the healthcare facility. The Administrator On-Call liaises with community leaders and designates a spokesperson for the healthcare facility.

Emergency Preparedness Information and Training

The CDC provides free tools for **emergency preparedness** at emergency.cdc.gov/preparedness/. The Safety Officer and facility's Incident Management System (IMS) must ensure that the facility has proper emergency training and equipment.

Medical assistants must recertify in CPR with the American Red Cross or the American Heart Association every two years at the Healthcare Provider Level. All staff must attend emergency preparedness training. This includes fire, natural disasters, severe weather, and CBRN (chemical, biological, radiation, and nuclear training against terrorism). The role of each person in the medical office during an emergency must be clearly identified in the job description. For example:

- The front desk receptionist phones EMS, notifies the doctor, directs traffic, and reschedules patients.
- The medical assistant obtains the crash cart, provides first aid, and assists the doctor with life support.
- The nurse administers drugs, first aid, and contacts the patient's next-of-kin and physician.
- The doctor leads two-person CPR and administers resuscitation drugs.

The medical assistant must rehearse and cross-train. Long-term inpatients and outpatients who are on the premises for extended periods (e.g., dialysis) and are capable of understanding and participating are required to have evacuation training.

First Aid, CPR, and Emergency Response

Standard Crash Cart Equipment

A standard crash cart contains a green oxygen tank, masks, airway options, a defibrillator, and resuscitation drugs. One crash cart should be available per floor. The location of each floor's crash cart should be known by all staff members. In an emergency, the medical assistant's duties are to:

- Tell the receptionist to call an ambulance (911) and notify the doctor, or if there is no receptionist, the medical assistant should handle these tasks directly.
- Place the patient in recovery position (side-lying) while retrieving the crash cart, or staying with the patient in recovery position while directing another staff member to retrieve the crash cart.
- Reposition the patient in the Trendelenburg position, lying on the back with feet raised above chest level if they are dizzy or briefly loss consciousness but are otherwise arousable.
- Apply direct pressure to a wound to stop bleeding, if necessary.
- Position the nasal cannula over the patient's ears, or into the nares, with tubing to the side. If utilizing a mask, it should fully cover the nose and mouth. Fasten the mask firmly. Administer oxygen immediately, from 2-4 L/min. If the patient is still conscious, encourage slow deep breaths, inhaling and exhaling fully.
- Try to calm and comfort the patient. Cover the patient with a blanket to help prevent shock. Screen the patient from public view.
- Palpate the radial pulse if the patient is not responsive. If no pulse is present and the patient is not breathing, initiate CPR, starting with 30 compressions, followed by 2 rescue breaths.
- The doctor or registered nurse will intubate the unconscious patient and administer resuscitation drugs. Assist as required.
- If there is no receptionist, wait at the door to guide the ambulance attendants to the patient.

AED

An **automated external defibrillator (AED)** can revive an individual that is in specific types of cardiac arrest, providing it is applied within four minutes and damage is not extensive. Continue CPR until the unit is charged. The patient must be on a flat, dry surface. Connect the pads of the AED to the patient, as illustrated on the unit. Press the "analyze" button first for a readout, to ensure the unit is ready and electroshock is appropriate. Announce, "stay clear of the patient" while the AED is analyzing the patient's rhythm. Restart chest compressions if defibrillation is contraindicated (in the case of asystole or ventricular tachycardia with a palpable pulse). The unit indicates by tone or light that it is ready to shock the patient. The AED display shows when defibrillation occurs. Check the pulse after the third shock. If there is a pulse, check the airway, breathing, and circulation and move the patient into recovery position. If there is no pulse, continue CPR. The defibrillator will continue to provide instructions through this process. When the defibrillator announces that it is analyzing, the patient must not be touched. Continue CPR as directed by the AED. The unit indicates when to stop defibrillation.

Choking Victim and Heimlich Maneuver

If a patient is reclined, anesthetized, or eating, a **foreign body airway obstruction** (FBAO) may occur. The universal distress signal for FBAO is clutching of the throat with both hands. If the patient does this, suspend treatment immediately. A choking patient cannot speak. Breathing is difficult or absent and the mouth may be blue (cyanotic). Ask the patient to sit up and cough. If he or she cannot force out the foreign body independently, call for help. Perform the **Heimlich maneuver** to open the blocked airway. If the patient is conscious, stand behind him or her. Wrap the arms around the patient's abdomen. Make one hand into a fist and grasp the other hand firmly over it. Deliver a series of swift subdiaphragmatic thrusts, until the airway is clear or the patient falls unconscious. The patient requires follow-up medical treatment in case the airway was damaged.

Abdominal Thrusts in Unconscious Patient with Airway Obstruction

If a patient with foreign body airway obstruction (FBAO) becomes **unconscious** during the standing Heimlich maneuver, phone Emergency Medical Services (EMS) immediately. Brain death occurs in 4-6 minutes. Place the patient on his or her back. Don gloves. Lift the tongue and jaw and if the object is visible, sweep the mouth with the fingers to remove the foreign body. If the object is not visible, it is no longer advised to do a blind sweep due to the risk of pushing the object further into the airway. Next, initiate CPR starting with 2 rescue breaths, and followed by 30 chest compressions, repeating this process until Emergency Medical Services arrive.

Single-Rescuer CPR for Adult Victim

Call emergency medical services (911) before beginning **cardiopulmonary resuscitation (CPR).** Only perform CPR on a patient with cardiac arrest, who is unresponsive, with no pulse or breathing. Don gloves, if possible. Place the patient supine on the floor. Look, listen, and feel for the patient's breathing and pulse. If there is no pulse, immediately start chest compressions at a 30:2 compression-breath ratio. If there is a pulse, but no breathing, open the patient's airway by inclining the head back and raising the chin. Place a resuscitation mouthpiece into the patient's mouth. Pinch the nose closed. Inflate the lungs with two breaths. Observe the chest's rise and fall. Check the carotid pulse after administering the rescue breaths. If the pulse has been lost, kneel beside the patient. Landmark the xiphoid process at the end of the sternum (breastbone), where the ribs meet. Place palms over the breastbone. Compress 30 times, followed by two breaths. After four cycles, check the carotid pulse again. Pulse checks should never be longer than 10 seconds. Continue until the patient regains a pulse/breathing or until a rescuer with higher training arrives to provide relief. Discard the mouthpiece. Document CPR in the patient's chart.

Bleeding

When direct pressure on an injury does not stop **bleeding**, exert indirect pressure with the flats of the fingers or thumb on the nearest pulse (pressure point). Compressing the artery against a bone where they are both close to the skin surface usually stops bleeding. If the fingers are insufficient, use the heel of the hand. Indirect pressure results in inadequate blood flow to an area and can cause tissue damage from ischemia. Use indirect pressure cautiously. Applying pressure to the carotid artery can cause cardiac arrest or stroke. The brachial artery is the pressure point to control bleeding in the forearm. The femoral artery is the pressure point to control bleeding from the leg. The subclavian artery controls upper chest and neck bleeding. The temporal artery and facial artery control bleeding in the face and neck.

Only use a tourniquet to control bleeding when all other methods have failed, and only on the extremities, not the trunk or head. Write the letters TK and the time the tourniquet was applied on the patient's forehead. Release the tourniquet every 5 minutes to allow circulation. The patient may lose the limb due to ischemia.

BURNS

The types of burns include thermal, chemical, electrical, radiation, and mechanical. There are also various degrees (representing severity) of burns:

- A **first-degree** (superficial) burn is damage to the epidermis with reddening and moderate pain.
- A **second-degree** (partial-thickness) burn involves the epidermis and dermis with reddening, blistering, and severe pain.
- A **third-degree** (full-thickness) burn extends through the epidermis, dermis, and deep tissues, such as muscle and bone. It may be leathery and white or charred, and is not painful where nerves are destroyed.

Take care to assess for signs of a respiratory tract burn (inhalation injury), which produces sooty nasal hairs, nostrils, or lips and a hoarse voice or stridor. Respiratory arrest may be impending and the patient should be treated accordingly.

To begin treatment for a first- or second-degree burn, remove the patient from the burning agent. Gently remove clothing and jewelry from the affected area, provided they are not sticking, because burns swell. If there is chemical powder, brush it from the patient with cardboard so it does not react with water. Flush the burn with cool water for 20 minutes. If skin is sloughing, immerse the burn in cold water. Do not use ice. If the burn cannot be flushed or immersed, wrap it in clean cloth soaked in cool water. After the burn has cooled, the wound should be loosely covered with sterile gauze. An over-the-counter pain reliever such as ibuprofen or acetaminophen should be given. For major burns, call 911 immediately. The patient needs an antibacterial silver bandage, an analgesic, and possibly IV fluid replacement therapy.

RULE OF NINES

The Rule of Nines is often used when transcribing burns:

- In an **adult**, each part of the body contributes the following percentage to the entire body surface area: Perineum, 1%; each leg, 18%; each arm, 9%; chest and abdomen, 18%; back and buttocks, 18%; and head, 9%.
- In a **child**, each part of the body contributes the following percentage to the entire body surface area: Each leg, 14%; each arm, 9%; chest, abdomen, and groin, 18%; back and buttocks, 18%; and head, 18%.
- In an **infant**, each part of the body contributes the following percentage to the entire body surface area: Each leg, 14%; each arm, 9%; chest and abdomen, 18%, back and buttocks, 18%, and head, 18%. The palm of the hand and groin are *each* 1% of the entire body surface.

The doctor uses the Rule of Nines to determine when to give fluid resuscitation (20-25%) and when to transfer the patient to the burn unit. Burns to the face and palms are usually critical.

Review Video: Rule of Nines
Visit mometrix.com/academy and enter code: 846800

Diabetic Coma and Diabetic Shock

Diabetic coma results from prolonged high blood sugar (hyperglycemia) caused by excessive sugar or carbohydrates and not enough insulin in patients with diabetes mellitus. Initially, the patient's mental status alters. He or she is confused, thirsty, and exhibits drunken behavior. The patient urinates frequently and may vomit. He or she complains of nausea and abdominal pain. The skin is flushed and dry. The patient snores when he or she eventually sinks into coma. Ketones will be present in the urine, the blood sugar level will be elevated, and the patient's breath may have a fruity odor. This patient requires immediate attention and insulin. Fluid replacement is required. The doctor should be informed immediately.

Diabetic shock is also known as insulin shock and results from sudden low blood sugar (hypoglycemia, glucose less than 70 mg/dL) through fasting, overexertion, alcohol ingestion, stress, or drug reactions. The patient displays nervousness, irritability, shaking, cold sweats, and complains of hunger. Loss of consciousness often follows. In this case, stop the procedure. The rule of 15 should be followed, where 15 grams of carbohydrate are administered (orally if the patient can tolerate it), then the blood glucose can be rechecked in 15 minutes. Give 4 ounces of orange juice, or a glucose drink, 3-4 glucose tablets, or 6-8 Lifesavers candies immediately. A delay may cause the patient to become unresponsive and require glucagon injections or hospital treatment for acidosis. If the blood glucose is still low after 15 minutes, this process should be repeated.

Fractures

A fracture is a break or disruption in the integrity of a bone that occurs when force or weight are applied to the bone that exceed the bone's ability to remain structurally intact. Fractures occur from direct or indirect trauma, or due to diseases (e.g., cancer and osteoporosis) and congenital states such as contractures. Fractures are frequently associated with adjacent soft tissue injuries. Fractures are classified as either **open** or **closed**.

Older fracture classifications still used in transcriptions include:

Transverse (right angled to the axis)	**Comminuted** (splintered)	**Greenstick** (twisted immature bones)	**Spiral** (twisted, as in a skiing accident)	**Displaced** (complete separation; ends no longer align)
TRANSVERSE	COMMINUTED	GREENSTICK	SPIRAL	DISPLACED

Additional terms used to describe fractures include:

- Simple (skin intact, no bone contact with air)
- Compound (bone protrudes through skin)
- Compacted (bone ends are jammed together)
- Compression (where the patient loses height because the spine fuses)
- Oblique (diagonal to the axis)
- Linear (parallel to the axis)
- Incomplete (bone is still joined at some points)
- Complete (bone fragments are completely separated)

Locating and Treating a Fracture

Observe the patient for:

- **Angulation**: bones shifted out of their normal position
- **Deformity** or swelling
- **Guarding**: holding the injured body part or favoring it
- **Inability** to use the part
- **Paradoxical breathing movements**
- **Rotation**: a bone fragment turned around its central axis

The goals of the medical assistant are to:

- **Immobilize** the area with bandages or splints to prevent further injury and pain
- **Identify** the mechanism of injury
- **Call EMS** for transportation to the nearest Emergency Room for x-ray

Look for associated injuries, such as flail chest and pneumothorax. If it is an open fracture, apply a dressing to control bleeding, prevent further contamination, and minimize psychogenic shock, because the patient does not have to look at the injury. Burns that cause fractures are critical. Fractures or dislocations involving the vertebral column can cause spinal cord injuries and paralysis so do not move the patient. Clear yellow cerebrospinal fluid or blood leaking from the ear, nose, or eyes indicates a skull fracture.

Poisoning

Rapid treatment of poisoning most commonly involves activated charcoal. Syrup of ipecac, a medication that used to be recommended by pediatricians to treat poisoning, induces vomiting. More recent studies have not been able to provide evidence that ipecac prevents impending poisoning, and have found frequent misuse in the home environment. For that reason, it is no longer recommended. Activated charcoal pills or slurry absorb poison and are more often recommended to treat poisoning.

- If it **burned** the esophagus on the way down (e.g., petroleum distillates or lye), then it will burn on the way up. Therefore, dilute the corrosive poison with 2 cups of water or milk. Do not induce vomiting.
- If the patient ingested **cyanide, a medication, or a non-corrosive substance** AND is completely **conscious**, then activated charcoal is administered to absorb and clear it from the body. The medical assistant may give water and multiple doses of charcoal (charcoal slurry) to dilute and absorb the residue.
- When the doctor arrives, assist him or her with gastric lavage and neutralizing the ingested substance, if required. Depending on the pH, the doctor may neutralize a base with vinegar or lemon juice, or neutralize an acid with baking soda.

Seizures

Epilepsy is an electric storm in the brain from uncontrolled, synchronized firing of neurons. Epilepsy can be acquired from head injury or innate, from neural membranes abnormally permeable to sodium and potassium. Anticonvulsants such as carbamazepine (Tegretol), phenobarbital (Luminal) and phenytoin (Dilantin) are used to control epilepsy.

An **absence seizure** is a generalized seizure, formerly called petit mal, with no specific focus in the brain. The patient stares, lip smacks, and blinks for a few seconds. Absences begin and end without warning and are difficult to discern because there is no after-effect. However, a 3 Hz spike and wave discharges result on an EEG. Absence seizures interfere with learning. The patient is unaware of what occurred during the seizure. Youths ages 7-19 are prone to seizures from flashing strobe lights at discos and flickering TV patterns. A famous case is the December 1997 Pokémon episode that sent 700 children to hospital; 500 had confirmed seizures.

Tonic-clonic seizure (formerly grand mal) is a convulsion involving the entire brain. An aura may precede the seizure (smell, lights, or other warning symptom). In the tonic phase, muscles contract, breathing is irregular, and skin is blue tinged from lack of oxygen (cyanosis). The patient loses bladder control. In the clonic phase, limbs jerk from quick muscle contraction and relaxation. After the seizure, the patient is limp, extremely drowsy, regains consciousness gradually, and is confused (referred to as the postictal phase). Recovery takes hours.

Stroke

Signs and symptoms of stroke (cerebrovascular accident or CVA) include the following:

- Disruptions in vision
- Trouble speaking or expressing thoughts
- Headache
- Weakness affecting one side of the body
- Difficulty walking
- Numbness or tingling on one side of the body

Loss of consciousness is rare. The patient may be having a transient ischemic attack (TIA or mini-stroke), which is a warning of an impending stroke. Call the EMS (911) immediately if a stroke is suspected. Do not administer anything orally, as this patient is at risk for aspiration. Place the patient in recovery position with the affected side down, the head slightly elevated, and cover him or her with a blanket. Retrieve the crash cart. Paramedics will ask the patient to smile, to extend the arms for 10 seconds with the eyes closed, and to repeat a phrase to assess the progression of the stroke. Approximately 33% of patients who experience a transient ischemic attack will have recurrent attacks.

Complete stroke (CVA) is diagnosed if neurological signs and symptoms last more than 24 hours. It is imperative to obtain medical care as soon as possible to improve outcome. Tissue Plasminogen Activator (tPA) should be started immediately if appropriate. It can only be given within 3-4 hours of symptoms starting (depending on specific exclusion criteria) to reduce the chance for long term disability, hence receiving medical attention as soon as possible. Approximately 5% of patients who have a transient ischemic attack will have a cerebrovascular accident within one month, and 30% will have a cerebrovascular accident within one year.

Review Video: Overview of Strokes
Visit mometrix.com/academy and enter code: 310572

Syncope

Syncope is characterized by fainting due to a temporary loss of consciousness caused by a disruption in the blood flow to the brain. The insufficiency of blood results in a lack of oxygen in the brain. When the patient falls into horizontal position, blood flow to the brain is restored and the problem corrects itself. After a patient regains consciousness, place the patient in recovery position. Alert the doctor and phone EMS (911) if necessary. Syncope may result from the following:

- Emotional stress/fear
- Physical pain
- Standing in one position for too long
- Overheating
- Dehydration
- Exhaustion
- Rapid changes in blood pressure
- Heart disease
- Neurological disorders
- Lung disease
- Adverse reaction to medication

If syncope occurs with exercise or is associated with irregularities in heart rhythm, it can indicate a serious health problem. Sharp muscle contractions called myoclonic jerks may occur with syncope. This is not true seizure activity. Bradycardia and increased vagal tone are often seen in cases of syncope.

Wounds

The following are different types of wounds and their proper treatment:

- **Contusion**: A raised bruise (hematoma). Treat contusions during the first 48 hours by applying cold packs for 15 minutes on and 15 minutes off, taking acetaminophen or ibuprofen, and elevating the area. Warm washcloths help after the second day.
- **Laceration**: A long break in the surface of the skin. The edges of a laceration may be linear (smooth) or stellate (irregular). A laceration is caused by a knife blow, glass, or a surgeon's scalpel and usually requires sutures.
- **Abrasion**: A scrape or scratch of the outer layer of the skin. Friction burns and rug burns are types of abrasions. Wash the wound and remove gravel with forceps.
- **Avulsion**: A flap of tissue that is torn away from the main body of tissue, which often requires sutures.
- **Puncture**: A small, deep perforation of the skin caused by teeth, needles, icepicks, small caliber bullets, and other narrow, sharp objects. The doctor irrigates and probes the puncture.
- **Amputation**: The body part is completely detached. Wrap the amputated part in a sterile dressing and place in a labeled plastic bag on ice. A surgeon may be able to reattach it.

Additional Miscellaneous Medical Emergencies

Condition	Response
Cold exposure	Remove from cold environment, remove any wet clothing, wrap in warm blankets, begin CPR if no pulse obtained after 30-45 seconds of assessment, and utilize AED if it indicates need to defibrillate. In the case of frostbite, remove jewelry and manually stabilize the affected area; do NOT break blisters, rub or massage the area, apply heat, rewarm the area if it may refreeze, allow the individual to walk, or give anything to the individual by mouth.
Heat exposure	Remove from heat; use evaporative cooling techniques or ice packs to axilla, groin, and neck; rehydrate (half glass of water every 15-20 minutes). Administer oxygen if needed.
Joint dislocations	Splint and immobilize area, apply cold compress, place in position of comfort. Do NOT force into correct position.
Asthmatic attack	Elevate head, monitor respiratory status, assist with inhaled bronchodilator (albuterol).
Hyper-ventilation	Reassure patient, encourage patient to slow their breathing and try to relax. If a paper bag is available, have the patient inhale and exhale into a paper bag to prevent alkalosis.
Animal bite	Control bleeding, flush with NS (100-200 mL of irrigant per inch of wound).
Concussion	Elevate head, monitor vital signs and level of consciousness.

Quality Assurance and Office Safety

QA Manager and Safety Officer

Every facility must comply with The Joint Commission's Standards Improvement Initiative to obtain accreditation. If a facility treats Medicare patients, then it must also comply with the federal Healthcare Quality Improvement Program (HCQIP), Quality Improvement Organization (QIO) projects, and Quality Improvement System for Managed Care (QISMC). The facility may want the prestige associated with the International Standards Organization (ISO) standard for quality management (9001:2015).

The **quality assurance (QA) manager** ensures that the facility follows best practices required by these standards. The QA manager uses tracer methodology to ensure the quality of patient care is excellent. Help the QA manager with data collection when asked.

The **safety officer** arranges for safety training at the employer's expense and informs the staff of pertinent changes OSHA makes. The safety officer checks waste disposal of radioactive, infectious, and chemically contaminated items. The safety officer devises a computerized error reporting system, focused on processes rather than individuals and punitive actions, and reviews errors to find trends and patterns. The safety officer establishes rapid response teams and investigates adverse incidents.

OSHA Bulletins

The US Department of Labor's Occupational Health and Safety Administration has a website that provides important **bulletins** that medical assistants are required to adopt as part of their standards of practice. The safety officer must check the site regularly, notify staff of any pertinent changes, and arrange for training at the employer's expense. Medical assistants need to check the site themselves in the following circumstances:

- Whenever they need a refresher about established safe practices, such as bloodborne pathogens
- Whenever a serious new threat develops, like an influenza pandemic
- When equipment or supplies change in the laboratory to make sure the current best practices for infection control and hazardous chemicals cover the change
- When contemplating a grievance against an employer for allowing unsafe practices to verify the correct standards before registering a complaint

Creating Safe Workplace Environments

The medical assistant should take an active role in creating a safe workplace environment and preventing accidents:

- **Slips**: Most slips occur when the floor is wet or lacks adequate traction. Common causes include spills (water, urine, soap), oily substances (leaking oil), loose rugs and mats, and excessive floor waxing. Slips are especially a risk during wet weather as people may track water or snow in from outside. Floors should be checked and kept clean and dry.
- **Trips**: Most trips occur when the foot encounters obstacles (wrinkled rugs, cables, cords, clutter), view/walkway is obstructed, or lighting is poor. Traffic areas should be kept clear of clutter and lighting checked. Uneven steps should have warning signs.
- **Falls**: Many falls result from slipping or tripping, but some occur from a height, such as from a ladder or stairs. Patients who are unstable should always be assisted when walking and assisted at an appropriate pace.

Needle Stick Injury

Most medical assistants perform phlebotomy (blood collection from a vein). Rarely does the phlebotomist contract bacterial, viral, or fungal infections, but it is possible. Keep immunizations up to date, particularly for Hepatitis B and tetanus, and follow OSHA bloodborne pathogens standards. If a **needle stick injury occurs,** follow these procedures:

1. Let the wound bleed freely.
2. Wash the wound immediately with povidone iodine.
3. Report the injury within 24 hours to the employer. The medical assistant is entitled to a confidential medical evaluation and follow up.
4. Fill out Workers' Compensation forms and keep copies.
5. If breastfeeding, stop until the doctor advises otherwise.
6. Request prophylactic Hepatitis B immune globulin (HBIG) to boost antibodies. This may help even if one's immunization did not include Hepatitis B.
7. Request disclosure of the disease status of the patient in contact with the sharp in question. If it is possible, the employer is legally obligated to determine whether the source was infected with hepatitis B or HIV. The medical assistant is also entitled to precautionary blood screening.
8. If the patient is HIV+, consider taking AZT and getting antibody tests at baseline, three months, and six months after exposure. There are health and insurance risks associated with this decision, so consult a doctor first.

Reporting Unsafe Activities and Behaviors in the Workplace

Each organization should have protocols in place for the **reporting of unsafe activities and behaviors**. In most cases, reports are made to the medical assistant's immediate supervisor. Unsafe activities and behaviors include:

- **Failure to follow standard procedures**: Taking shortcuts to save time often increases risk to staff and patients.
- **Lack of understanding/information**: Carrying out tasks without completely understanding what is expected or needed can result in doing the task incorrectly. Overconfidence can lead to attempting activities for which the person is not adequately trained.
- **Inadequate housekeeping**: Improper cleaning can lead to risk of falls (from clutter) and infection (from improper disinfection).
- **Noncompliance with safety protocols**: Ignoring safety rules (oxygen storage, smoke alarms) can put everyone at risk.
- **Distractions**: Emotional upset, pain, and illness can all increase risk of errors.
- **Inadequate planning**: Last minute assignments, constantly changing assignments and duties, and inadequate preparation all can lead to unsafe behaviors.

Disclosure of Errors in Patient Care

Each healthcare facility/office should have established protocols for **disclosure of errors in patient care**, and the medical assistant must always immediately report any error to a supervising nurse or physician so that steps can be taken to prevent further problems or injury to the patient involved. An incident report should be filled out to document the error, initiated by the person involved or closest to the patient when the incident occurred. The report should be detailed, listing the date, time, and exact sequence of events as well as any witnesses. The report should be reviewed by a supervisor. If the patient is aware of the error (such as when a medical assistant accidentally strikes a patient), the medical assistant should immediately apologize and ensure that the patient is examined by a nurse or physician. For more serious errors or those for which the patient may be unaware, risk management may have protocols in place that preclude discussing the error for liability reasons.

Physical Examination

Physical Examination/Health Assessment

Collect subjective data: Subjective data is the personal information that is given by the client, such as symptoms, feelings, perceptions, preferences, beliefs, values, and ideas. Subjective data includes biographical information, physical symptoms related to each body system, past health history, family health history, and personal health and lifestyle practices.

Collect objective data: Objective data is directly observed by the examiner, such as physical characteristics, measurements (blood pressure, heart rate, respiratory rate, temperature, height, weight), range of motion of joints, appearance, behavior, and results of laboratory testing. Objective data is obtained by general observation and by using the four physical examination techniques.

The **four physical examination techniques** include the following:

- **Inspection**: Involves looking at the patient and patient's body and determining color, shape, size, and abnormalities (such as scars, birthmarks, bruises, swellings, and other injuries)
- **Palpation**: Using the hands and fingers to touch and feel body parts, such as palpating the abdomen to feel for the liver margins
- **Percussion**: Tapping a part of the body with fingers or an instrument to test reflexes or to assess hollow organs (such as the lungs)
- **Auscultation**: Using a stethoscope to listen to the heart, the lungs, and the abdomen in order to assess for abnormalities

Examination Positions

The following are positions for examination:

- **Supine**: A lateral/horizontal lying position, where the patient is lying on the back, face up. This position is utilized when examining the patient's abdomen.
- **Fowler's/Semi-Fowler's**: A sitting position where the patient is sitting upright at 90° (Fowler's) or leaning back slightly (Semi-Fowler's). This position is used when examining the patient's ears, nose, and throat, in addition to during dental procedures and the auscultation of the posterior lung lobes.
- **Trendelenburg**: Also known as shock position, where the patient is supine (face up) with the feet elevated and the head down. If the patient faints when his or her blood is drawn, then place him or her in a left side-lying Trendelenburg position to increase blood flow to the brain and reverse syncope. Place a patient with an air embolism from an IV in the Trendelenburg position to decrease the chance that the embolism will push further into the pulmonary circulation.
- **Sims**: A left side-lying position that often benefits the patient suffering with abdominal distension or ascites from liver disease.
- **Orthopneic**: Also known as the tripod position, the patient is seated upright and leaning forward to allow easy respiration. Avoid placing a patient with breathing difficulty (dyspnea) in the supine position (reclining on the back). The orthopneic position is good for EKG patients with labored breathing to minimize artifacts on the tracing.

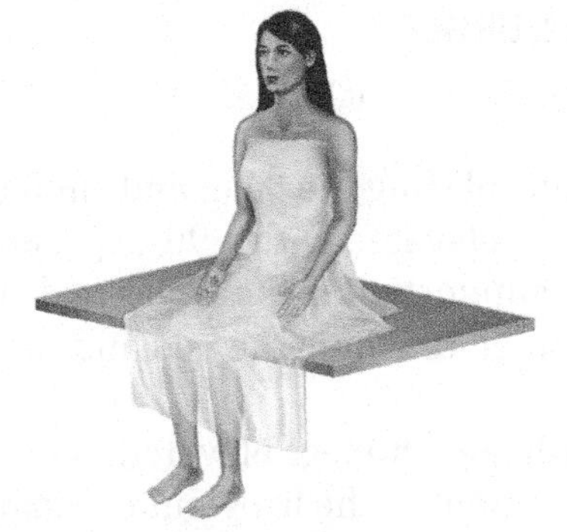

SEATED POSITION

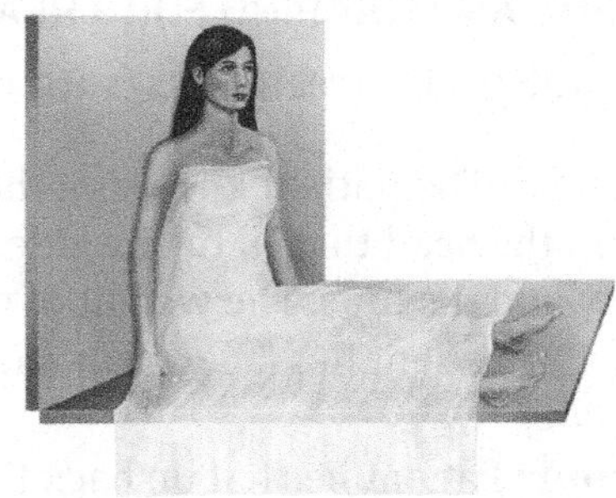

HIGH FOWLER'S POSITION

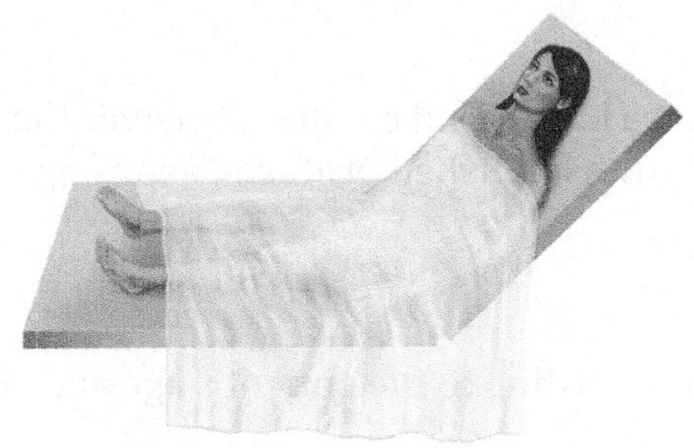

SEMI FOWLER'S POSITION

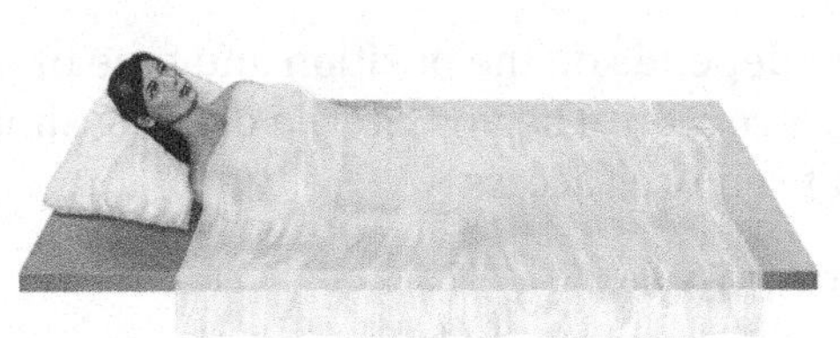

SUPINE POSITION

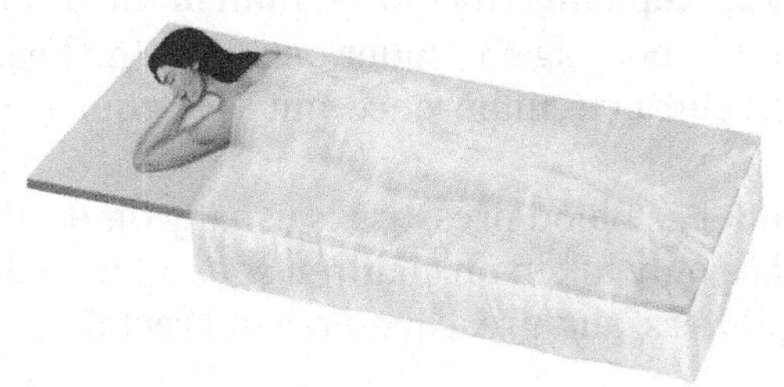

PRONE POSITION

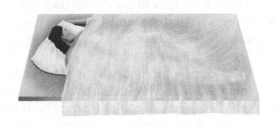

SIMS POSITION

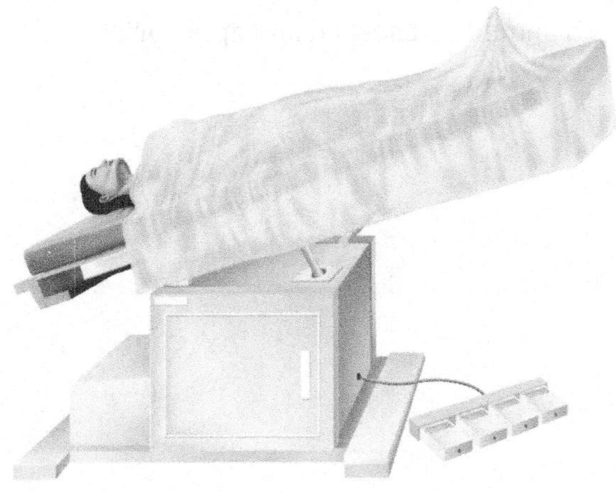

TRENDELENBURG POSITION

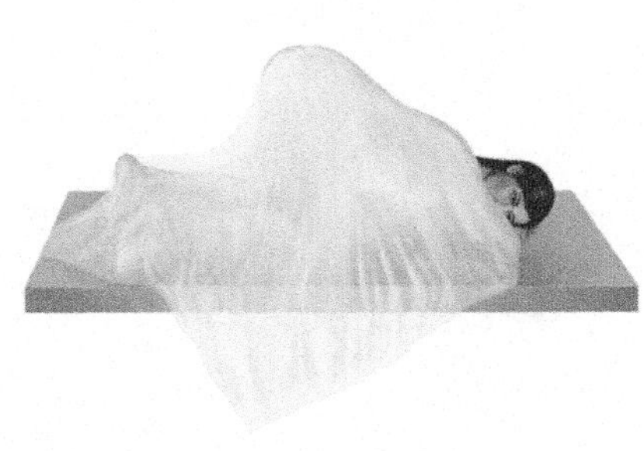

KNEE-CHEST POSITION

Body Positions and Draping for Treatments/Surgery

Body positions utilized for treatments/surgical procedures may include:

- **Knee-chest**: The patient kneels on the exam table, placing the head and shoulders on the bed, with the head turned to one side. The trunk is elevated with a 90-degree angle between the body and the hips. The weight of the body is supported by the knees and chest.
- **Prone**: The patient lies face down with the abdomen touching the bed and the head turned to one side.
- **Lithotomy**: Patient lies flat on back (supine) with feet and legs elevated in stirrups, exposing the genital area for examination or treatment of the urogenital organs and anus. The arms are extended alongside the trunk.
- **Dorsal recumbent**: The patient lies flat on the back with the knees bent and the feet resting flat on the bed so that the knees are elevated.

Draping depends on the position and type of procedure but should completely cover the patient until the procedure begins. Sterile draping should follow established protocol, exposing only the area that requires access.

Pediatric Exam

Components of a pediatric exam may vary somewhat according to the patient's age and size:

- **Height and weight**: The infant's height will be measured according to length with the infant lying in supine position.
- **Head circumference**: This is measured on infants and children until about 3 years of age to assess growth of the skull and indications of hydrocephalus (increased fluid in the brain).
- **Chest circumference**: This is also measured until about age 3. Under one year, the head circumference is usually 2-3 inches greater than chest circumference, but they equalize between ages 1 and 2.
- **Vital signs**: Apical pulse is used for children under 5; blood pressure is usually omitted on infants and small children. Oral temperatures are only taken on children ages 5 and older; tympanic or axillary temperature on infants, toddlers, and preschoolers; and rectal temperature on infants when necessary.
- **Eye examination**: A special Snellen Eye Chart with pictures or the letter E is used for small children.
- **Scoliosis exam**: Conducted between ages 8 and 10.
- **Immunizations**: The immunization record should be checked and appropriate immunizations administered.

Child's Height, Weight, and Head Circumference

The child's height, weight, and head circumference are compared to a standard growth chart to obtain the child's percentile. For example, if the child's measurements fall within the 60th percentile for height, then he or she is taller than 60% of American children of the same age and he or she is shorter than 40% of American children of the same age. To collect the data, use the following techniques:

- If the child struggles, the medical assistant should hold him or her and step on the scale. The medical assistant can then subtract his or her weight from the total to obtain the child's weight in pounds or kilograms. One kilogram equals 2.2 pounds.
- For an infant or child unable to stand, lay the child face up on a measuring mat with his or her head gently touching the headpiece. Gently straighten the infant's leg and place the sliding foot positioner on the sole of the foot. If no adjustable measuring device is available, gently place the child's head against the wall, straighten the legs, and then place a tape measure against the wall and measure to the child's heels to obtain the height in inches or centimeters. One centimeter equals 0.39 inches.
- Always record occipital-frontal circumference (OFC) in centimeters. Place a non-stretchy tape measure above the eyebrows, extend it above the ears, and note the place where the ends meet at the back of the child's head.

OB-GYN Exam

Pelvic Exam/PAP Smear

The supplies needed for pelvic exam and Pap smear include the following:

- Gloves
- Vaginal speculum
- Lubricant
- Cervical brush, spatula, and/or combination cytobrush
- ThinPrep solution or slide with fixative.

The **procedure** is as follows:

1. Explain the procedure and verify that the patient is not menstruating and has not had a douche or sexual intercourse for at least 24 hours, as these activities may interfere with test results.
2. Ask the patient to empty bladder and undress below the waist or completely (if breast exam included) and put on a gown. Instruct the patient into lithotomy position with feet in stirrups and to cover with draping.
3. Warm the speculum and provide supplies to the physician/nurse practitioner, who will insert the vaginal speculum and scrape some cells from the cervix and place them in the ThinPrep solution or on a slide for examination.

The patient may experience slight discomfort and should be advised she may have slight bleeding after the procedure. The Pap smear will be normal (negative) or abnormal (positive), meaning that abnormal cells were found. The Pap smear may also be used to test for human papillomavirus but cannot be used to detect other sexually transmitted infections.

PRENATAL EXAMS

Supplies needed for prenatal exams (initial and subsequent) are same as for Pap smear and also include:

- Venipuncture supplies: tourniquet, collection tubes, syringe, gloves
- Pregnancy test, urine specimen container

The **procedure** is as follows:

1. Obtain height, weight, and vital signs.
2. Obtain a clean-catch urine specimen and carry out dipstick urinalysis for glucose and protein.
3. Collect blood samples (if done in-house) for complete blood count; blood typing/Rh factor; syphilis; rubella titer; HIV, hepatitis B, and possibly hepatitis C titers; and blood chemistry. Complete pregnancy test.
4. Prepare, position, and drape patient and assist with pelvic exam, Pap smear, pelvimetry, vaginal cultures for STIs, and assessment of fetal heart rate and gestational age.

The physician/nurse practitioner should discuss fetal screening (triple or quad screen), timing of subsequent examinations, and procedures. At **subsequent visits** (usually every 4 weeks until month seven and then every 2-3 weeks), the fundal height, fetal heart rate, and fetal development will be assessed along with the mother's weight and urine for protein and glucose.

- Elevate head of examining table 15-25° to prevent hypotension.
- Assist with vaginal exam if discharge or spotting has occurred.
- Set up ultrasound if used to assess fetus.

POSTNATAL EXAM

Supplies needed for postnatal exam (usually at 6 weeks postpartum) include:

- Gloves
- Venipuncture supplies
- Vaginal speculum
- Lubricant
- Contraceptive supplies (if indicated)

The **procedure** is as follows:

1. Obtain height, weight, and vital signs.
2. Ask patient about lochia and cramping or other discomfort.
3. Collect blood sample (if done in-house) for hemoglobin and hematocrit.
4. Ask the patient to undress from the waist down or completely (if doing a breast exam), put on a gown, and position on examining table with drape.
5. Assist physician/nurse practitioner with pelvic exam.
6. Assist physician/nurse with insertion of contraceptive device if the patient wishes either procedure:
   a. **Contraceptive implant device**: Expose upper arm, and set up sterile field with antiseptic, syringe with needle, local anesthetic, contraceptive implant trocar kit, gauze pads, and tape.
   b. **IUD**: As for pelvic exam but with sterile field and antiseptic, uterine tenaculum, uterine sound, sterile scissors, and IUD kit.

Proctology Exam

Examination of the anus, rectum, sigmoid, and colon is generally carried out after a GI prep that typically includes laxatives and sometimes enemas to cleanse the bowel of fecal residue. Patients are typically positioned in the left Sims position. Elements of **proctology** include:

- **Proctoscopy**: A 10- to 12-inch instrument 1 inch in diameter is used to examine the anus and rectum. It is commonly used to examine for the cause of rectal bleeding, presence of hemorrhoids and indications of rectal cancer. It may also be used to obtain a biopsy and identify or remove polyps or other abnormalities.
- **Sigmoidoscopy**: Longer (extends about 20"), thinner (1/2") and more flexible than the proctoscope, the sigmoidoscope is used to examine the rectum and the sigmoid colon. The sigmoidoscope includes a distal light and camera. Use is similar to proctoscope.
- **Colonoscopy**: Similar to the sigmoidoscopy but longer (50-64 in) so that examination of the entire colon is possible. Used for diagnostic purposes and for removal of polyps.

Cystoscopy

Cystoscopy assesses the urethra, bladder, and associated structures using an endoscope. It is used to diagnose urinary problems, such as cancer, retention, infections, obstruction, strictures, and bleeding. Tissue biopsy as well as irrigations or instillations may be done through the endoscope. The patient may be asked to fast or have a special diet before the test, and may also need to stop taking anticoagulants or aspirin for a period of time. The procedure may be done under a local anesthesia or with conscious sedation.

The **procedure** is as follows:

1. An intravenous line is inserted.
2. Patient is positioned in supine position with feet in stirrups.
3. A topical anesthetic gel is placed in urethral meatus with a catheter.
4. The cystoscope is inserted through the urethra into the bladder.
5. Sterile water or saline may be instilled in the bladder to allow better visualization.
6. A biopsy or urine specimen may be obtained.
7. Cystoscope is removed.

Visual Acuity Testing

To test an individual's visual acuity, both distance and near vision must be assessed. Start with the assessment of **distance vision**. Tape a line on the floor exactly 20 feet from a well-lit eye chart. Place the Snellen chart at the patient's eye level. Perform the test first with the patient's glasses or contact lenses in place. Position the patient at the floor line. Give the patient an eye pad or paper cup. Tell the patient to keep both eyes open, but to cover the right eye with the pad or cup. Stand beside the eye chart and point to the letters. Ask the patient to read the letters aloud, line by line, from the top down. The line on which a patient makes an error is his or her visual acuity for distance. Record the reading beside the line in the patient's chart (e.g., 20/50). The top number is the distance the patient stands from the chart, 20 feet. The bottom number indicates the distance from which a person with normal vision could read the same line. For example, a patient with 20/40 vision can read the line 20 feet away that a person with normal sight can see clearly from 40 feet away. Repeat with the left eye. Tell the patient to remove his/her glasses or contact lenses. Provide a sink, soap, towel, lens case and saline, if the patient with contacts requires them. Repeat the test without glasses or contact lenses.

To test **near vision**, repeat the test with a Jaeger card held 14 inches from the patient's face.

Refractive Errors of Vision

Normal visual acuity (VA) is 20/20, meaning the patient can read the eighth line down on a Snellen eye chart from a distance of 20 feet away. The **refractive errors of vision** that may obstruct this vision include the following:

- **Myopia**: The patient sees nearby objects clearly but objects in the distance are blurry because the eye is too long. The patient can read the Jaeger card but not the Snellen wall chart and requires glasses for driving and distance vision.
- **Presbyopia**: Around age 45, the aging patient's lenses become inelastic and his or her eyes do not focus well on nearby objects. The patient can see the Snellen wall chart well, but not the Jaeger card, and requires reading glasses.
- **Hyperopia**: The eye may be too small or the focusing power too weak, so the patient is unable to see objects nearby (far-sighted). The patient can read the Snellen chart, but not the Jaeger card, and requires glasses.
- **Astigmatism**: The patient's cornea and/or lens are not smooth; they have irregular curvatures, with flat and steep sections that blur sections of the visual field.

Color Blindness and Ishihara Test

Color blindness is an inherited condition affecting 12% of men of European descent and 0.5% of women. There is no treatment, but the patient can wear glasses with red-orange filters to see cooked meat and ripe fruit. An **Ishihara test** measures Color Vision Deficiency (CVD) in a patient's sight. Color blindness is an inaccurate term because there are degrees of color loss. Many people with excellent visual acuity can see some colors but cannot distinguish differences in complementary colors, such as red and green or blue and yellow. Some people see colors well in one eye but not in the other. Seeing totally in shades of gray is a very rare condition. The U.S. Army uses colorblind people to detect camouflage. At night, colorblind people tend to see better than people with normal vision. To test for color blindness, the medical assistant seats the patient in a well-lit room and holds 10 Ishihara plates 75 centimeters (almost 30 inches) from the patient's eyes. The plates look like dotted discs from a distance. A number is hidden in the dots that colorblind people cannot see. The individual is asked to read the number on each plate in order to determine which colors, if any, the individual is unable to see.

Audiology Testing

Audiology testing measures the ability of the patient's inner ear to hear sounds through varying degrees of loudness (intensity) and vibration speed (tone). The audiometer measures **intensity** in decibels (dB) and **tone** in hertz (Hz or cycles per second).

A whisper is 20 Hz and 20 dB. Prolonged sounds louder than 85 dB cause hearing loss. A loud concert is 100 dB. The bass plays at 50 Hz, and the high violin plays at 10,000 Hz. Normal hearing range is 20-20,000 Hz. Speech ranges from 500-3,000 Hz.

If an adult cannot hear a ticking watch or a whisper, he or she needs an audiology test, which takes about 10 minutes. The doctor taps a tuning fork and holds it on the sides of the patient's head to find if the sound conducted through air is heard. The tuning fork is also held behind the patient's ear on the mastoid bone and tapped to find if the sound conducted by vibration through bone is heard. The medical assistant conducts the portion of the hearing test with the audiometer by placing earphones on the patient, connecting them to the audiometer, and attaching a bone oscillator to the patient's mastoid bones. Pure tones are emitted through one earpiece at a time, and the intensity is controlled by the medical assistant. The patient either raises one hand or presses a button when he or she hears a tone. The minimum intensity the patient needs to hear each tone is recorded on a graph. The patient should be able to hear 250-8,000 Hz at 25 dB or lower. If he or she cannot hear below 25 dB, then hearing loss is present.

Pulmonary Function Tests

Pulmonary function tests (PFTs) measure how much air the patient's lungs can hold, how fast air can be moved in and out of the patient's lungs, and how well the lungs retain oxygen and discard carbon dioxide. Use an interpretation table, because PFT varies by age, body mass, gender, and race. Seat the patient. Place a clip over his or her nose. The patient inhales to full capacity and exhales completely into a spirometer for 6 seconds. Repeat twice and take the best reading out of three, measured in liters.

- **Tidal volume** (TV) is the volume of one normal inhalation and exhalation.
- **Inspiratory reserve volume** (IRV) is the most volume the patient can inhale after a complete breath.
- **Expiratory reserve volume** (ERV) is the most volume a patient can exhale forcefully after one normal exhalation.
- **Residual volume** (RV) is the amount of air remaining in the lungs after the patient exhales forcefully.
- **Minute volume** (MV) is the air inhaled and exhaled in one minute of normal breathing.
- **Vital capacity** = TV + IRV + ERV
- **Total lung capacity** = TV + IRV + ERV + RV

Intradermal Skin Testing

Intradermal skin testing is often done to test for TB and allergies. Injections are given with the needle bevel facing upward and inserted slowly at a 10-15° angle under the skin without aspiration. When the fluid is injected, a wheal should form and then the needle slowly withdrawn, leaving the wheal intact. The skin may be gently patted with a swab but pressure should not be applied to the wheal.

Allergy Testing

When preparing to do an allergy skin test on a patient, wait until the patient's serology results come back from the lab because skin pricking could cause an antibody reaction that would result in a false positive outcome. Check the patient's existing allergy alerts recorded in the chart, particularly for latex and contrast dye, before proceeding. Keep an Epi-pen handy, in case the patient has an anaphylactic reaction. Ask the patient if he or she is taking antihistamines (e.g., Benadryl), which invalidate the results. Use a drop of normal saline on the skin as a negative control and histamine as a positive control. Follow a template for applying allergens to the skin (pollen, dander, mold, etc.) so they are recognizable after application. Scratch each application site gently with a separate needle. Wait 15 minutes. If the skin reddens at a scratch site, there is an IgE antibody on mast cells and the patient is allergic to the substance.

Allergy Injections

Allergy injections are administered to build tolerance to the substance causing an allergic response. Dosages of allergens are calculated individually and administered in slowly increasing dosages. Injections are subcutaneous with a 28-gauge, 1/2-inch allergy syringe because IM injection increases the risk of severe reaction. Patients must be observed for 20-30 minutes after injections so that emergency treatment can be administered if an allergic reaction occurs (rash, edema, itching, shortness of breath). Injections are usually administered 2 times weekly for about 15 weeks and then monthly for about 5 years.

Procedures

Eye Irrigation

The **supplies** required for eye irrigation include the following:

- Gloves
- Sterile irrigant solution
- Irrigating syringe or water pick
- Basin
- Disposable underpad
- Sterile gauze
- Towel

The following is the **procedure** for performing eye irrigation:

1. Wash hands.
2. Ask the patient to remove glasses or contact lenses.
3. Position the patient lying down and turned to the side of the eye to be irrigated or, if sitting, with the head turned to the affected side. Place a disposable underpad and towel under the patient's head or on the patient's shoulder if sitting.
4. Place a curved basin beside or beneath the affected eye (ask patient to help hold in place if sitting).
5. Wash hands again and apply gloves.
6. Cleanse eye from inner canthus to outer with damp gauze.
7. Prepare irrigating syringe or water pick and hold eye open with thumb and index finger.
8. Ask the patient to look upward or stare at fixed point and begin the irrigation from the inner to the outer canthus, allowing the solution to flow over the eye and into the basin, usually using about 500 mL solution.
9. Wipe eyelids with dry gauze from inner to outer canthus.
10. Discard supplies.

Ear Irrigation

The **supplies** required for ear irrigation include the following:

- Gloves
- Irrigating syringe or Elephant ear wash
- Curved basin
- Irrigating solution
- Disposable underpad
- Towel
- Cotton balls
- Otoscope

The following is the **procedure** for performing ear irrigation:

1. Wash hands and apply gloves.
2. Warm the prescribed solution to body temperature.
3. Check ear with otoscope if indicated to check location of earwax.
4. Position the patient in sitting position with their head tilted to affected side.
5. Place a disposable underpad and towel on the patient's shoulder.

6. Prepare the syringe or elephant ear wash and check that the solution is as prescribed (may contain hydrogen peroxide and alcohol with water).
7. Hold a curved basin under the ear.
8. Insert the irrigating tip and begin irrigation, aiming solution toward the roof of the ear canal and catching the solution as it returns in basin.
9. Continue for the duration prescribed or until the earwax is removed.
10. Dry the outer ear with cotton balls.
11. Use the otoscope to check ear for irrigation effectiveness.
12. Assess the patient for dizziness or nausea.
13. Properly dispose of supplies and gloves.

Nebulizer Treatments

A nebulizer is a therapeutic device that allows the patient to inhale medication in mist form. The purpose of **nebulizer treatments** is to alleviate difficulty breathing (dyspnea) associated with lung diseases such as asthma, emphysema, lung cancer, and Chronic Obstructive Pulmonary Disease (COPD). Examples of nebulizer medication are Pulmicort Repsules (budesonide) and Atrovent (ipratropium). The medical assistant must check the regulations in the state in which they practice, as some states do not permit medical assistants to administer medication. Assist the RN in nebulizer administration by preparing the patient for treatment. Position the patient, clean and assemble the nebulizer apparatus, and encourage the patient in deep breathing and coughing exercises before and after treatment. Recognize side-effects of nebulizer therapy, including a rapid heart rate, dry mouth, and headache.

Dressing Change

The **supplies** required for a dressing change include the following:

- Gloves (non-sterile)
- Gloves (sterile)
- Sterile dressings
- Tape
- Bandage scissors

The following is the **procedure** for performing a dressing change:

1. Wash hands and apply non-sterile gloves.
2. Place disposable underpad under the area of the wound if on an extremity or under the body if the wound is located on the chest, abdomen, or back.
3. Inspect the dressing for soiling, discharge, and loosened edges.
4. Cut the outer dressing with bandage scissors if necessary, loosen tape, and remove the dressing by pulling toward the center of the wound and lifting. Note any drainage on the inner dressing.
5. Examine the wound.
6. Remove gloves and wash hands.
7. Set up sterile field with all required dressing supplies.
8. Wash hands or use alcohol rub, and apply sterile gloves.
9. Cleanse the wound if prescribed.
10. Place the sterile dressing over the wound and utilize bandaging as appropriate for the site, securing the dressing with tape or other wrapping.
11. Dispose of all supplies, removed dressings, and gloves in a biohazard container.

Suture/Staple Removal

The **supplies** required for a suture/staple removal include the following:

- Gloves
- Suture removal kit or staple removal device
- Antiseptic as prescribed or NS
- Steri-strips, if necessary

The following is the **procedure** for performing a suture/staple removal:

1. Verify the type and number of sutures or staples in the patient's record.
2. Wash hands and apply non-sterile gloves.
3. Set up suture/staple removal kit and dressings if needed on sterile field.
4. Position the patient so that the wound is easily accessible.
5. Remove the dressing, if present.
6. Remove gloves, wash hands or use alcohol rub and apply sterile gloves.
7. Cleanse the incision with the prescribed solution or NS by wiping with dampened gauze or premoistened swabs.
8. Using forceps, lift the suture knots upward and hold them with one hand while slipping scissors underneath and clipping sutures with other hand.
9. Pull the sutures out using straight forceps and lay the removed sutures on gauze for counting.
10. If removing staples, slip the staple remover under the staples and press handle to compress and remove. Lay the staples on gauze for counting.
11. Cleanse the incision as prescribed and apply Steri-strips if indicated.
12. Apply a dressing if necessary, to protect the area; otherwise, leave open to air.
13. Verify the suture/staple count and dispose of all supplies, removed dressings, and gloves in a biohazard container.

Surgical Procedures

Surgical Tray Preparation

The **supplies** required for a surgical tray preparation include the following:

- Mayo stand
- Sterile surgical pack
- Sterile gloves or sterile transfer forceps

The following is the **procedure** for performing a surgical tray preparation:

1. Wash hands.
2. Adjust the height of Mayo stand.
3. Place the surgical pack on the Mayo stand and check its sterilization tape for color change and date.
4. Remove tape and pull the first flap away from body (the outer inch of wrap is considered unsterile). Pull the side flaps, grasping the corners only, and then pull the last flap toward the body. Do not allow the corners to fall back over the sterile field as they are now contaminated and any flap that has been below the sterile field is considered unsterile.

5. If adding liquid to a container in the sterile field, open the bottle before donning sterile gloves. Grasp the bottle by the label side, remove the lid and place it open side up on counter. If the bottle was opened previously, pour a small amount of liquid into a waste container, such as an emesis basin.
6. Apply sterile glove to non-dominant hand and pick up sterile container into which liquid is to be poured and step back from the sterile field.
7. Pour liquid into container holding the bottle 2-6 inches above container, being careful not to touch the container or splash. Replace the sterile container onto the sterile field.
8. Recap the bottle with non-gloved hand.
9. Apply other sterile glove or open sterile pack of transfer forceps to move supplies about the sterile field.
10. Cover sterile field with sterile drape if not using immediately.

Antiseptic Skin Prep

Infection control prior to surgical procedures is critical in preventing dangerous postoperative complications. The procedure for **antiseptic skin preparation** includes the following:

1. Wash hands and ensure surgical attire covers arms. Open a sterile basin and pour solution or open package of pre-moistened antiseptic swabs.
2. Wash hands (again) or use alcohol rub and apply sterile gloves.
3. Prep the skin with the solution in circular motions from incision site outward or from the least contaminated area to most (such as toward anus) in a large enough area to accommodate any extension of incision.
4. Prep all surfaces of surgical site.
5. Allow the prepped surfaces to dry completely.
6. Remove the prep solution from the skin with sterile water and gauze sponge unless it is to be left on the tissue and dry with gauze sponge.
7. Apply draping, framing the surgical site on all four sides and placing a fenestrated (windowed) drape over the incision site.

Surgical Assisting in Non-Sterile Procedures

Responsibilities of the medical assistant when assisting in **non-sterile procedures** include the following:

- Reassure the patient
- Assist others in fastening gowns
- Obtain supplies and place them on the sterile field (using appropriate technique)
- Adjust lighting, facemasks, glasses for others
- Hold specimen containers

Surgical Assisting in Sterile Procedures

When assisting with sterile procedures, first the medical assistant must be familiar with sterile field boundaries. Areas with sterile drapes are sterile fields and anything within that field is sterile. The individual's sterile field, including hand position, is limited to above the waist and below the neck. Anything below the level of the operating table or sterile field is unsterile.

Responsibilities of the medical assistant when **assisting in sterile procedures** include the following (the assistant may be gloved and gowned or just gloved, depending on the procedure):

- Ensure sterile field is not contaminated
- Pass instruments to physician and receive instruments
- Hold retractors
- Pass sponges to physician
- Take used sponges from physician and lay out for later counting
- Suction or sponge blood or drainage from surgical field
- Prepare suture/staple materials
- Apply dressing

Common Surgical Instruments

Common surgical instruments that the medical assistant should be familiar with include the following:

Forceps	Tools used to hold, grasp, or pull tissue, supplies, or other instruments (such as a needle). The jaws may be blunt, sharp, or toothed. Hemostats are forceps with narrow jaws used to grasp blood vessels and control bleeding. Needle holders grasp needles during suturing. Foerster and Bozeman forceps grasp gauze sponges. Tissue and dressing forceps (like giant tweezers) grasp tissue or sponges. Splinter forceps with very sharp tips remove foreign bodies from tissue; ear forceps remove foreign bodies from ears. Tenaculum forceps have sharp curved points to grasp tissue. Biopsy forceps have a long rod that can pass through an endoscope and a cutting instrument at the end to take a tissue sample.
Scissors	Tools used to cut tissue and supplies. Metzenbaum and Mayo scissors have sharp straight blades. Spencer suture scissors have one straight blade and one curved at the end to hook sutures for removal. Lister bandage scissors are angled to slide under bandages with a blunt tip on the bottom blade.
Scalpels/ Blades	Surgical knives used to cut tissue. A straight scalpel/blade is used to make an incision and a curved scalpel/blade to excise tissue. Scalpels may be disposable or have reusable handles with disposable blades.
Retractors	Tools used to hold wounds open with smooth, toothed, or rake-like tips. Retractors come in various sizes and shapes and some are self-retaining.
Probes/ Sounds	Long thin tools used to probe a wound to show depth and identify foreign objects.
Curettes	Instruments with a metal loop at the end to scrape tissue, such as to remove fetal tissue or to remove earwax.
Endoscopes	Instruments used to examine the interior of a body cavity or hollow organ. There are many different types, but they generally have a long flexible tube with a light source and camera at the end. A laryngoscope examines the throat; a cystoscope, the bladder; and a colonoscope, the colon.

Common Medical Instruments

The medical assistant must have knowledge of the use of the following **medical instruments**:

Catheter	Used to insert into a body part for drainage, most often into the bladder to drain urine or to obtain a urine specimen
Endoscope	Inserted into body openings (mouth, nose, urethra, rectum) to examine and to obtain a biopsy or carry out a minor operative procedure
IV start kits	Used to prepare the skin and insert an intravenous line
Kidney dish/basin	Used to collect fluids used in irrigations (such as of ear or eye) and for emesis
Nasogastric tube	Inserted through the nose and to the stomach for decompression and drainage; may also be used for gastric lavage
Otoscope	Used to examine the ear canal, the tympanic membrane, and the nares
Nebulizer	Nebulizers convert liquid medication into an aerosol that can be inhaled, such as for treatment of asthma and COPD
Sphygmo-manometer	Used to monitor patients' blood pressure, usually applied to the upper arm
Stethoscope	Used to listen to the heart, the lungs, the bowel sounds, and the carotid arteries

Preparing Patient for Safe Medical Imaging

Medical imaging includes x-rays (radiographs), CAT scan (computerized axial tomography), MRI (magnetic resonance imaging), ultrasound, and contrast and barium studies. **Preparing the patient for safe medical imaging** includes the following considerations:

- Check the patient's allergy alerts recorded in the chart, particularly for latex and contrast dye, and alert the radiology technologist (RT) if necessary.
- If the patient may be pregnant, perform a pregnancy test before imaging and inform the patient and RT if it is positive.
- Tell the patient to wear loose, comfortable clothing. Explain that he or she may need to don a gown because metal snaps, zippers, buttons, and fasteners interfere with imaging.
- Dentures, hearing aids, eyeglasses, hairpins, credit cards, watches, jewelry, and keys must be placed in the locker provided or left with an attendant because they interfere with imaging.
- Metal jewelry worn in body piercings and new tattoos are dangerous because they heat up during MRI scans. The patient must remove the jewelry and may need to wait until the dye of a new tattoo becomes safe before imaging.
- Contact the RT for specific directions that vary by test and relay them to the patient (e.g., fast 8 hours, drink a liter of water, take a laxative and enema the night before).

Electrocardiography

ELECTROCARDIOGRAPH

An electrocardiograph machine records the heart's electrical activity on an **electrocardiogram** (EKG or ECG). The EKG monitors heart rate, patterns of heartbeats, the size and location of the chambers of the heart, and helps to diagnose heart conditions. The EKG is a non-invasive, painless, inexpensive way to determine if there is any damage to the heart muscle (myocardium) or electrical conduction system. The cardiologist uses the EKG to determine if drug therapy or pacemaker implants are having the desired effect. The P wave on an EKG corresponds to the atria contracting. The QRS complex corresponds to the ventricles contracting. The T wave is repolarization.

For a resting EKG, position the patient lying down, face up. If the patient has difficulty breathing (dyspnea), prop the patient's head up with pillows. For a stress test, 12-15 leads are attached to the patient, who runs on a treadmill. For a Holter monitor, 3-5 leads are used, and the results of the EKG are recorded on a telemetry device worn around the patient's neck for 24-48 hours.

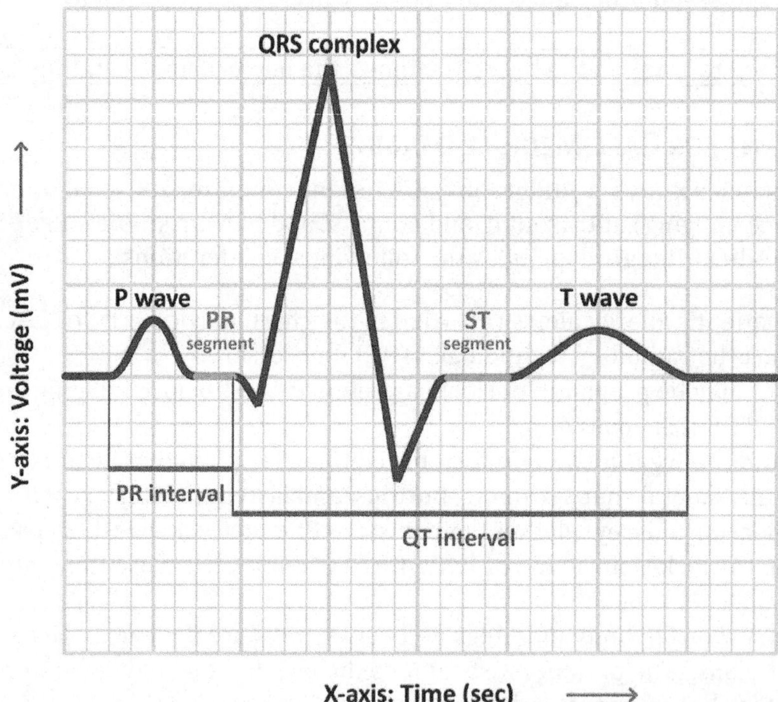

Review Video: EKG Rhythms – Reading the Graph
Visit mometrix.com/academy and enter code: 872282

Section of Heart Monitored in Each EKG Lead

An EKG lead is the wire and electrode that connects the patient to the electrocardiograph machine (also abbreviated ECG). A standard 12-lead EKG actually has only 10 wires and electrodes, which record 12 electrical vectors:

- **Unipolar Leads**:
  - Augmented Vector Right (AVR) [right atrial view]
  - Augmented Vector Left (AVL) [lateral view]
  - Augmented Vector Foot (AVF) [inferior view]
  - Precordial chest lead V1 [anterior view]
  - Precordial chest lead V2 [anterior view]
  - Precordial chest lead V3 [septal view]
  - Precordial chest lead V4 [septal view]
  - Precordial chest lead V5 [lateral view]
  - Precordial chest lead V6 [lateral view]
- **Bipolar Leads**:
  - Limb lead I [lateral view]
  - Limb lead II [inferior view]
  - Limb lead III [inferior view]

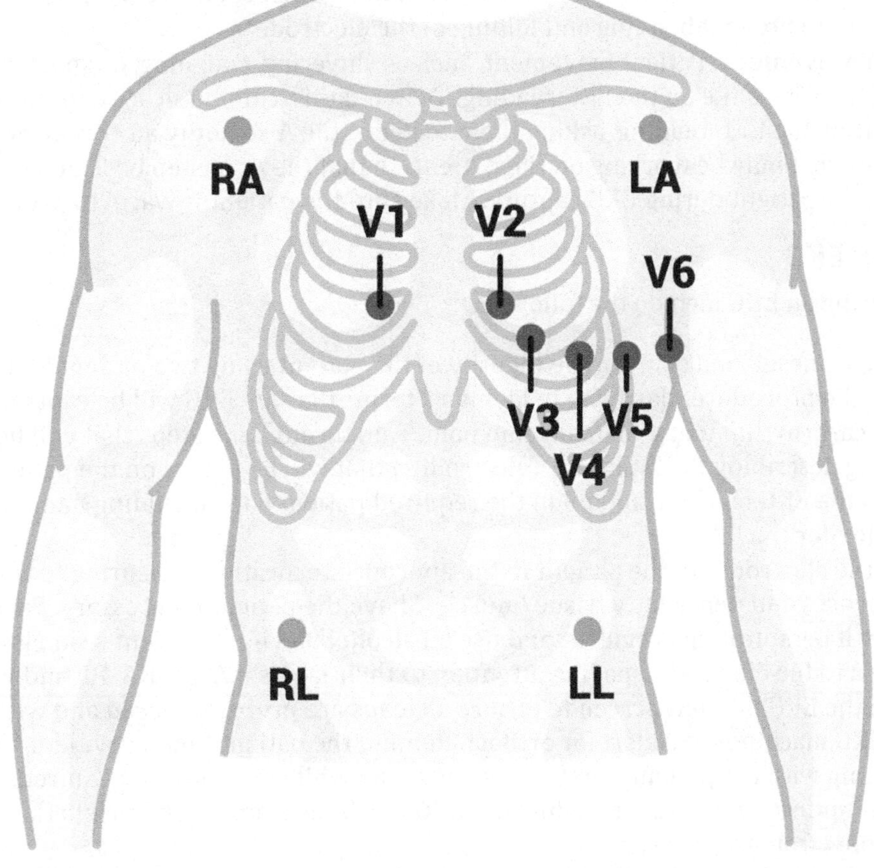

Techniques for Patients with Special Conditions

Capturing an EKG on a patient with special conditions requires the following considerations:

- **Amputee**: If the patient has an amputated limb, or a limb is not accessible for an electrode due to a dressing or wound, the priority is that the EKG leads are placed symmetrically on the body. For instance, if the right wrist of a patient is amputated, place the RA and LA electrodes on the soft tissue below the shoulder joint.
- **Pacemaker**: If a patient has a pacemaker, be sure not to place the electrode directly atop the pacemaker to avoid interference with the EKG reading. Place the electrode 3-5 inches from the pacemaker and place the RA electrode symmetrically on the other side of the body.
- **Piercings**: It should be advised that patient's remove all jewelry possible. Body piercings present a particular risk during EKG's and may be ripped out unintentionally after being snagged on the lead wires.

Artifacts on the EKG Tracing

The two most common **causes of artifact** on the EKG tracing are easily preventable:

- **Loose Leads**: Electrodes may not have sufficient adhesion to the body, due to body hair, perspiration or oil on the skin, or lead location. To avoid this problem, quickly shave heavy body hair and wipe the skin of any perspiration or dampness. Use alcohol pads to effectively remove oil from the skin and allow the alcohol to dry. Select flat locations for electrode placement to prevent bending and folding of the electrode.
- **Patient Movement**: Patient movement, such as shivering, coughing, or speaking, can cause a wandering baseline on the EKG reading. To avoid this, communicate with the patient prior to initiating the EKG reading, asking them to keep still. Also notify any of the health care members that may be working on the patient, so that they can step back and refrain from moving the patient during EKG capture. Make sure the patient is warm to prevent shivering.

Capturing an EKG

Steps for capturing an EKG include the following:

1. Introduce oneself and confirm the identity of the patient using two patient identifiers.
2. Explain the procedure, clarifying in layman's terms that the EKG will be capturing a picture of the heart rhythm that will involve no pain. Talk through the steps that will be taken, including describing the "stickers" (electrodes) that will be placed on the patient.
3. Turn on the EKG machine and fill in the required patient data, including name, age, sex, and indication for the EKG.
4. Attach the electrodes to the patient in the appropriate locations, ensuring to avoid bony prominences and dense fatty tissue/muscle. Shave the patient if necessary. Pat the patient's skin dry if perspiration is evident and use an alcohol pad if the patient's skin is oily. Attach the leads to the electrodes, paying attention to their labels: LA, LL, RA, RL and V1-V6.
5. Review the EKG preview screen to ensure all leads are properly placed and without artifact. Some EKG machines will alert for artifact. Remind the patient (and providers who are interacting with the patient) not to move or speak while the image is acquired.
6. Initiate capture. Wait patiently while the EKG machine acquires and prints the EKG. Tear the EKG report from the printer.
7. Review the EKG for artifact or malfunctioning leads.
8. Clean the EKG machine with the proper disinfectant based on the precautions required by the patient's condition. Remove the EKG and the EKG machine from the patient's room, and return to proper location.

Cleaning and Storage of the EKG Machine

Following the EKG, the medical assistant must disinfect the EKG machine. The EKG machine is used across patient rooms; therefore, all bacteria must be removed prior to removing the EKG machine and using it on another patient. While wearing gloves, disinfect the machine using the proper disinfectant identified for this patient based on their level of isolation. Wipe down the entire machine, being sure to wipe each wire and lead. Remove gloves, wash hands, and exit the patient room with the EKG machine. Every unit should have a docking station for their EKG machine. It is the responsibility of the medical assistant to know where this docking station is located. Return the EKG machine to the docking station and plug it in to the power source to ensure power is available for the next EKG ordered. Apply a "clean" tag to the EKG machine to confirm that it has been properly disinfected after patient use.

Permanent Record of EKG for Patient's Chart

While **recording the EKG**, mark the leads on the top while changing the dial to different lead settings. To make a permanent record of a strip EKG, cut it to fit an 8.5" x 11" mounting card that fits in the chart. Examine the recording, and find one accurate representative example of each lead for the permanent record (I, II, III, AVR, AVL, AVF, V1, V2, V3, V4, V5, and V6). The example must not wander from the baseline, should contain any ectopic beats, and must contain a 1-milivolt standard deflection for comparison to the wave height. If there is a run of irregular beats, include it as a fold-over. Cut the example to fit the appropriate section of the mounting card. Peel back the cover over the adhesive, and press the cutting onto the card. Include a long rhythm strip from Lead II. Note if the patient is taking cardiac drugs, such as digoxin, or if he or she had difficulty breathing (dyspnea) or complained of chest pain during the recording.

Wound Classification Systems

Classification of Wounds by Cause

Wounds can be classified in various ways. The most common classification of wounds is that according to cause:

- **Vascular wounds:** Vascular changes can result in wounds that occur most commonly in the lower extremities, such as those that result from arterial insufficiency and ischemia, those that relate to changes in the lymphatic system, and those related to venous insufficiency.
- **Neuropathic wounds:** Neuropathic changes that occur with chronic diseases, such as diabetes, and chronic alcoholism can decrease sensation and circulation, resulting in ulcerations.
- **Pressure ulcers:** Shear friction and pressure, especially over bony prominences such as the sacral area and heels, causes erosion of the tissue.
- **Traumatic wounds:** Trauma often results in contaminated wounds.
- **Surgical wounds:** Surgery can result in wounds that are originally contaminated or originally clean, depending upon the type of surgery and the reason.
- **Infected wounds:** Inflammation and infection may result in deteriorating wounds or fistulas.
- **Self-inflicted wounds:** Vary widely, from minor cuts to traumatic gunshot wounds.
- **Dysfunctional healing wounds:** Hypergranulation/keloid formation can change the character of a wound and prevent adequate healing.

Modified Wagner Ulcer Classification System for Foot Ulcers

The modified Wagner Ulcer Classification System divides foot ulcers into six grades, based on lesion depth, osteomyelitis or gangrene, infection, ischemia, and neuropathy:

- **Grade 0**: At risk but no open ulcers
- **Grade 1**: Superficial ulcer, extending into subcutaneous tissue; superficial infection with or without cellulitis
- **Grade 2**: Full-thickness ulcer to tendon or joint with no abscess or osteomyelitis
- **Grade 3**: Full-thickness ulcer that may extend to bone with abscess, osteomyelitis, or sepsis of joint and may include deep plantar infections, abscesses, fasciitis, or infections of tendon sheath
- **Grade 4**: Gangrene in one area of foot, but the foot is salvageable
- **Grade 5**: Gangrene of entire foot, requiring amputation

While this classification system is useful in predicting outcomes, it does not contain information about the size of the ulcer or the type of infection, so it should be only one part of an assessment, as more detailed information is needed to fully evaluate an ulcer.

S(AD) SAD Classification System

S(AD) SAD stands for Size (Area and Depth), Sepsis, Arteriopathy, and Denervation. The S(AD) SAD classification system for lower-extremity neuropathic disease is one of many that builds upon the original or modified Wagner classification system and assigns a 0-3 grade based on 5 categories: area, depth, sepsis, arteriopathy, and denervation.

- **Grade 0**: No pathology is evident.
- **Grade 1**: Ulcer is <10 mm^2, involving subcutaneous tissue with superficial slough or exudate, diminution or absence of pulses, and reduced sensation.
- **Grade 2**: Ulcer is 10-30 mm^2, extending to tendon, joint, capsule, or periosteum with cellulitis, absence of pulses except for neuropathy dominant ulcers that have palpable pedal pulses.
- **Grade 3**: Ulcer is >30 mm^2, extending to bones and/or joints; seen with osteomyelitis, gangrene, and Charcot's foot.

This grading system is useful, but as with most other classification systems, it doesn't provide a simple way to distinguish those wounds that follow an atypical pattern or may be consistent with the grade in some areas and inconsistent in others.

CEAP Classification for Chronic Venous Disorders

Clinical (C0-C6)

- 0: No apparent venous disease
- 1: Telangiectasia/reticular veins
- 2: Varicose veins
- 3: Edema
- 4: Skin changes
- 5: Healed ulcer
- 6: Active ulcer

Etiologic

- E_C: Congenital
- E_P: Primary
- E_S: Secondary
- E_N: No cause identified

Anatomic distribution

- A_S: Superficial veins
- A_D: Deep veins
- A_P: Perforating veins
- A_N: No location identified

Pathophysiological classification

- P_R: Reflux
- P_O: Obstruction
- $P_{R,O}$: Reflux and obstruction
- P_N: No pathophysiology identified

Staging System for Pressure Ulcers

The National Pressure Injury Advisory Panel developed a staging system to ensure that definitions for pressure ulcers were standardized.

- **Stage I—non-blanchable erythema**: Intact, reddened area that does not blanch.
- **Stage II—partial thickness**: Destruction of the epidermis and/or dermis. This type of injury may be an intact blister, ruptured blister, or an open ulcer if it has a pinkish or a reddish wound bed.
- **Stage III—full thickness skin loss**: Epidermis and dermis have experienced loss and the injury now extends through to the subcutaneous fat tissue.
- **Stage IV—full thickness tissue loss**: Damage has progressed to the bone, muscle, or tendons.
- **Unstageable/unclassified**: Injury is present and involves full thickness, but cannot be staged until slough is removed.
- **Suspected deep tissue injury**: Discolored skin that is still intact but has been damaged. The injury is likely deeper than a stage one injury, but the epidermis is still intact, and therefore the depth cannot be visualized.

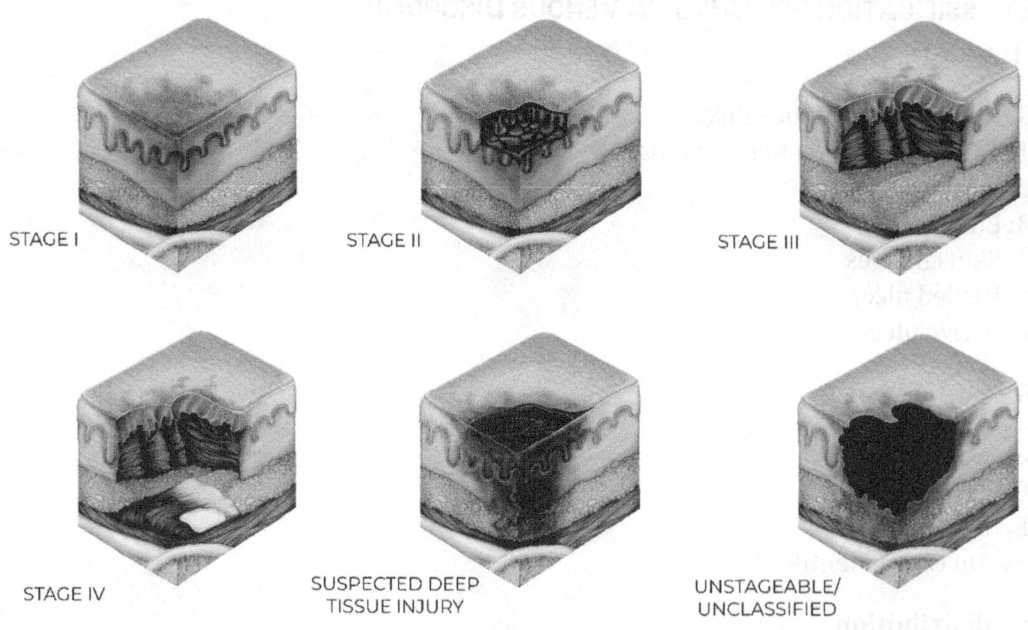

Wound Healing

PRIMARY, SECONDARY, AND TERTIARY HEALING

Primary healing (healing by first intention) involves a wound that is surgically closed by suturing, flaps, or split or full-thickness grafts to completely cover the wound. Primary healing is the most common approach used for surgeries or repair of wounds or lacerations, especially when the wound is essentially "clean."

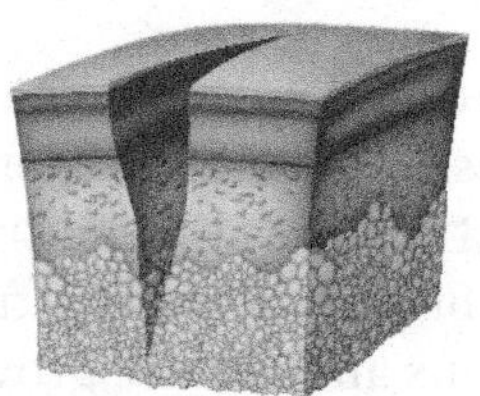
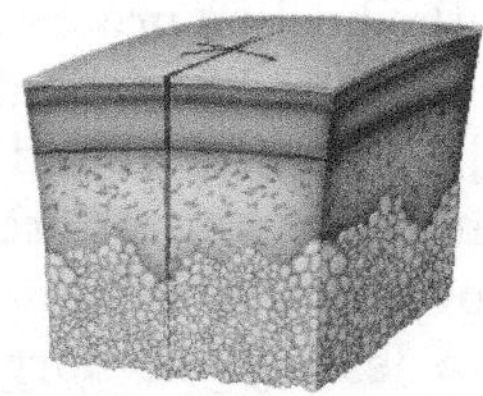
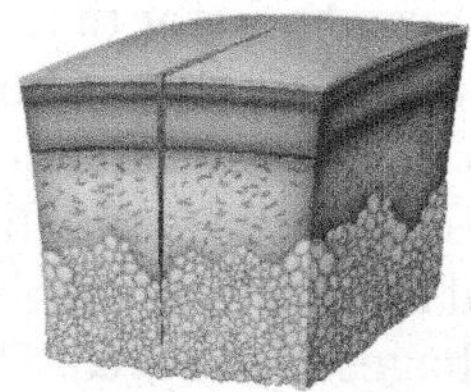

Secondary healing (healing by second intention) involves leaving the wound open and allowing it to close through granulation and epithelialization. Debridement of the wound is done to prepare the wound bed for healing. This approach may be used with contaminated "dirty" or infected wounds to prevent abscess formation and allow the wound to drain.

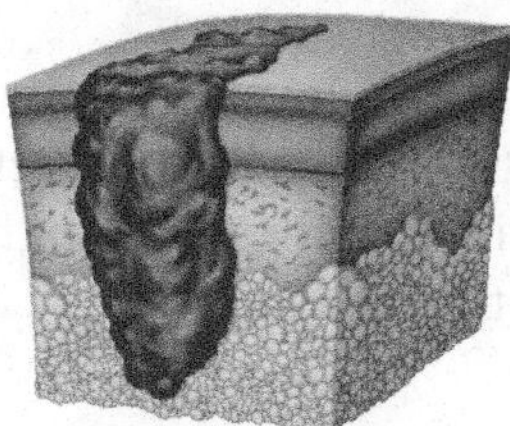
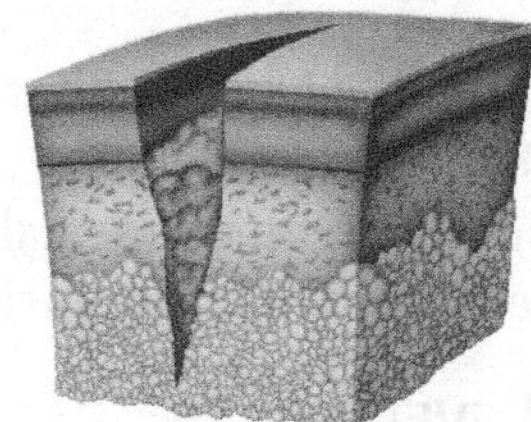
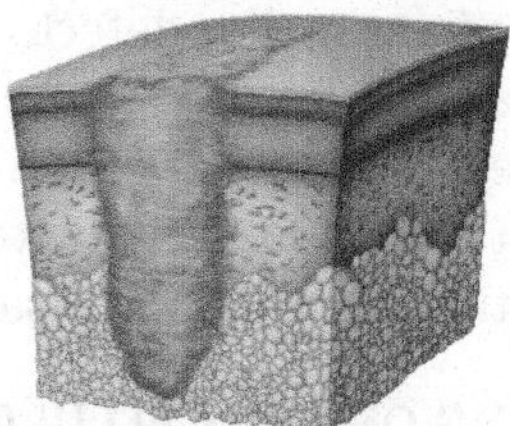

Tertiary healing (healing by third intention) is also sometimes called delayed primary closure because it involves first debriding the wound and allowing it to begin healing while open and then later closing the wound through suturing or grafts. This approach is common with wounds that are contaminated, such as severe animal bites, or wounds related to mixed trauma.

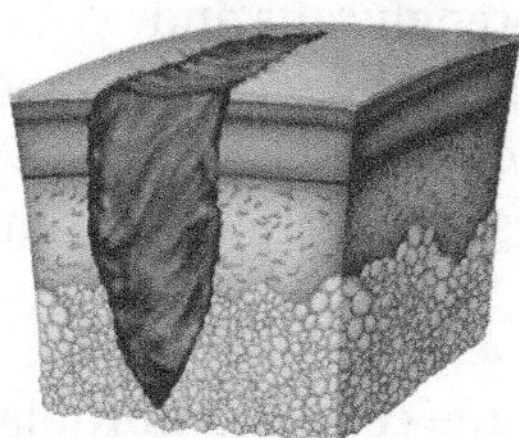
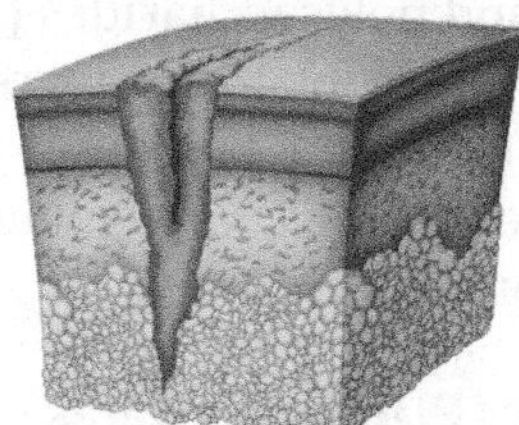
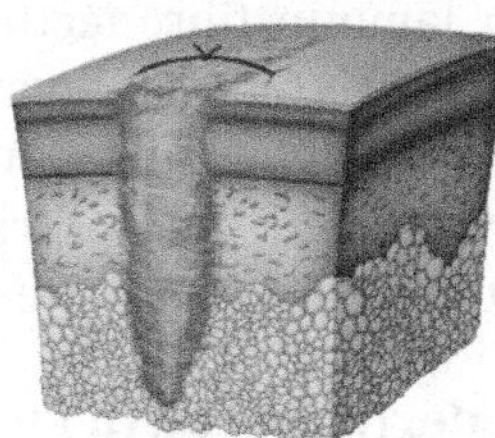

Phases of Wound Healing

There are **four phases of wound healing**:

1. **Hemostasis** is the first phase of wound healing, occurring within minutes of injury. After the wound occurs, the blood vessels constrict to decrease bleeding. Platelets gather to form a clot and then secrete factors, which cause the production of thrombin. This stimulates fibrin formation from fibrinogen. The resultant clot is a strong one, which becomes the serosanguinous crust (scab) for the wound. Platelets secrete cytokines, including platelet-derived growth factor that begins the healing process.
2. The **inflammation phase** occurs next and lasts about four days normally. Blood vessels in the area leak plasma and neutrophils into the wound, causing erythema, edema, and increased warmth. Any debris or microorganisms are destroyed by the neutrophils and localized mast cells through phagocytosis. When fibrin is broken down, it attracts macrophages to the area. They also destroy microorganisms and secrete growth factors to stimulate the next phase of healing.
3. The **proliferative phase** occurs over about days 5-20 in normal healing. During the proliferative phase, fibroblasts secrete collagen to manufacture a framework within the wound. New capillaries sprout from damaged vessel ends in a process called angiogenesis. Keratinocytes cause epithelialization in which new skin cells form at the edges of the wound, migrating inward to meet in the center of the defect. Approximately five days after a wound occurs, the fibroblasts and myofibroblasts contract to bring the wound edges closer, resulting in a smaller defect.
4. **Remodeling or maturation** of a wound begins about 21 days after the wound occurs and continues over the next year. Collagen is deposited, eventually resulting in a stiff, strong scar that has 70-80% of the tensile strength of normal skin. Blood vessels in the newly formed tissues gradually disappear from the scar during this phase.

Wound Healing on the Cellular Level

Cytokines are proteins that serve as soluble mediators and are essential to wound healing. They include growth factors, tumor necrosis factors, interferons, and interleukins. Cytokines are produced from platelets, fibroblasts, monocytes, endothelial cells, and macrophages and facilitate communication between cells and regulate cell proliferation and inflammatory reactions as part of healing. Cytokines also attract neutrophils and macrophages. Cells in the wound produce extracellular matrix proteins. The extracellular matrix includes fibrous and adhesive proteins (collagen, elastin, laminin, fibronectin) and polysaccharides (proteoglycans and glycosaminoglycans [GAGs]). Following injury, platelets aggregate and degranulate, activating factor XII (Hagerman), which promotes formation of a fibrinous clot, which then activates fibrinolysis to break down the clot triggering the complement system. Platelet degranulation triggers release of cytokines into the wound, including:

- **Platelet-derived growth factor (PDGF)**: Activates immune cells and fibroblasts, promotes formation of extracellular matrix and angiogenesis.
- **Fibroblast growth factor (FGF) and epidermal growth factor (EGF)**: Increases proliferation/migration of keratinocytes and extracellular matrix deposition, epithelial cell proliferation, angiogenesis, and formation of granulation tissue.
- **Transforming growth factor (TGFα and TGFβ)**: Promotes formation of extracellular matrix, reduces scarring, increases collagen and tissue inhibitors of metalloproteinase synthesis, decreasing collagen and fibronectin.
- **Tumor necrosis factor α**: Expressed by macrophages to stimulate angiogenesis.

Partial-Thickness and Full-Thickness Wound Healing

Partial-thickness wounds involve only the epidermis and the upper parts of the dermis, so the underlying structures that repair skin and provide nutrients, such as the vasculature, and protection, such as the glands, remain intact. Bleeding activates hemostasis and provides a temporary bacterial barrier. Coagulation occurs and fibrin is formed with the clot sealing disrupted vessels. This is followed by fibrinolysis, during which the clot breaks down and repair begins with the inflammatory stage. Healing phase's progress and wounds usually heal within about 2 weeks.

Full-thickness wounds involve the loss of the epidermis and dermis and may also involve loss of underlying tissues, through the fascia, muscle, and to the bone. Full-thickness wounds may be acute or chronic and heal by primary or secondary intention. Those healing by secondary intention are usually surgical wounds that have dehisced or those resulting from underlying morbidities that interfere with normal healing. Bleeding and hemostasis do not occur with healing by secondary intention, compromising the healing process.

Acute and Chronic Wound Healing

Acute wounds are usually related to an injury and bleed freely because circulation is unimpaired. They heal quickly and continuously, going through the phases of healing in a predictable manner for the size of the wound. There are few if any complications in the healing process.

Chronic wounds are associated with problems in healing, often because of underlying arterial insufficiency. There may not be normal functioning of the components in the healing process or the components may be delayed. For example, the inflammatory phase of healing is usually prolonged. Normal regulatory signals that cause growth to occur may be ignored by the body. There may be repeated injuries to the area, increased inflammation, and poor supply of oxygen and nutrients to the wound. There may be host factors, such as smoking and malnutrition that hamper healing. Genetic and systemic disease can both result in chronic wounds that fail to heal.

Microenvironmental Factors That Affect Wound Healing

Wound microenvironment refers to the condition of the wound bed. One problem is that there is often insufficient bleeding in the wound microenvironment initially, so there is less thrombin produced and this impairs production of fibrin. There may be an inadequate supply of growth factors. The lack of growth factors prevents the proliferation of new cells. Lack of innervation may further impair healing. The inflammatory phase is often prolonged, and there is inadequate debridement as phagocytosis is impaired. The presence of infection competes with newly forming skin cells for adequate oxygen and nutrients. The toxins from bacteria further pollute the microenvironment. Moisture is necessary for repair but the presence of excess exudate can restrict cell growth and introduce harmful proteases that further break down growth factors.

Signs of Wound Healing

The wound bed must be examined to determine the color of the tissues, amount of moisture present, and degree of epithelialization to demonstrate **signs of healing**:

- Granulation tissue has a granular appearance, is beefy red, feels soft and sponge-like to the touch, bleeds readily when probed, and exhibits no twitch when pinched. It must be distinguished from non-granular tissue, which is smooth and red, and not healing, and hypergranulation, which is soft and spongy and rises above the level of the wound and interferes with epithelialization.
- Epithelialization migrates out from the edges of the wound towards the center. Tissue is usually dry and appears light pink or violet-colored.

The wound bed may show a combination of slough, necrotic tissue, and granular tissue at the same time, so the percentage of each should be determined so that the progress of epithelialization can be demonstrated over time. Pain should be assessed as it may indicate infection.

SCARRING

FACTORS INFLUENCING THE AMOUNT OF SCAR TISSUE FORMED

Deeper wounds produce more scar tissue because a larger amount of granulation tissue is deposited over a longer period of time. The amount of inflammation in a wound also helps to determine the amount of scar tissue formed. Highly pigmented skin produces more scar tissue as does a genetic propensity towards scarring. Tension on a wound during healing causes tissue damage and increased inflammation. This tension is increased in the young versus an older person due to tighter skin and more activity, so children form larger scars than elderly people. Wound location also contributes to scar formation.

EXCESSIVE SCARRING

Excessive scarring includes hypertrophic and keloid scars, which are characterized by raised scars that are erythematous and itchy. Excessive scarring is more common in darkly pigmented skin or in areas where the tissue may stretch, such as over joints. Young or pregnant patients or those with a family history of excessive scarring are at increased risk. There are some distinctions between hypertrophic and keloid scars:

- **Hypertrophic scars** most frequently occur over joints where there is tension on the wound (dorsum of the feet, buttocks, shoulder and upper arms, and upper back). They remain localized to the area of the original wound and may spontaneously regress. Scars that form over joints can cause limited mobility as they contract and may need surgical revision to allow more normal movement.
- **Keloid scars** most frequently occur on the upper back and chest as well as the deltoids and earlobes. They extend beyond the original wound and rarely regress. They usually arise after the wound has healed as raised, shiny, rope-like fibrous scars. They do not result in contracture of the wound. Keloids are most common in those with darker skin and occur due to excess collagen deposition, causing increased growth.

SCARLESS HEALING

Scarless healing occurs in the early-gestation fetus, during the first 2 trimesters, but this ability to heal without scars is lost during the 3rd trimester. This is important for intrauterine surgical procedures, commonly performed during the second trimester when abnormalities become evident. The fetus heals without scarring for a variety of reasons:

- Platelet aggregation is lessened, resulting in less growth factor, such as PDGF.
- The inflammatory response is lessened because of immaturity of the immune system and lack of inflammatory cytokines.
- Wounds move quickly from the inflammatory to the proliferative stage of healing. Fibroblasts, keratinocytes, and endothelial cells, critical to tissue formation, rapidly cover the wound bed. There is no contraction or scarring of the wound.
- Growth factors are balanced so they stimulate growth of connective tissue but prevent excess from forming.
- New and native collagen is indistinguishable, so the new tissue remains flexible.

Non-Healing Wounds

Characteristics of non-healing wounds include:

- **Infection**: Infection increases pro-inflammatory cytokines and prolongs the inflammatory phase of wound healing, sometimes resulting in a non-healing chronic wound. Growth factors may degrade. With infection, granulation tissue may appear dusky. Common pathogens include *Staphylococcus aureus, Pseudomonas aeruginosa,* and β-hemolytic *streptococci.*
- **Biofilm**: A dense thin layer of bacteria in a moist adhesive matrix of secreted polymers that clings to the surface of wounds. Multiple bacteria may be present in a biofilm. The biofilm is resistant to antibiotics and to phagocytosis by white blood cells, resulting in degrading and/or non-healing wounds. Biofilms on the surface of wounds may be mechanically removed.
- **Closed edge**: The wound edges become rolled/curled, dry, and hyperkeratotic and fail to advance, a condition referred to as epibole. Epibole appear light-colored in comparison to surrounding tissue, rounded, and firm. Causes include impaired wound bed, infection, hypoxia, drying, and trauma.

Factors That Affect Skin's Ability to Heal

Age

Age is an important consideration when evaluating the skin because the characteristics of the skin change as people age.

- An **infant's** skin is thinner than an adult's because, while the epidermis is developed, the dermis layer is only about 60% of that of an adult and continues to develop after birth. The skin of premature infants is especially friable, allowing for transepidermal water loss and evaporative heat loss.
- During **adolescence**, the hair follicles activate, the thickness of the dermis decreases about 20%, and epidermal turnover time increases, so healing slows.
- As people **continue to age**, Langerhans' cells decrease in number, making the skin more prone to cancer, and the inflammatory reactions decrease. The sweat glands, vascularity, and subcutaneous fat all decrease, interfering with thermoregulation and contributing to dryness and irritation of the skin. The epidermal-dermal junction flattens, resulting in skin that is prone to tearing. The elastin in the skin degrades with age and solar exposure. The thinning of the hypodermis can lead to pressure ulcers.

Review Video: Integumentary System
Visit mometrix.com/academy and enter code: 655980

Lotions, Oils, and Soaps

Lotions, oils, and soaps all have an effect on the skin. Many oils and lotions are used to increase hydration of the skin. These can include oil baths, which have a minimal effect on hydration but do increase the skin-surface lipids. Lipids are the fatty substances that surround skin cells, and those in the outer layer of skin, the stratum corneum, with fatty acids form the water barrier to retain skin hydration and soften skin. Sebum, produced by the sebaceous glands, is also a lipid. Applying lotion increases the hydration of the epidermis, giving the skin a smoother appearance, and moisturizing lotions also increase the lipids, providing some protection. Alkaline soaps, on the other hand, removes the lipid coating of the skin for about 45 minutes after a normal washing and may increase dryness and susceptibility to bacterial infection. Alcohol and acetone also remove the lipid coating and can increase dehydration of the skin. Acidic cleaners are less irritating than either neutral or alkaline cleaners.

Sun Exposure

Sun exposure is one of the primary factors in aging of the skin, referred to as photoaging or dermatoheliosis. Tanning occurs when ultraviolet radiation (UVR) damages the epidermis and stimulates the production of melanin as a protective mechanism to prevent damage to deeper layers of skin. When the melanin is overpowered, sunburn results, damaging the outer layers of the skin and sometimes the DNA of the skin cells, which can lead to cancer. There are several effects of photoaging that should be noted in assessment:

- Decrease in elasticity and strength
- Dry, rough, wrinkled skin
- Fine veins on face and ears
- Freckles and large brown macules (solar lentigines, liver spots) on face, and exposed areas, such as hands and arms and white macules on exposed areas of upper and lower extremities
- Benign lesions, such as actinic and seborrheic keratoses
- Malignant lesions, such as basal cell and squamous cell carcinoma

Medications

Medications are a frequent cause of dermatologic effects that can impair the integrity of the skin:

- **Photosensitivity** can be either photoallergic with exposure to ultraviolet radiation causing an allergic reaction, usually with rash, erythema, edema, and pruritis or phototoxic with the drug being converted into a toxin that causes edema, pain, and pronounced erythema. Thiazide diuretics and conjugated estrogens often cause photosensitive reactions.
- **Allergic reactions** may involve rash, urticaria or more complex reactions, such as serum sickness. Amoxicillin alone or with clavulanate causes a high rate of these reactions.
- **Erythema multiforme** has been caused by nifedipine, verapamil, and diltiazem (calcium channel blockers).
- **Toxic epidermal necrolysis** with full-thickness loss of epidermis can be caused by ciprofloxacin.
- **Thinning or atrophy of the skin** because of a loss of collagen and telangiectasia (spider veins) are associated with oral, topical, and inhaled corticosteroids.

Local Factors

Local factors that may impact the healing process include:

- **Local infection**: Invasion of the wound by microorganisms, such as *Staphylococcus aureus, MRSA, Pseudomonas,* and *Escherichia coli,* not only slows healing but may cause the wound to erode and increase in size, increasing the risk of systemic infection. Inflammation is a normal part of the healing process, but prolonged inflammation delays healing.
- **Repeat trauma**: If a wound is not adequately protected or if the patient is not positioned correctly, further erosion of the wound may occur.
- **Impaired tissue oxygenation**: Conditions that result in vasoconstriction or low blood flow to the area (such as PAD, blood clot, and hypotension) of the wound can impair healing or worsen the wound. Wounds are typically hypoxic initially because of disruption of blood flow and increased need for oxygen, but this triggers angiogenesis and release of growth factors, which should increase oxygenation unless other factors are present.

Systemic Factors

Systemic factors that may impact the healing process include:

- **Inadequate nutrition**: A diet with adequate nutrition and protein is necessary for healing, so an inadequate diet may slow the healing process.
- **Obesity**: Patients who are overweight are at increased risk of pressure sores because of compression of tissues, and have slower rates of healing as well as increased risk of infection.
- **Chronic disease**: Some diseases, such as diabetes mellitus and hypertension may impair healing.
- **Systemic infection**: Whether originating from the wound or elsewhere, a systemic infection impairs healing.
- **Decrease in sex hormones** (usually associated with age): Low levels of androgens and estrogen slow healing of wounds.
- **Stress**: Emotional stress increases glucocorticoids and reduces cytokines at the wound, impairing healing.

Wound Preparation

Closure of Dead Space

Dead space is the defect of soft tissue left behind after debridement or excision of a space-occupying lesion. Dead space may also occur if portions of the wound separate beneath the skin after primary closure, leaving an open pocket if air/fluid becomes trapped between tissue layers. Closure of the dead space is essential because it promotes healing and decreases the risk of infection. Treatment options vary depending on the location, extent of the dead space, and the cause, but may include application of a compression bandage (using care not to apply excessive pressure that may impair oxygenation), insertion of a drain (open or closed, active or passive), and/or aspiration of fluid contents (seroma) of the dead space. Negative pressure wound therapy may be utilized for large wounds. Dead spaces open to the surface should be completely filled with suitable wound packing material (depending on the extent of drainage) but should be lightly packed so as to avoid pressure on healthy tissue. Patients may need to restrict activity during treatment for dead space.

Wound Edge Optimization

Chronic wounds may take weeks or months to heal, so wound edge optimization is essential to healing. If the wound edges are not advancing or there are indications of undermining or deterioration, this may indicate that the wound cells are nonresponsive and that there are abnormalities of protease activities. Wound optimization methods include careful wound assessment and adequate debridement of the wound to remove necrotic tissue through sharp excision or enzymatic debridement, such as with collagenase, which debrides and promotes epithelialization. Maintaining appropriate moisture balance is also important as excessive moisture may cause maceration and deterioration of the wound, while inadequate moisture may result in desiccation of the wound and slowed epithelialization. The choice of dressing, therefore, may affect the healing process. If infection occurs appropriate antimicrobials (systemic or topical) may be necessary. In some cases, bioengineered skin or skin grafts may be appropriate. Additionally, edema slows healing, increases the risk of bacterial colonization, and must be controlled, such as through compression therapy. Wound exudate should be controlled because exudate, especially with chronic wounds, depresses cell proliferation (fibroblasts, keratinocytes).

Maintaining a Warm and Moist Wound Environment

One of the basic principles of current wound care is the use of occlusive dressings that keep the wound warm and moist. There are a number of reasons for keeping a healing wound warm and moist:

- **Reduction in dehydration** allows cells such as neutrophils and fibroblasts to carry out their functions in wound repair, as they require a moist environment. This also results in less cell death.
- **Angiogenesis** requires a moist environment and low oxygen tension, which is found in occlusive dressings.
- **Autolytic debridement** with proteolytic enzymes is enhanced in a moist environment.
- **Re-epithelization** of tissue occurs because the epidermal cells are able to spread across the surface of the wound.
- **Reduction in microorganisms** because of the seal provided by occlusive dressings decreases infection.
- **Pain reduction** results from the protection of the nerve endings and the need for fewer dressing changes.

Periwound Skin Protection

The area extending about 4 cm from the wound edges is the periwound tissue, and it is especially vulnerable to irritation from drainage and adhesive. The periwound tissue should be evaluated for increased warmth and erythema as well as signs of maceration from exposure to exudate. Moisture-associated and adhesive associated skin damage can be prevented and treated by gentle cleansing of the periwound tissue with NS or water and application of a skin barrier. Moisture-retentive dressings help to keep the wound surface moist while avoiding excessive wetness and can wick fluid away from the periwound tissue. Dressing changes should be minimized to prevent stripping of periwound skin. Barriers may include:

- **Alcohol-based skin sealants**: Provide a sticky surface to help adhesives adhere and provide some skin protection. Available in wipes and spray.
- **Creams/Ointments**: May contain petrolatum, zinc oxide, or dimethicone and are applied in a thin layer to the skin and covered with absorptive dressings or applied in the perineal area to prevent skin irritation from incontinence.
- **Topical corticosteroids**: Used for allergic reactions, such as to adhesives.

Wound Cleansing

Wound Cleansing with Each Dressing Change

Microorganisms, contaminants, and cellular debris in a wound can significantly delay healing and increase inflammation. Antiseptics such as hydrogen peroxide, acetic acid, povidone-iodine, or sodium hypochlorite (Dakin solution) are toxic to developing fibroblasts and interfere with healing over time. They are sometimes used and rinsed with saline for a short period of time to control heavily infected wounds. The current standard is to use irrigation to deliver normal saline in a manner forceful enough to break the adhesion of debris to the wound bed yet gentle enough to prevent injury to developing cells. Pressures of at least 5-15 psi delivered by mechanical irrigators are needed for effective cleansing. Higher pressures can cause penetration of the fluid into tissues. Irrigation using a 12 mL syringe and a 22 G needle will deliver a force of 13 psi. The use of a 35 mL syringe and a 19 G needle will deliver 8 psi and is more effective than using a bulb syringe when mechanical irrigation is not available.

Cleansing a Wound by Soaking

Soaking is a beneficial way to cleanse a wound that has a large amount of necrotic debris or contamination. Contamination must be removed from new wounds to avoid excess inflammation that will delay wound healing. Soaking softens any necrotic tissue and helps to ease it away from the healthy tissue at the bottom of the wound bed. It also helps to loosen contaminants that are embedded in the wound. Antiseptic agents should not be used in the soaking solution. Soaking may be accomplished using any container that will hold the wound area, or by whirlpool. The container must be disinfected well prior to and after the soaking. It may take several soaks to remove tough, dry eschar, and once the necrotic material has been removed, soaking should be discontinued, as it will then delay healing.

Irrigating a Wound for Cleansing Purposes

When **irrigating a wound** for cleansing purposes, the area beneath the wound should be covered to prevent contamination of the bed linens:

1. Place a basin beneath the wound to catch the returned solution.
2. Wash hands and wear gloves.
3. Use pulsatile lavage or a syringe to deliver water or saline with a force of 5-15 psi to the wound bed. Using pressure >15 psi forcefully injects irrigating fluid into newly formed tissues and risks inoculating microorganisms into deeper tissues. Highly contaminated or infected wounds may require pressure at the higher range of 15 psi to cleanse. Use low pressure (5-8 psi) to cleanse healthy wounds so new capillaries are not damaged.
4. Flush undermined, tunneled areas well, and then massage over the area of tunneling or undermining to dislodge debris and encourage the fluid to return.
5. Repeat as needed until the return fluid is free of debris.
6. Finish by packing these areas as ordered.

Cleansing a Shallow Wound by Scrubbing

Scrubbing is sometimes combined with a cleansing solution to initially cleanse a wound to remove debris. It is best performed using a very porous, soft sponge and a nonionic surfactant cleansing solution to avoid damaging the wound bed as much as possible. Even so, damage to the wound bed is often unavoidable, so scrubbing may be done initially to a traumatic wound, but the practice should not be continued after the wound is clean and beginning to heal because it can disrupt the development of granulation tissue and damage areas of epithelialization. When scrubbing, one should begin cleansing in the center of the wound and work in a circle toward the edges of the wound, avoiding recleansing an area to prevent recontamination of the center of the wound.

Pulsed Lavage

Pulsed lavage (pulsatile high-pressure lavage) is irrigation of an infected or necrotic wound under pressure, using an electrically powered device. Normal saline is commonly used for lavage treatments with the amount varying according to the size and amount of exudate on the wound. It is recommended that the pressure be 8-15 psi. The pressure can be varied as needed. While there is concern that higher pressure may inoculate tissue with bacteria, studies have not indicated this. Exposed blood vessels, graft sites, and muscle tissue should be avoided with the lavage treatments, and treatments should be discontinued if bleeding occurs with patients taking anticoagulants. Treatment is usually done 1-2 times daily. Both the hose and irrigating nozzle are intended for one-time use, so treatments can be expensive.

Wounds Requiring Pulsed Lavage

Pulsatile lavage can be used on almost any type of wound but is particularly indicated for the following:

- Clean wounds to encourage granulation and healing
- Wounds with delayed healing to encourage granulation and stimulate epithelialization
- Severely contaminated or infected wounds to reduce microorganisms in the wound bed
- Pre-graft wound preparation to remove any contamination, foreign material, or necrosis and provide an optimal graft surface
- Diabetic neuropathic ulcers to treat without damaging callus or fragile areas
- Sacral wounds to allow easy access and comfort (as opposed to sitting in whirlpool)
- Wounds with undermining and tunneling to effectively irrigate (using smaller, flexible irrigation wands)

Patients who have cardiac monitoring, urinary catheters, IV lines, or other invasive monitoring avoid compromise to these areas when they have bedside irrigation of wounds. Febrile patients do not experience core warming as they do in whirlpools.

Precautions

Aerosolization of microorganisms is possible during the use of pulsatile lavage with suction to cleanse wounds. The patient should wear a facemask, and all areas of the body, except for the wound, should be covered. The cleansing should be done in a ventilated private room with cupboards, drawers, and doors closed with no one else present. Waterproof mattresses or pads without surface tears should be used. Unnecessary equipment in the room should be stowed during irrigation since all exposed areas of the room must be disinfected after irrigation is done. Wheelchairs or transport stretchers should be removed from the room. The person performing pulsatile lavage should have full personal protective gear on, including hair and shoe coverings, face shields, mask, gown, and gloves. Suctioned fluids should be emptied into a toilet or designated commode. Disposable equipment should be disposed of as hazardous waste. Suction canisters should be disposable or sterilized after use if made of glass. Bed linens and towels used during lavage should be double bagged and laundered.

Hydrotherapy

Hydrotherapy, often in the form of whirlpool treatments to a limb or the whole body, is used to cleanse and debride wounds that are large with significant necrosis. Hydrotherapy is frequently used to treat burn injuries. Water is used at a temperature of 37 °C. Antiseptics are sometimes added to the water but can interfere with healing. Hydrotherapy has been implicated in a number of outbreaks of wound infections caused by cross-contamination; so many facilities have discontinued the use of whirlpools. Additionally, they are contraindicated for venous ulcers because vasodilation can increase edema. Diabetic patients may be insensitive to temperature, so therapy must be used cautiously. Wounds related to arterial insufficiency may not benefit. Whirlpool treatments do not appear to reduce surface bacteria of wounds, but rinsing the tissue after the treatment does. Equipment must be thoroughly disinfected between patients to prevent spread of infection.

Patient Safety Measures During Whirlpool Treatments

Whirlpools are used to cleanse wounds with a large amount of contamination or necrotic tissue. Small whirlpools are best for extremity wounds so the entire body does not need to be immersed. Water used in whirlpools should first be tested for the presence of microorganisms. If antiseptics are used in the water, the patient should wear a mask to avoid allergic reactions to aerosolized antiseptic or pneumonia from water vapor droplets. Additional **patient safety measures** include:

- Transfer the patient into and out of the whirlpool cautiously if a large whirlpool is used.
- Monitor vital signs before, during, and after whirlpool treatments and observe for fainting, dizziness, or altered mental status.
- Position the patient away from the jets to avoid damage to the wound or other tissues from the high pressure.
- Adjust or discontinue agitation if tissues are fragile.
- Rinse all body surfaces and the wound after whirlpool to remove antiseptics, contamination, and cellular debris. This is best done by a vigorous warm water rinsing or by showering.

Periwound Cleansing

The stratum corneum of the **periwound skin** is not as stable as normal skin. Periwound skin has more skin debris, such as water-insoluble proteins, amino acids, urea, ammonia, microorganisms, and cholesterol, than other tissue. Microorganisms up to 10 cm away from the wound edge can be more numerous and differ from those found in the wound bed, so cleansing prevents wound contamination. The microorganism level increases when the amount of protein on the periwound surface is increased. This area must be cleansed along with the wound when dressing changes are done. Cleansing reduces bacterial counts within and around the wound for about 24 hours. Normal saline may not remove these substances adequately. A skin cleanser that is mild and will not harm skin or strip away intercellular lipids may be used on the periwound area.

Dressings

Basic Dressing Requirements

The **basic dressing requirements**, regardless of the type, are the following:

- Maintain a moist environment in order to promote healing.
- Absorb wound drainage and prevent leakage.
- Increase wound temperature to promote healing.
- Provide a protective barrier to prevent mechanical injury to the wound.
- Provide a protective barrier to prevent colonization and infection with microorganisms.
- Allow exchange of gases and fluids.
- Retain and absorb odor of the wound or drainage.
- Remove easily without causing additional trauma to the wound or disrupting the healing process.
- Debride wound of dead tissue and exudate.
- Provide protection without toxicity or causing sensitivity reactions.
- Provide a sterile protective covering for the wound.

The dressing that directly covers the wound may be inadequate to absorb large amounts of drainage, so sometimes additional secondary dressings are needed.

Wound Dressing Selection

The proper **dressing** for a wound may change over time depending on wound characteristics:

- The wound environment's moisture content may call for a dressing that either wicks away too much moisture or provides moisture to a dry wound to enhance epithelialization.
- Slough and dry eschar calls for a dressing that will enhance debriding.
- The presence of tunneling or undermining will require a packing material.
- Some wounds need dressings that are absorbent and deodorizing to control exudate.
- Control and prevention of infection is important in some wounds.
- Dressings must allow oxygen, water, and carbon dioxide to be exchanged between the environment and the wound.
- Dressings need to provide warmth as well.
- Dressings must not adhere to or harm the wound tissues but must be kept in place reliably without harming the skin around the wound.

Categories of Dressings and Methods of Securing Dressings

Dressings are considered primary if they are next to the wound surface and secondary if they are used to cover the primary or to secure the dressing. There are **three main types of dressings** to consider when determining which will be the most effective for a particular type of wound:

- **Traditional topical dressings** are used primarily to cover the wound, such as gauze and tulle.
- **Interactive dressings**, such as polymeric films, are generally transparent so that the wound can be observed and are permeable to water vapor and oxygen but provide an effective barrier for microorganisms, such as hyaluronic acid, hydrogel, and foam dressings.
- **Bioactive dressings** provide substances that directly promote wound healing, such as hydrocolloids, alginates, collagens, and chitosan.

Securing a dressing depends on the health of the surrounding skin and the type of dressing. Skin protection and tape may be appropriate. Some are self-adherent. Tubular dressings or wraps can help to secure dressings with fragile skin.

Gauze Dressings

Gauze dressings are made from cotton, rayon, or polyester, and are frequently used with primary closure where there is little or no exudate. The purpose of these dressings is to provide protection of the partial or full-thickness wounds or those with cavities or tracts. They may be sterile or non-sterile. In the past they were used for wet to dry dressings. Wet to dry dressings have little use in current wound care unless the wound is very small because the gauze adheres to the wound and can disrupt granulation or epithelization. Wet to moist saline gauze dressings are sometimes used to treat wounds but are less effective than hydrocolloid dressings. Gauze dressings may be used as secondary dressings with another type of dressing in direct contact with the wound or as packing to fill dead space in combination with amorphous hydrogel or other dressings. When used to fill space, the gauze should be fluffed to avoid causing excess pressure.

Tulle or Impregnated Gauze Dressings

Tulle dressings, also known as paraffin gauze, (Jelonet, Paranet) are open weave gauze that are coated with paraffin so they do not adhere to the wound. They are suitable only for flat or shallow wounds. They may be useful for people with sensitive skin. When these are placed in contact with the wound, secondary dressings may be used to absorb exudate.

Impregnated gauze may contain antimicrobials, medications, nutrients, and moisture (such as normal saline). Commonly used gauzes are impregnated with petrolatum, zinc oxide, and iodoform. They are used for partial or full-thickness wounds or those with cavities, tracts, or infection. The choice of gauze depends upon the needs of the wound. They should be loosely packed into cavities and avoid contact with intact skin as they may cause maceration because of the moisture content of the dressing. Exudate should be carefully monitored so dressings can be changed as needed.

Foam Dressings

Foam dressings are made of semi-permeable hydrophilic foam, and sheet forms may have an impermeable barrier. They come in a wide variety of sizes and shapes (wafers, rolls, pillows, films) depending upon the manufacturer. Some types have a charcoal layer to control odor. Foam dressings provide a warm, moist environment and provide cushioning. Foam dressings may be used for partial and full-thickness wounds. Non-sheet forms are used as packing and are appropriate for minimal to heavy exudate. When used as packing, a secondary non-occlusive dressing is secured over the foam. They are used for leg ulcers as well as pressure sores. Because they are intended for wounds with exudate in order to provide the appropriate environment for healing, they are not suitable for dry epithelializing wounds or those with eschar. Sheet forms can be used as secondary dressings with alginates, pastes, or powders. Some have adhesive borders. Foam dressings are changed every 2-7 days, depending on the dressing type and the wound.

Semi-Permeable Film Dressings

Semi-permeable film (OpSite, Tegaderm, Polyskin II) dressings are composed of polyurethane with a coating of acrylic adhesive so the dressing will adhere to the skin. These types of dressings are frequently used over intravenous sites to allow observation of tissue. They are suitable only for shallow partial-thickness wounds that have little or no exudate because they are not able to absorb; therefore, they are not suitable for infected wounds. They are permeable to air and water vapor but provide a barrier to pathogenic agents and liquid. The tissue under the dressing is maintained in a warm moist environment, encouraging autolysis. The dressings are comfortable and may be left in place for up to 1 week although some people may develop local irritation from the adhesive. Semi-permeable film may be used as a protective dressing and is often used for stage I and II pressure ulcers.

Alginates or Other Fiber Gelling Dressings

Alginates (AlgiSite M, Sorbsan, Aquacel, Hydrofiber) are very absorbent dressings made from brown seaweed. Through ion exchange, they absorb drainage and form a hydrophilic gel that conforms to the size and shape of the wound. They are useful for full-thickness wounds with moderate to heavy exudate or slough, such as pressure ulcers and cavity wounds, especially if there is undermining or tunneling. They are effective for infected and foul-smelling wounds. Alginates are sold in sheet form or fibers for packing. Alginate dressings or packing fibers are loosely packed into the wound to allow for swelling and then secured with a secondary dressing. They are usually changed once daily. Alginates serve to cushion and protect the wound as well as contain exudate. They are easier to remove than gauze dressings used for packing and cause less discomfort. Alginates need differing times to gel with some requiring 24 hours, so they are not interchangeable.

Hydrocolloid Dressings

Hydrocolloids (DuoDerm, Restore, Tegasorb) are sheets or wafers of absorbent adherent material with an occlusive coating so that they provide a barrier to moisture. They are used for clean granulating wounds that are partial and full thickness with minimal to moderate amounts of drainage. They may be used with pastes or alginates. Hydrocolloids come in various sizes and shapes and can be cut to fit, overlapping the wound by 2-3 cm. They are usually changed about every 2-5 days. Hydrocolloid material may be stiff and should be warmed between the hands to soften before application. Some hydrocolloids emit an unpleasant odor when active. Because the dressings are occlusive, infected wounds should be observed carefully for signs of infection with anaerobic bacteria. They may be used with compression for venous ulcers but are not recommended for third degree burns. Hydrocolloids may cause hypergranulation tissue to form.

Hydrogel Dressings

Hydrogel dressings (AquaForm, Curasol, Hypergel, Elastogel, Vigilon, Intrasite gel) are produced in amorphous form, supplied in tubes, or impregnated in packing strip materials. They are also produced in sheet form, with or without an adhesive border. They have a high moisture content with water or glycerin with hydrophilic sites allowing them to absorb exudate and provide a warm, moist wound environment. Hydrogels are used for partial and full-thickness wounds, dry to small amounts of exudate, necrotic wounds, and infected wounds. They are applied directly to the wound and provide rehydration and autolysis, effectively and quickly debriding the wound. They are usually used with a secondary dressing, such as gauze or films. Dressings may be changed every 1-3 days, depending upon the type of product used. Hydrogels are contraindicated for wounds with heavy exudate, as the leakage may cause maceration of periwound tissue or candidiasis.

Contact Layer Dressings

Contact layers (Dermanet, Mepitel, Tegapore) are composed of woven polyamide net and may be coated with silicone (Mepitel). They adhere lightly to the wound but have pores that allow exudate to pass through to absorbent secondary dressings. They are particularly useful in wounds in which adherence of dressings to the tissue may pose problems, such as with abrasions, second degree burns, grafts, full-thickness granular wounds, and skin damaged by radiotherapy or steroids. They may be used with negative pressure wound therapy. They protect the wound base but are not recommended for shallow or dry wounds. Usually, the contact layer stays in place for up to a week while the secondary absorbent dressings are changed more often. If exudate is extremely viscous, it may not penetrate the net and can build up beneath the contact layer. Some types of contact layers may need to be kept moistened with normal saline so they don't adhere to the wound base.

Composite Dressings

Composites are combination dressings that are frequently used to secure primary dressings or with other dressings, such as alginates. The material in composites varies from one dressing to another, but usually consists of some type of impermeable exterior barrier to prevent leakage of exudate, an absorptive layer (*not* alginate, foam, hydrocolloid, or hydrogel), a semi-adherent or non-adherent surface for covering the wound, and an adhesive rim to secure the dressing to the periwound tissue. Used alone, they are most suitable for partial or shallow full-thickness wounds but used with other dressings they are suitable for larger wounds with minimal to large amounts of exudate. A paper backing must be removed prior to application. They are usually changed about 3 times a week or more often if needed for wounds with larger amount of exudate.

Absorptive Dressings and Wound Fillers

Absorptive dressings (Surgipad, Tendersorb, ABD pad, Exu-dry) are composed of cellulose, cotton, or rayon fibers. Some have adhesive borders. They are highly absorptive and are intended for wounds that have moderate to heavy drainage. They are changed every 1-2 days.

Wound fillers (Biafine WDE, DuoDerm Sterile Hydroactive Paste, Multidex Maltodextrin Wound Dressing) are composed of starch copolymers in numerous different forms, such as pastes, granules, beads, gels, and powders. They fill dead space in shallow wounds, hydrate, provide a warm, moist environment, and absorb exudate. They soften necrotic tissue and aid debridement. Wound fillers are indicated for partial and shallow full-thickness wounds with minimal to moderate exudate and can be used for both infected wounds and uninfected wounds. They are used with secondary dressings, such as films and hydrocolloids. Wound fillers are not recommended for use in dry, eschar-covered, or tunneled wounds. Dressings are usually changed daily.

Wound Pouches

Wound pouches (Convatec Wound Manager, Hollister Wound Manager) are adapted from ostomy appliances and work in a similar way to contain heavy exudate from fistulas, wounds, drains, and tubes. The pouches provide a skin barrier to protect the skin and a drainage spout so that the pouch can be attached to straight drainage and a bedside bag. The pouch provides odor control as well. The opening in the pouch is cut to fit around the wound and paste, such as Stomahesive, is applied about the cut opening to ensure seal. The skin is usually wiped with a skin barrier prior to application, and any skin crevices are filled with paste. Forceps are used to feed drains or tubes through the opening of the pouch. Pouches are usually changed about every 4-7 days or when there is leakage or drainage under appliance.

Anatomy and Physiology

Body Systems

Functions of the human body can be divided into the following body systems:

- **Cardiovascular**: Pumps blood throughout the body via the heart and blood vessels
- **Digestive**: Transforms food into energy and eliminates solid waste
- **Endocrine**: Releases hormones into the bloodstream to control metabolism, growth, and reproduction
- **Immune**: Defends against all foreign substances
- **Integumentary**: Skin prevents moisture loss, regulates temperature, protects from sunburn, and senses pain, pressure, touch, hot and cold
- **Musculoskeletal**: Skeletal muscles move the body, smooth muscles control the physical functioning of internal organs, and cardiac muscle pumps blood. The skeleton supports and shapes, protects internal organs, stores minerals, and produces blood cells
- **Nervous**: Controls movement, memory, and senses and communicates with the outside world
- **Reproductive**: Allows continuation of the human species through reproduction and childbearing and differentiates the sexes
- **Respiratory**: Regulates gas exchange (oxygen intake and carbon dioxide expulsion)
- **Urinary**: Removes waste and toxins from the blood and expels them from the body through urine

Cardiovascular System

The cardiovascular system controls blood flow throughout the body and to the tissues, controls gas exchange (carbon dioxide and oxygen) by transporting oxygenated blood from the lungs, serves as a reservoir for blood, maintains blood pH through a buffer system, responds to infections, and facilitates coagulation (blood clotting). The cardiovascular system has the following components:

- **Heart**: The heart has four chambers, two upper (right atrium, left atrium) and two lower (right ventricle and left ventricle). The heart muscle receives blood from four major coronary arteries (right, left main, left anterior descending, and left circumflex) and their branches, and then distributes blood via the aorta and pulmonary arteries.
- **Vessels**: The venous system includes veins, venules, and venous capillaries and returns blood back to the heart via the inferior and superior vena cava. The arterial system, (including the coronary arteries) branches from the aorta after it leaves the heart and includes arteries, arterioles, and arterial capillaries.
- **Blood**: Blood consists of red blood cells (erythrocytes), white blood cells (leukocytes including monocytes, lymphocytes, basophils, neutrophils, and eosinophils), platelets (thrombocytes), and plasma, the liquid portion of the blood (which contains clotting factors). Blood carries oxygen from the lungs and distributes it to the rest of the body.

The cardiovascular system is responsible for oxygenation of cells, perfusion (carrying of blood with oxygen, glucose, and nutrients to cells) and removing waste products, such as carbon dioxide.

Review Video: Cardiovascular System
Visit mometrix.com/academy and enter code: 376581

Anatomy of the Heart

The human heart is about the size of a fist and weighs 7–15 ounces. It is located in the middle of the chest, behind the sternum, and leans slightly left. The heart is covered by a double-layered membrane called the **pericardium**. The outer layer, called the parietal pericardium, is fibrous and surrounds the roots of the major blood vessels of the heart. The inner layer, called the visceral pericardium, is attached to and covers the heart muscle. The two layers of membrane are separated by fluid. The heart itself has **four connecting chambers**. The two upper chambers are the **right atria and left atria**; the lower chambers are the **left ventricle and right ventricle**. The left and right atria and the left and right ventricle are separated by a muscular structure called the septum.

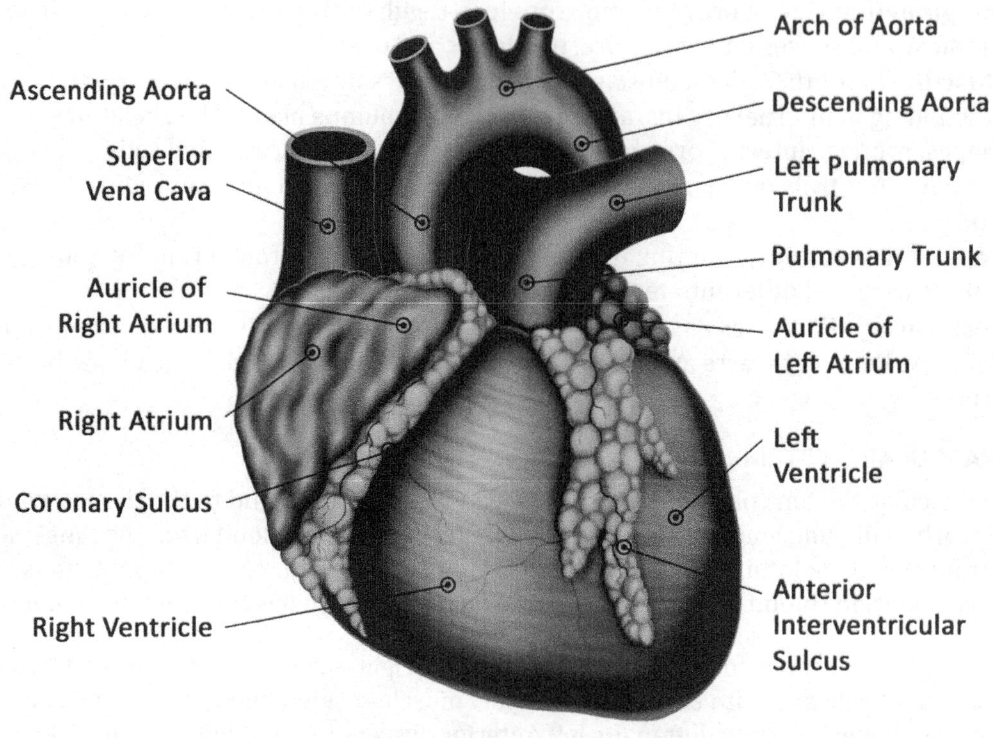

> **Review Video: Heart Anatomy and Physiology**
> Visit mometrix.com/academy and enter code: 569724

Heart's Conduction System

The **sinoatrial node (SA)** is referred to as the pacemaker of the heart because electrical impulses normally originate in the SA, within the wall of the right atrium. The SA produces electrical impulses that are transmitted to the **atrioventricular node (AV)** by specialized conducting tissue. The AV node is found between the atria and ventricles. From here, the electrical impulse is relayed down the conducting tissue called the Bundle of His. The **Bundle of His** splits into a right bundle branch (RBB) and a left bundle branch (LBB), which serve the right and left ventricles, respectively, through both sides of the intraventricular septum. The bundle branches then split to form the **Purkinje fibers**, which transmit electrical impulses to the myocardium.

> **Review Video: Electrical Conduction System of the Heart**
> Visit mometrix.com/academy and enter code: 624557

A **normal sinus rhythm** on an EKG (the expected result in a healthy individual) denotes that the electrical impulses start in the sinoatrial node (SA) first. The intrinsic rate of the SA node is 60–100 beats per minute (bpm), which reflects the normal range for an adult's pulse rate. If the SA node does not initiate the electrical impulse, the atrioventricular node (AV) can do so. However, the AV node is not as capable of increasing the heart rate, with an intrinsic rate of only 40-60 beats per minute. The patient may require a pacemaker to address the slow heart rate. All of the cells of the heart are capable of generating the electrical impulses necessary to trigger a heartbeat (automaticity). Signal conduction problems (block) can occur at any site along the conduction pathway, causing alterations in the normal rhythm (arrhythmia).

Heart Valves and Blood Flow

Four heart valves regulate the flow of blood through the heart.

- The **tricuspid valve** controls the flow of deoxygenated blood from the right atrium to the right ventricle.
- The **pulmonary semilunar valve** controls the flow of blood from the right ventricle to the pulmonary artery. The pulmonary artery carries the blood into the lungs where it is oxygenated.
- The blood then flows through the pulmonary vein back to the heart, and the **mitral valve** controls the flow of the now oxygenated blood from the left atrium to the left ventricle.
- The **aortic semilunar valve** regulates blood flow from the left ventricle to the aorta. From the aorta, the oxygenated blood is conducted to the rest of the body. The deoxygenated blood travels through the venules, then the veins, and then the inferior vena cava and superior vena cava back to the right atrium.

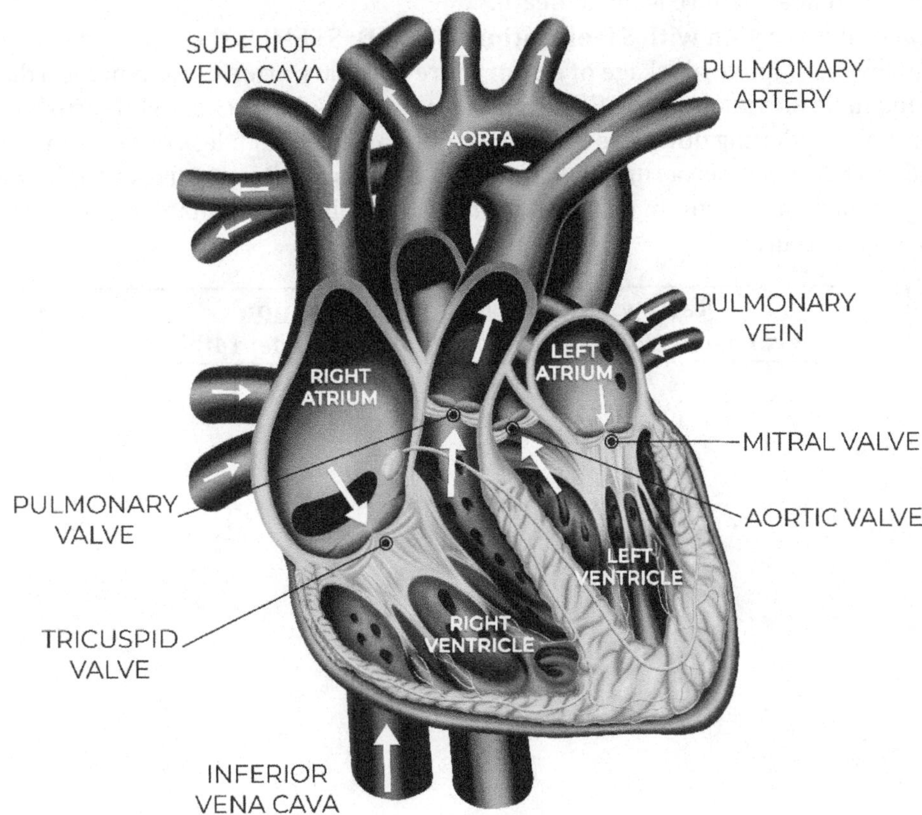

Review Video: Heart Blood Flow
Visit mometrix.com/academy and enter code: 783139

CARDIOVASCULAR DISORDERS

Cardiovascular disorders include the following:

- **Atherosclerosis**: Atherosclerosis is characterized by fatty deposits that build up inside of arteries, resulting in decreased blood flow because of narrowing and stiffening of the arteries, which in turn leads to high blood pressure and increased risk of thrombi (blood clots) and emboli (moving clots).
- **Edema**: Edema is swelling from fluid retention. Edema may occur because of heart failure (weakness of the heart muscle) that causes fluid to build up in the legs and feet and/or in the lungs (causing shortness of breath). Edema (often involving the whole body) may also occur with kidney disease and severe allergic (anaphylactic) reaction.
- **Thrombophlebitis**: Thrombophlebitis is inflammation of a vein that occurs as the result of a thrombus (blood clot) forming in the vein. The vein appears red, swollen, and tender and is at increased risk of spreading emboli to other areas of the body, such as the brain (stroke) and heart (heart attack).
- **Heart failure**: Heart failure is cardiac disease that includes disorders of contractions (systolic dysfunction) or filling (diastolic dysfunction) or both and may include pulmonary, peripheral, or systemic edema. The most common causes are coronary artery disease, systemic or pulmonary hypertension, cardiomyopathy, and valvular disorders. The incidence of chronic heart failure correlates with age. Heart failure progresses through Class I to Class IV, involving congestion in the lungs, limitations of activity, and discomfort. Uncontrolled heart failure leads to death.
- **Myocardial infarction with ST-elevation (STEMI)**: STEMI is the more severe type of MI that involves complete blockage of one or more coronary arteries with myocardial damage, resulting in ST elevation on the EKG. Symptoms are those of an acute MI (crushing pain substernally, radiating down the left arm or both arms, though less obvious in women and the elderly). As necrosis occurs, Q waves often develop, indicating irreversible myocardial damage, which may result in death, so treatment involves immediate reperfusion before necrosis can occur.

Review Video: Myocardial Infarction
Visit mometrix.com/academy and enter code: 148923

ENDOCRINE SYSTEM

The major glands that comprise the endocrine system, the hormones they secrete, and diseases resulting from their dysfunction include the following:

Gland	Hormones	Disease
Adrenal Cortex	Aldosterone Cortisol Androgens	Addison's Disease Cushing's Disease
Adrenal Medulla	Epinephrine Norepinephrine	Anxiety Attacks Depression
Anterior Pituitary	Adrenocorticotropic hormone (ACTH) Follicle-stimulating hormone (FSH) Gonadotropic hormones Growth hormone (GH) Luteinizing hormone (LH) Prolactin Thyroid Stimulating Hormone (TSH)	Dwarfism Gigantism
Hypothalamus/ Posterior Pituitary	Inhibiting hormones (stop the release of other hormones) Antidiuretic hormone (ADH) Oxytocin Releasing hormones (trigger the release of other hormones)	Diabetes Insipidus
Kidneys	Calcitriol Erythropoietin	Hypertension
Ovaries	Estrogen Progesterone	Endometriosis Menometrorrhagia
Pancreas	Insulin Glucagon	Diabetes Mellitus
Parathyroid	Parathyroid hormone	Tetany Renal calculi
Pineal	Melatonin	Alzheimer's Disease
Testes	Testosterone	Gynecomastia Klinefelter Syndrome
Thymus	Thymic factor (TF) Thymosin Thymic humoral factor (THF) Thymopoietin	DiGeorge Syndrome
Thyroid	Calcitonin Thyroxine (T4) Triiodothyronine (T3)	Cretinism Hypo/Hyperthyroidism Goiter Myxedema
Digestive tract	Gastrin Cholecystokinin Secretin Ghrelin Motilin	Gastritis Gastroesophageal reflux

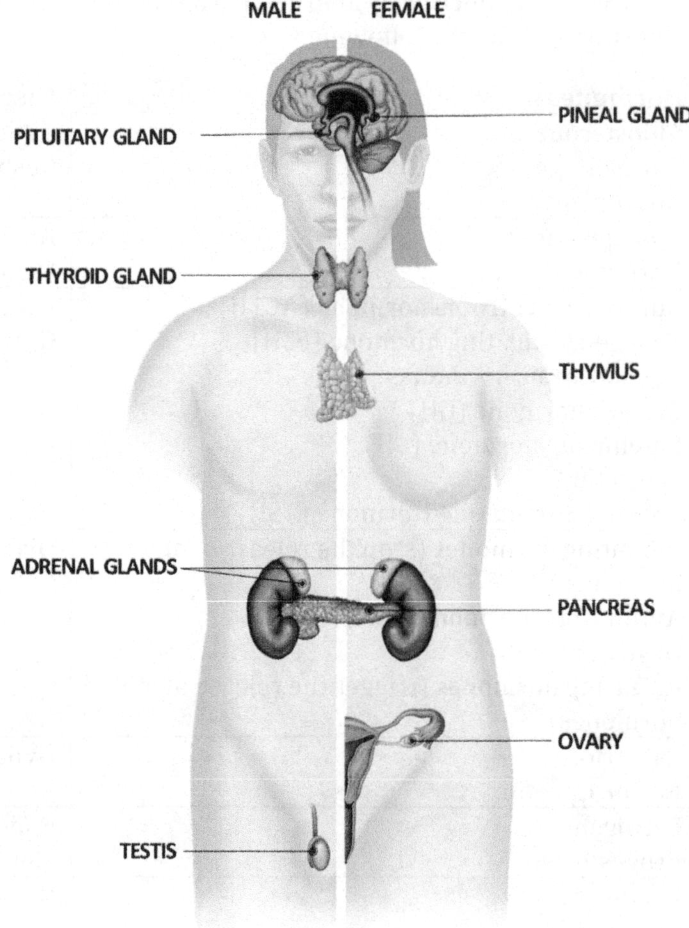

Review Video: Endocrine System
Visit mometrix.com/academy and enter code: 678939

Gastrointestinal System

Digestive Tract

The gastrointestinal tract (GI tract) is divided into upper and lower sections:

- The **upper GI tract** consists of the mouth (buccal mucosa, tongue, and teeth), pharynx, esophagus, and stomach.
- The **lower GI tract** is comprised of the small intestine (duodenum, jejunum, ileum, and ileocecal valve) and the large intestine (ascending, transverse, and descending colon, sigmoid flexure, rectum, and anus).

The vermiform appendix is attached to the cecum, the first section of the ascending colon, closest to the ileocecal valve. The sigmoid flexure leads into the rectum, which terminates in the anus. An internal and external sphincter control the anus. The liver, gall bladder, and pancreas secrete digestive enzymes into the GI tract through various ducts that aide in the breaking down of food and absorption of nutrients.

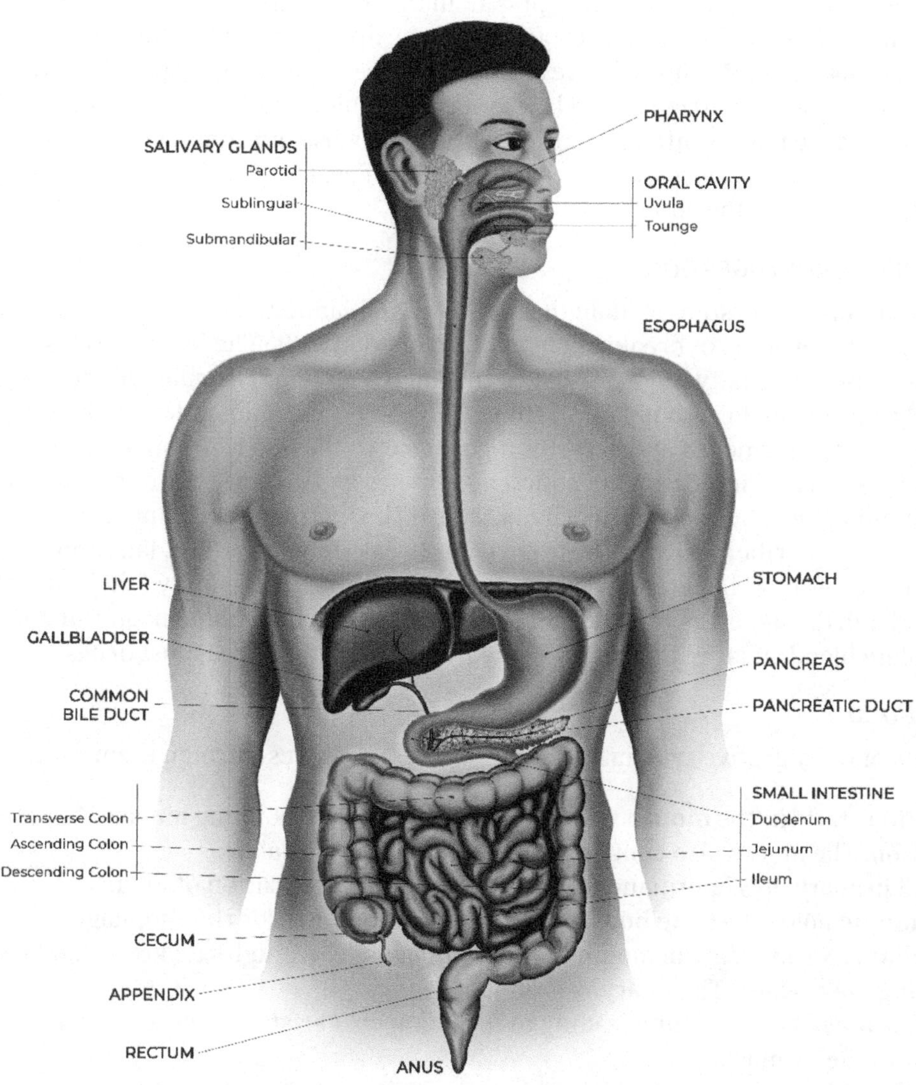

Review Video: Gastrointestinal System
Visit mometrix.com/academy and enter code: 378740

Functions

The gastrointestinal tract is a system of organs responsible for the:

- Ingestion of food
- Digestion of food
- Absorption of nutrients and medications
- Production of Vitamins B_{12} and K
- Elimination of waste products

The process begins at the mouth with ingestion and ends at the anus with excretion. The GI tract breaks down and reabsorbs nutrients using ptyalin in the mouth, hydrochloric acid in the stomach, bile from the gall bladder, and insulin, glucagon, amylase, lipase, and other chemicals from the pancreas. Food is digested into slurry in the stomach, where B_{12} is manufactured to prevent anemia. The small intestine absorbs nutrients. The large intestine (colon) reabsorbs water and salts and turns semi-liquid waste matter into firm, formed stools. Bacteria, normally found in the large intestine, produce Vitamin K, necessary for blood clotting. Fecal waste matter is held temporarily in the rectum and expelled by the anus.

Accessory Organs of Digestion

The accessory organs of digestion include the liver, the gallbladder, and the pancreas. The liver produces bile as a by-product of breaking down old red blood cells. The liver excretes bile into the small intestine to break up fatty foods by way of the biliary system. The gallbladder's only function is to store and concentrate bile, so if painful stones form in it, the gallbladder can be safely removed. The pancreas secretes hormones and excretes digestive enzymes, so it is both an endocrine and an exocrine gland. As an exocrine gland, the pancreas releases an isosmotic fluid into the small intestine containing the enzymes trypsin, chymotrypsin, lipase, pancreatic amylase, deoxyribonuclease, and ribonuclease. These enzymes break down proteins, fats, and starches. The pancreatic duct makes bicarbonate to decrease the acidity of the food slurry (chyle and chyme). As an endocrine gland, the pancreas regulates blood sugar with the hormone insulin, and the pancreas and liver regulate blood sugar with glucagon. The liver also metabolizes most drugs.

Passage of Food

The main parts of the digestive system in order of how food passes through them are as follows:

1. Digestion starts in the **mouth** with the action of saliva containing amylase to start starch digestion. The mouth also contains the hard and the soft palates.
2. The 20 primary or 32 permanent **teeth** are used for mastication of food.
3. The **tongue** holds the taste buds and moves the food towards the esophagus.
4. The **pharynx** connects the mouth to the esophagus. The **epiglottis** keeps food from entering the trachea. The pharynx is about 5" long.
5. The **esophagus** is a 12" tube leading to the stomach. Peristaltic waves start here and move food into the stomach.
6. The **stomach** sac is controlled by the lower esophageal sphincter (at the top) and the pyloric sphincter (at the bottom). Food mixes with hydrochloric acid in the stomach to make chyme. Food stays in the stomach for 2–4 hours.
7. The **small intestine** contains the duodenum (10"), jejunum (8'), and ileum (12'). The majority of digestion takes place in the duodenum. The small intestine receives bile, produced by the liver and stored in the gall bladder, to digest fats, and amylase and insulin from the pancreas to break down starches and sugars. Digestion in the small intestine can take between 3 and 10 hours.
8. The **large intestine** absorbs water and salts. The large intestine consists of the cecum (with vermiform appendix), ascending, transverse, descending, and sigmoid colon, the rectum, and anus for defecation. The ileocecal valve prevents food from reentering the small intestine.

Total digestion can take between 24 hours and 3 days.

Hematologic System

Components

Blood is the liquid that moves through the circulatory system. The average adult has about 5 liters of blood. Bone marrow produces red blood cells (RBC or erythrocytes), white blood cells (WBC or leukocytes), and platelets (thrombocytes).

- **Red blood cells** transport oxygen and carbon dioxide, **white blood cells** fight infection, and **platelets** clot blood after an injury. These blood cells travel through the circulatory system suspended in plasma: 55% of blood is yellow, liquid plasma, and 45% is cells. **Blood plasma** carries nutrients, proteins, hormones, and waste products.
- White blood cells that absorb Wright stain are classified as **granulocytes**, because there are granules in the cytoplasm, and agranulocytes, with no granules present. There are three different kinds of granulocytes: neutrophils, basophils, and eosinophils. The **agranulocytes** include lymphocytes (T and B cells) and monocytes. Each type of WBC proliferates to combat a different type of pathogen. For example, increased eosinophils (eosinophilia) can indicate allergies, whereas increased monocytes (monocytosis) can indicate tuberculosis (TB).

Red Blood Cells

A red blood cell **(erythrocyte, RBC)** is a doughnut-shaped raft that transports oxygen to cells through hemoglobin. The RBC offloads its oxygen, takes on carbon dioxide from the cells, and changes color, turning a bluish-purple. The RBC then returns to the lungs, where it takes on oxygen again during gas exchange. Red blood cells typically have a life span of 120 days and require the nutrients iron, protein, B_{12}, and folate. If a patient has too few erythrocytes from heavy bleeding or lacks the nutrients, then he or she is considered anemic.

Platelets

Platelets **(thrombocytes)** clot the blood when a vessel is damaged by converging on the area to seal the leak. Platelets have a life span of nine days and work in conjunction with clotting factors in the blood, the proteins that work with platelets to produce a clot. If a patient lacks a clotting factor, then the platelets alone are unable to seal an injury adequately. This occurs in hemophiliacs, who lack Factor VIII. This disease and others that lead to decreased platelets put individuals at high risk for bleeding. Bone marrow produces red blood cells and platelets daily to replace dead or lost circulating cells.

Immune System

The immune system is the body's main defender against disease. The immune system is comprised of the spleen, thymus, bone marrow, and a series of transparent tubes that run throughout the body, parallel to the blood vessels. The tubes are lymph vessels, and carry 4 liters of clear lymphatic fluid, or lymph. Lymph circulates throughout the body in the same manner as blood, with valves opening and closing to move the liquid along. There are hundreds of small glands, called lymph nodes, stationed at intervals along the lymphatic vessels. The lymphatic fluid carries invaders to the nodes to be destroyed by lymphocytes, a type of white blood cell. Antibodies are also found in lymphatic fluid. Nodes swell during infections. Plasma from the blood vessels seeps out of the capillaries, immerses body tissues, and then drains off into the lymph vessels. Once in the lymphatic system, the plasma is called lymph. Lymph travels through the lymphatic vessels until it reaches the thoracic duct, the largest lymph vessel, extending from L2 to the neck. The lymph drains from the thoracic duct into the blood and is then carried to the kidneys and liver by the cardiovascular system where the waste is removed.

Review Video: Immune System
Visit mometrix.com/academy and enter code: 622899

The Complement System

The complement system consists of proteins produced by the liver that work with an individual's antibodies to clear the body of pathogens. Complement proteins are a part of the immune system that burst (lyze) pathogens and alert the phagocytes that the dead pathogen must be removed. If the patient is hypersensitive, the complement system may work against its own body. An exaggerated inflammatory response may occur, called a cytokine storm. Young people are most prone to cytokine storm if they have pandemic influenza, rheumatoid arthritis, sepsis, bronchitis, bird flu, or pneumonia. Complications from the COVID-19 pandemic also included the overreaction of the immune system, leading to excessive fluid accumulation in the lungs and excessive clotting. In a cytokine storm, the complement system calls too many immune cells to defend the site of infection, which can cause the blockage of small arteries with clumped white cells (aggregate). The inflammatory response may be so extreme that gangrene develops in the fingers and toes or the patient dies from the cytokine storm.

White Blood Cells

The white blood cells of the immune system include the following:

WBC	Type	% of WBCs	Causes of Increase	Causes of Decrease
Basophils (black or purple)	Granulocyte	1%	Asthma, chronic myelocytic leukemia, Crohn's disease, dermatitis, estrogen, hemolytic anemia, Hodgkin's disease, hypothyroidism, polycythemia vera, and viruses	Allergies, corticosteroids, hyperthyroidism, pregnancy, and stress.
Eosinophils (orange-red, double-lobed nucleus)	Granulocyte	1-3%	Allergy, asthma, or parasitic infestation	Cushing's disease or glucocorticoids use
Lymphocytes (dark, large nucleus surrounded by thin cytoplasm rim)	Agranulocyte	15-40%	Antigens or chronic irritation	AIDS
Monocytes (lavender)	Agranulocyte	2-8%	Myeloproliferative process, like an inflammatory response or chronic myelomonocytic leukemia (CMML)	Hairy cell leukemia
Neutrophils (pink cytoplasm, dark nucleus)	Granulocyte	50-70%	Burns, kidney failure, heart attack, cancer, hemolytic anemia	Leukemia and abscess

Lymphocytes make proteins for immunoglobulins and cytokine production. Small B and T cells secrete antibodies and regulate the immune system. Large Natural Killer cells lyze tumors and virus-infected cells. Children, aged four months to four years, normally have inverted differential (relative neutropenia and increased lymphocytes). **Neutrophils** are phagocytic. A segmented nucleus (seg) indicates a mature cell. A banded nucleus (band) indicates an immature cell.

Integumentary System

The largest organ of the body is the skin, which forms the **integumentary system**, along with cutaneous glands, hair, and nails. It has three layers: epidermis, dermis, and hypodermis (subcutaneous or superficial fascia). The functions of the integumentary system are to:

- Excrete salts and nitrogenous wastes
- Metabolize vitamin D
- Prevent bacteria, parasites, and other invaders from entering the body
- Protect the body from chemicals
- Produce melanin as sunscreen
- Protect the body from water loss
- Regulate body temperature through perspiration, fat storage, and radiating heat from capillaries
- Serve as a sensory communication tool through temperature, touch, pain, and pressure receptors

Skin can be damaged by chemicals, sharp or blunt instruments, heat, friction, pressure and radiation. Among the injuries that can happen to the skin are abrasions, burns, contusions, crushing injuries, decubitus ulcers (bedsores), gunshots, hematomas, incisions, lacerations, and punctures.

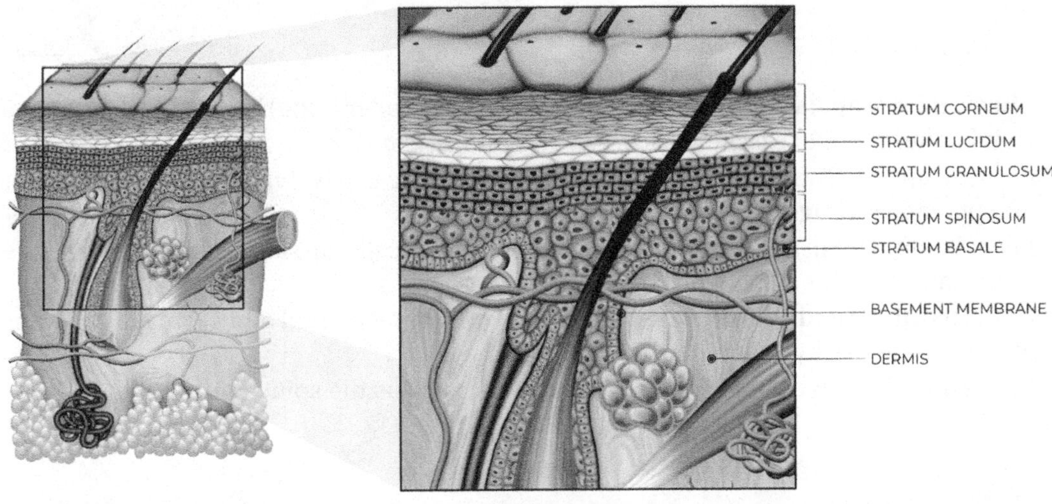

Review Video: Integumentary System
Visit mometrix.com/academy and enter code: 655980

Musculoskeletal System

Bones and Joints

The bones of the musculoskeletal system include the following:

- **Head**: The cranium includes frontal (forehead), parietal (back), temporal (side), mandibular (lower jaw), maxillary (upper jaw), nasal conchae and septum (nose), and zygomatic (cheek) bones; the ear includes the malleus (hammer), incus (anvil) and stapes (stirrup) bones.
- **Spine**: Comprised of seven cervical (neck), 12 thoracic (upper back), and five lumbar (lower back) vertebrae, the sacrum, and the coccyx (tail bone).

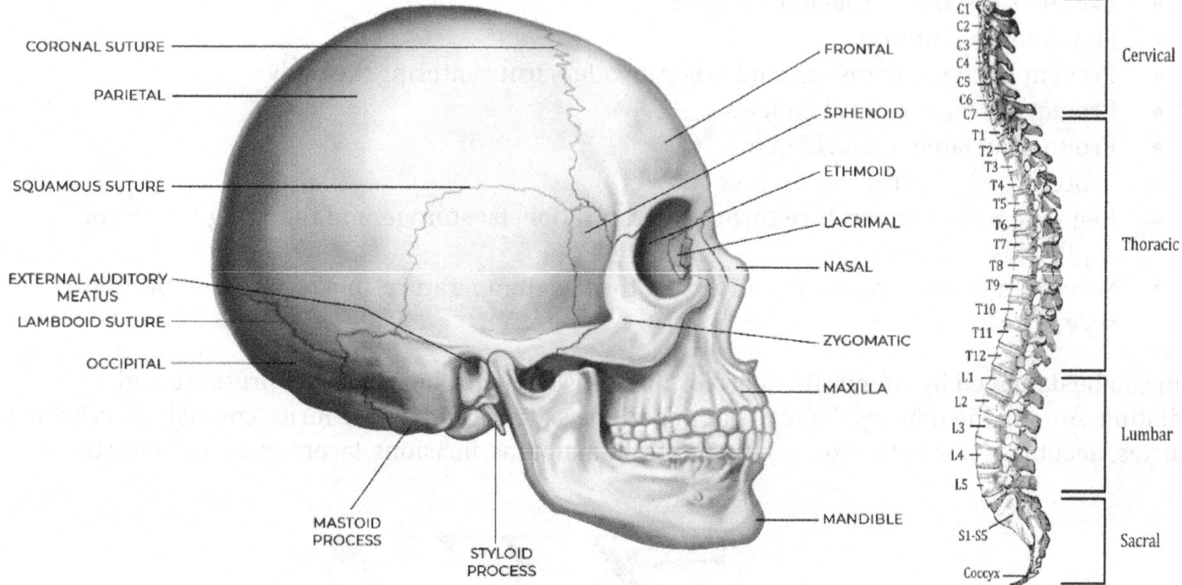

- **Chest**: Ribs, scapula (shoulder blade), and clavicle (collar bone).
- **Pelvis**: Ilium (upper), ischium (lower), and pubis (front).
- **Arms**: Humerus (upper), radius and ulna (forearm), carpals (wrist), metacarpals (hand), and phalanges (fingers).
- **Legs**: Femur (thigh), patella (knee), tibia and fibula (calf), tarsals (ankle), metatarsals (front foot), calcaneus (heel), and phalanges (toes).
- **Diarthrotic articulations**: Moveable joints with synovial fluid and cartilage cushions that are held together by ligaments, like the limbs.
- **Synarthrotic articulations**: Immovable joints, such as the spine and skull.

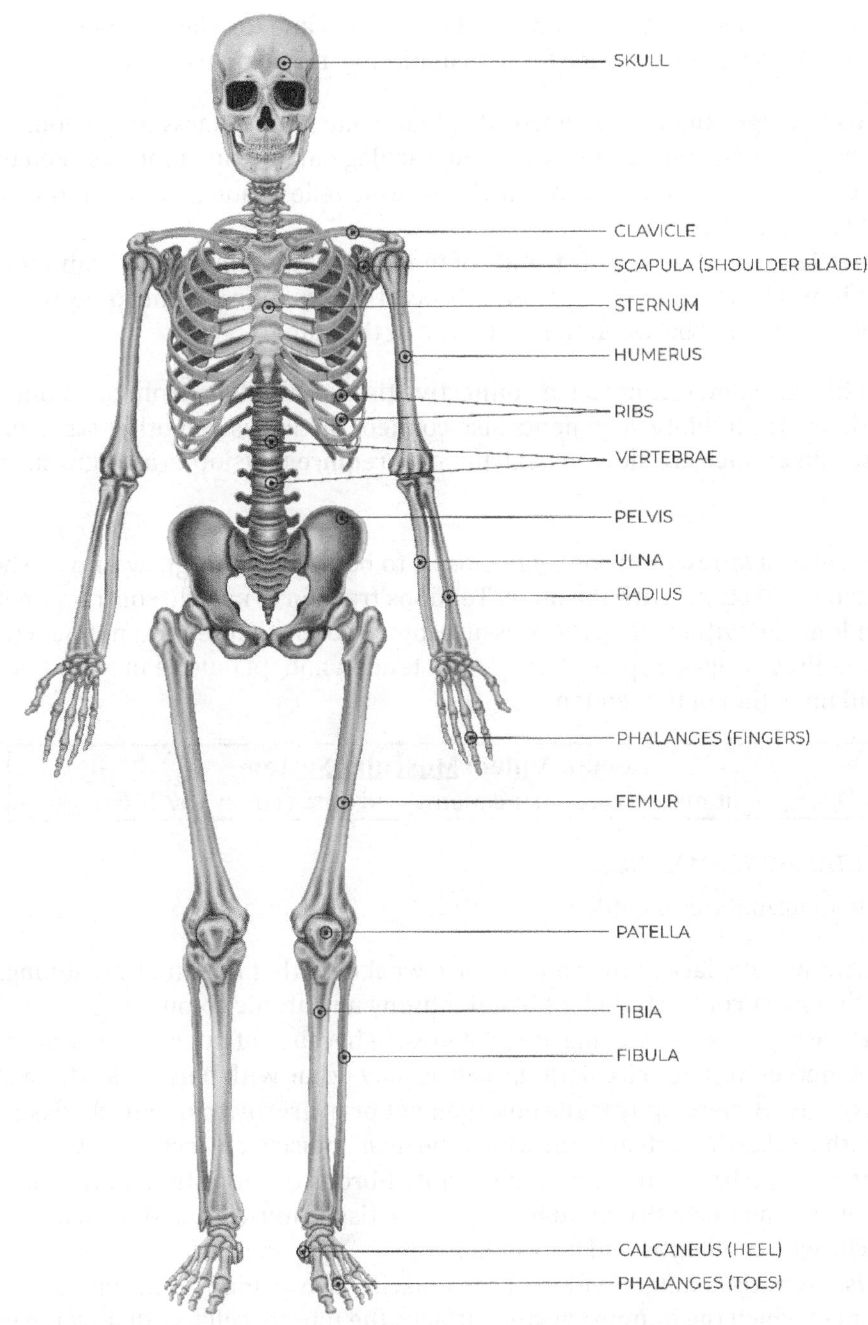

Review Video: Skeletal System
Visit mometrix.com/academy and enter code: 256447

Cartilage and Ligaments

Cartilage is a dense connective tissue composed of collagen and/or elastin fibers on the end of bones, which provides a smooth surface for articulation by reducing friction.

- **Hyaline cartilage** contains chondrocytes that make it look glassy and is found in the nose, larynx, trachea, ribs, and sternum. Hyaline cartilage makes an embryo's skeleton.
- **Elastic cartilage** contains elastin, which makes it yellow, and is found in the outer ear (pinna) and epiglottis.
- **Fibrocartilage** is composed of strands of fibers that function to help limit movement and prevent bones from rubbing together. Fibrocartilage is found in the knee, the pubic bones in the pelvic region and between the vertebrae in the spine.

A **ligament** is a fibrous band composed of connective tissue stretching from one bone to another in a joint to provide lateral stability. Ligaments also connect cartilages and other structures. Injuries to ligaments are sprains, which are slow to heal and may require physiotherapy and surgery.

Tendons

A tendon is also called a **sinew**, and connects muscle to bone. Tendons grow into the bone and make mineralized connections with the bone. Tendons transform muscle contraction into joint movement. Tendons can withstand great pressure, but tendons that tear do not heal well. A complete tear requires surgical repair. Damage to a tendon and its muscle in a joint is a strain. Tendonitis is inflammation of the tendon.

Review Video: Muscular System
Visit mometrix.com/academy and enter code: 967216

Musculoskeletal Abnormalities

Musculoskeletal abnormalities include:

- **Atony**: Atony is the lack of tone and muscle weakness that impairs functioning, especially of organs that must contract, such as bladder atony and atonic colon.
- **Atrophy**: Atrophy is the wasting away of muscle because of poor nourishment, lack of use, impaired nerves, or poor circulation, such as may occur with paralysis after a stroke.
- **Hypertrophy**: Hypertrophy is the enlargement or overgrowth of muscle tissue, such as may occur with cardiac hypertrophy in which the heart muscle enlarges and weakens.
- **Fibrositis**: Fibrositis is inflammation of white fibrous tissue with hyperplasia (enlargement caused by cell overgrowth) found in connective tissue muscles, and muscle sheaths, such as may occur with tendonitis and fibromyalgia.
- **Myositis**: Myositis is inflammation of the muscle, such as may occur with autoimmune disorders in which the immune system attacks the muscle cells, with adverse effects of drugs, and with infection. Disorders include polymyositis, dermatomyositis, and infectious myositis.

Musculoskeletal Diseases

Osteoporosis is a condition with thin porous bones that break easily because of low bone mass and structural deterioration, with more bone lost than gained. Osteoporosis is most common in post-menopausal women, although men >65 lose bone at the same rate as women. Osteoporosis is one of the leading causes for vertebral fractures and femur (hip) fractures in older adults, often associated with falls that break the brittle bones.

Osteoarthritis is a degenerative joint disease in which joints become inflamed, stiff, and painful as cartilage (which covers bone ends) deteriorates. Osteoarthritis may affect any joint and often results from a previous injury to a joint, so it may affect only one joint. Joints most commonly affected include the knees, hips, neck, and lumbar (lower) back as well as finger joints. Osteoarthritis usually has a slow onset with symptoms appearing after age 60. Pain tends to increase with weight bearing. Osteoarthritis is the primary reason for joint replacement surgery.

Gait Disorders

Functional movement disorders are defined as an involuntary, abnormal movement of part of the body in which pathophysiology is not fully understood. Functional tremors are the most frequent type of functional movement disorder. Dystonia, myoclonus, and Parkinsonism are other types of functional movement disorders. Functional gait disorders are another type of functional movement disorder and are common in the elderly. Gait disorders can manifest as a dragging gait, knee buckling, small slow steps or "walking on ice," swaying gait, fluctuating gait, hesitant gait, and hyperkinetic gait in which there is excessive movement of the arms, trunks and legs when ambulating. Patients with gait disorders are at an increased risk of falling. Gait disorders are diagnosed by a thorough clinical examination (including a neurologic assessment) and health history. Treatment for functional gait disorders includes strength and balance training. Assistive devices such as walkers and canes may also be utilized.

Nervous System

The human nervous system is divided into the central nervous system (CNS) and the peripheral nervous system (PNS).

- The **CNS** is composed of the brain and spinal cord and is located in the dorsal cavity. The brain is protected by the skull, while the spinal cord is protected by the vertebrae.
- The **PNS** is made of those structures of the nervous system not contained in the dorsal cavity, such as long nerves (neuron axons). The PNS is divided into the somatic nervous system and the autonomic nervous system. The autonomic nervous system is further divided into the sympathetic nervous system and the parasympathetic nervous system.

Review Video: Nervous System
Visit mometrix.com/academy and enter code: 708428

Somatic Nervous System

The somatic division of the peripheral nervous system is involved in the coordination of body movements. It is comprised of peripheral nerve fibers that receive sensory information and carry this information into the spinal cord. It also contains motor nerve fibers that connect to skeletal muscle. The somatic system employs an afferent nerve network to carry sensory information to the brain and an efferent nerve network with motor nerves that transmit information from the brain to the skeletal muscles. The somatic nervous system regulates activities that are under the individual's conscious control, processes sensory information, and executes voluntary movements. The somatic nervous system does not control reflex arcs.

Autonomic Nervous System

The **sympathetic division** of the peripheral nervous system is involved in the "fight-or-flight" response and is activated in times of danger or stress. Signs and symptoms of sympathetic stimulation are an increased heart rate (tachycardia), vasoconstriction and rise in blood pressure, dilation of the pupils (mydriasis), goose bumps on the skin (piloerection or cutis anserine), increased sweat secretion (diaphoresis), and feelings of excitement. These reactions are due to the release of adrenaline (epinephrine).

The **parasympathetic nervous system** is in charge when the individual feels relaxed or is resting. The parasympathetic system is responsible for constriction of the pupil, slowing of the heart rate, dilation of blood vessels, and stimulation of the digestive tract and genitourinary system. The neurotransmitter at work is acetylcholine.

Dorsal Cavity

The dorsal cavity contains the brain and spinal cord, which are the organs of the central nervous system (CNS). Like the ventral cavity, the dorsal cavity is divided into two smaller cavities: the cranial cavity and the spinal cavity. The cranial cavity contains the brain, eyes, and ears, while the spinal cavity holds the spinal cord. The brain and spinal cord are covered by three layers of connective tissue called the meninges. The outermost layer is the dura mater; the middle layer is the arachnoid mater; and the innermost layer is the pia mater. The space between the arachnoid mater and the pia mater is filled with cerebrospinal fluid (CSF), which flows throughout the CNS. If an injured patient has clear yellow fluid leaking from the ears, nose, eyes, or mouth, it is probably CSF and indicates a skull fracture.

Neurons

Neurons are nerve cells that transmit nerve impulses throughout the central and peripheral nervous systems. The basic structure of a neuron includes the cell body, the dendrites, and the axons. The **cell body**, also called the soma, contains the nucleus. The nucleus contains the chromosomes. The **dendrite** of the neuron extends from the cell body and resembles the branches of a tree. The dendrite receives chemical messages from other cells across the synapse, a small gap. The **axon** is a thread-like extension of the cell body, which varies in length, up to 3 feet in the case of spinal nerves. The axon transmits an electro-chemical message along its length to another cell. Peripheral nervous system (PNS) neurons that deal with muscles are myelinated with fatty Schwann cell insulation to speed up the transmission of messages. Gaps between the Schwann cells that expose the axon are **nodes of Ranvier** and increase the speed of the transmission of nerve impulses along the axon. Neurons in the PNS that deal with pain are unmyelinated because transmission does not have to be as fast. Some neurons in the central nervous system (CNS) are myelinated by oligodendrocytes. If the myelin in the CNS oligodendrocytes breaks down, the patient develops multiple sclerosis (MS).

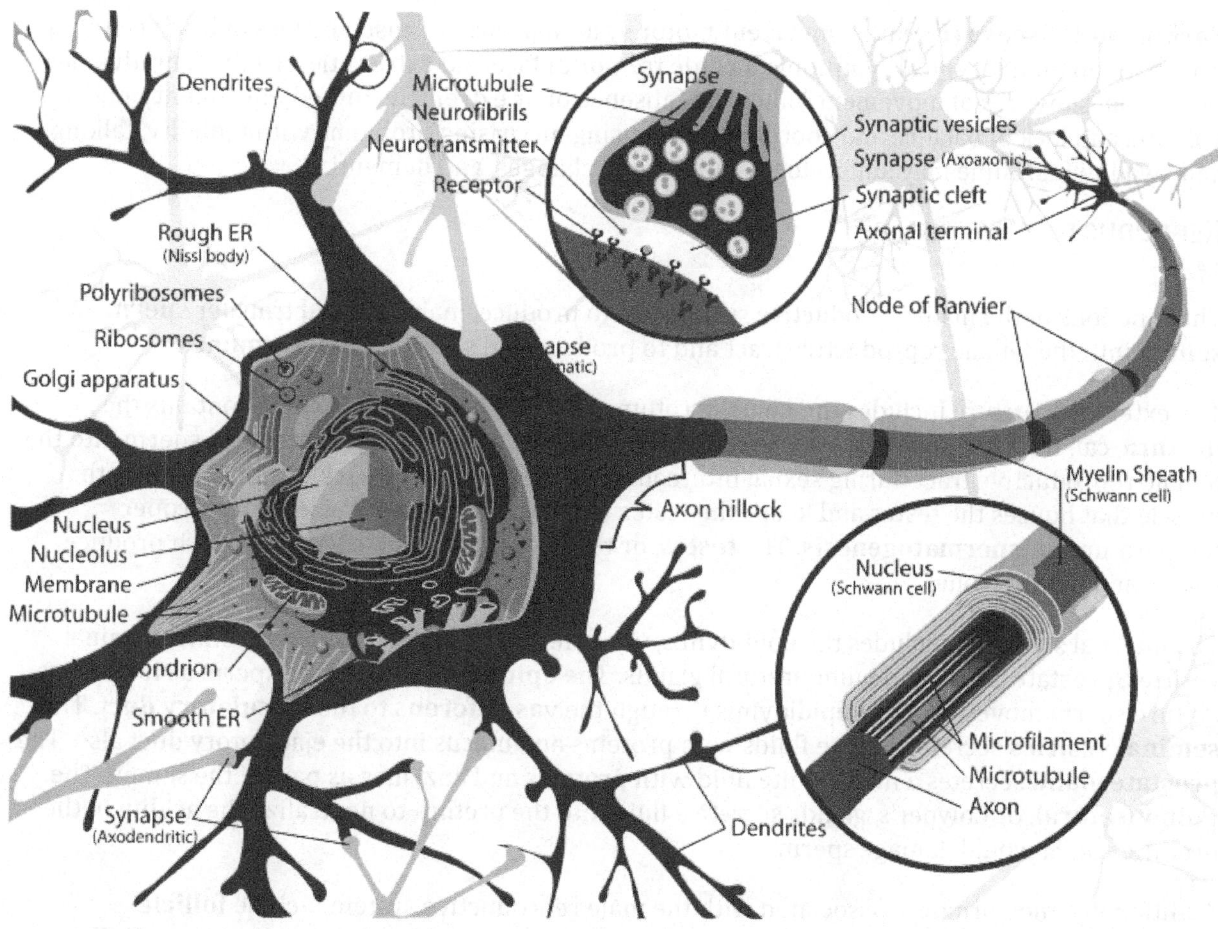

The three **categories of neurons** are as follows:

- **Afferent neurons** carry sensory impulses from the environment to the brain and spinal cord and are also called sensory neurons or receptor neurons. Afferent neurons are found in the skin, muscles, joints, and sensory organs. They permit the perception of pressure, pain, temperature, taste, odor, sound, and visual stimuli.
- **Efferent neurons** transmit motor impulses from the brain and spinal cord to effectors, such as muscles and glands. Efferent neurons are involved in motor control and stimulate movement throughout the body.
- **Interneurons** connect sensory and motor neurons. Also called connection neurons or relay neurons, interneurons are located in the CNS; sensory and motor neurons are found in both the CNS and PNS.

Nervous System Diseases

Epilepsy is a seizure disorders with sudden involuntary abnormal electrical disturbances in the brain that can manifest as alterations of consciousness, spastic tonic and clonic movements, convulsions, and loss of consciousness. Following seizures, patients may have confusion, disorientation, and impairment of motor activity, speech, and vision for several hours and headache, nausea, and vomiting may occur. During the seizure, the patient should be turned to the side and the head and body protected from injury, but no attempt should be made to insert anything into the mouth or restrain the person.

Parkinson's disease (PD) is a movement motor system disorder caused by loss of brain cells that produce dopamine. Typical symptoms include tremor of face and extremities, rigidity, bradykinesia (abnormal slowness of movement), akinesia (absence of or extremely limited movement), poor posture, and lack of balance and coordination, causing increasing problems with mobility, talking, and swallowing. Some may suffer depression, mood changes, and dementia.

Reproductive System

Male

The functions of the male reproductive system are to produce, maintain, and transfer **sperm** and **semen** into the female reproductive tract and to produce and secrete **male hormones**.

The external structure includes the penis, scrotum, and testes. The **penis**, which contains the **urethra**, can fill with blood and become erect, enabling the deposition of semen and sperm into the female reproductive tract during sexual intercourse. The **scrotum** is a sack of skin and smooth muscle that houses the testes and keeps the testes outside the body wall at a cooler, proper temperature for **spermatogenesis**. The **testes**, or testicles, are the male gonads, which produce sperm and testosterone.

The internal structure includes the epididymis, vas deferens, ejaculatory ducts, urethra, seminal vesicles, prostate gland, and bulbourethral glands. The **epididymis** stores the sperm as it matures. Mature sperm moves from the epididymis through the **vas deferens** to the **ejaculatory duct**. The **seminal vesicles** secrete alkaline fluids with proteins and mucus into the ejaculatory duct also. The **prostate gland** secretes a milky white fluid with proteins and enzymes as part of the semen. The **bulbourethral**, or Cowper's, glands secrete a fluid into the urethra to neutralize the acidity in the urethra, which would damage sperm.

Additionally, the hormones associated with the male reproductive system include **follicle-stimulating hormone (FSH)**, which stimulates spermatogenesis; **luteinizing hormone (LH)**, which stimulates testosterone production; and **testosterone**, which is responsible for the male sex characteristics. FSH and LH are gonadotropins, which stimulate the gonads.

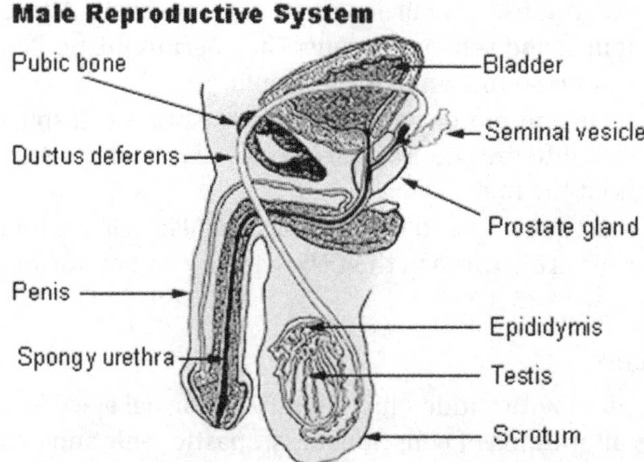

FEMALE

The functions of the female reproductive system are to produce **ova** (oocytes or egg cells), transfer the ova to the **fallopian tubes** for fertilization, receive the sperm from the male, and provide a protective, nourishing environment for the developing **embryo**.

The external portion of the female reproductive system includes the labia majora, labia minora, Bartholin's glands, and clitoris. The **labia majora** and the **labia minora** enclose and protect the vagina. The **Bartholin's glands** secrete a lubricating fluid. The **clitoris** contains erectile tissue and nerve endings for sensual pleasure.

The internal portion of the female reproductive system includes the ovaries, fallopian tubes, uterus, and vagina. The **ovaries**, which are the female gonads, produce the ova and secrete **estrogen** and **progesterone**. The **fallopian tubes** carry the mature egg toward the uterus. Fertilization typically occurs in the fallopian tubes. If fertilized, the egg travels to the **uterus**, where it implants in the uterine wall. The uterus protects and nourishes the developing embryo until birth. The **vagina** is a muscular tube that extends from the **cervix** of the uterus to the outside of the body. The vagina receives the semen and sperm during sexual intercourse and provides a birth canal when needed.

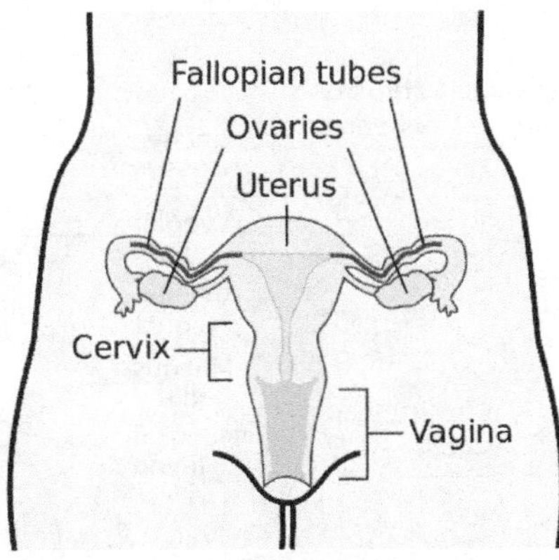

Review Video: Reproductive Systems
Visit mometrix.com/academy and enter code: 505450

REPRODUCTIVE CYCLE

The female reproductive cycle is characterized by changes in both the ovaries and the uterine lining (endometrium).

The ovarian cycle has three phases: the follicular phase, ovulation, and the luteal phase. During the **follicular phase**, FSH stimulates the maturation of the follicle, which then secretes estrogen. Estrogen helps to regenerate the uterine lining that was shed during menstruation. **Ovulation**, the release of a secondary oocyte from the ovary, is induced by a surge in LH. The **luteal phase** begins with the formation of the corpus luteum from the remnants of the follicle. The corpus luteum secretes progesterone and estrogen, which inhibit FSH and LH. Progesterone also maintains the thickness of the endometrium. Without the implantation of a fertilized egg, the corpus luteum begins to regress, and the levels of estrogen and progesterone drop. FSH and LH are no longer inhibited, and the cycle renews.

The uterine cycle also consists of three phases: the proliferative phase, secretory phase, and menstrual phase. The **proliferative phase** is characterized by the regeneration of the uterine lining. During the **secretory phase**, the endometrium becomes increasingly vascular, and nutrients are secreted to prepare for implantation. Without implantation, the endometrium is shed during **menstruation**.

RESPIRATORY SYSTEM

The respiratory system is made up of the nasal cavity, pharynx, larynx, trachea, right and left bronchi, and lungs, which branch into bronchioles and alveoli. The respiratory system has two divisions. The upper respiratory tract is comprised of the nasal cavity and pharynx and their associated structures. The lower respiratory tract consists of the larynx, trachea, bronchi, and lungs.

The diaphragm and muscles of the thoracic wall are responsible for the bellows movements necessary for breathing. The process of external respiration (breathing) involves the inspiration of oxygen and the exhalation of carbon dioxide. Normally, respiration occurs through the nasal cavity. Patients who are congested or under exertion breathe through their mouths. Those with airway blockages are neck-breathers with stomas.

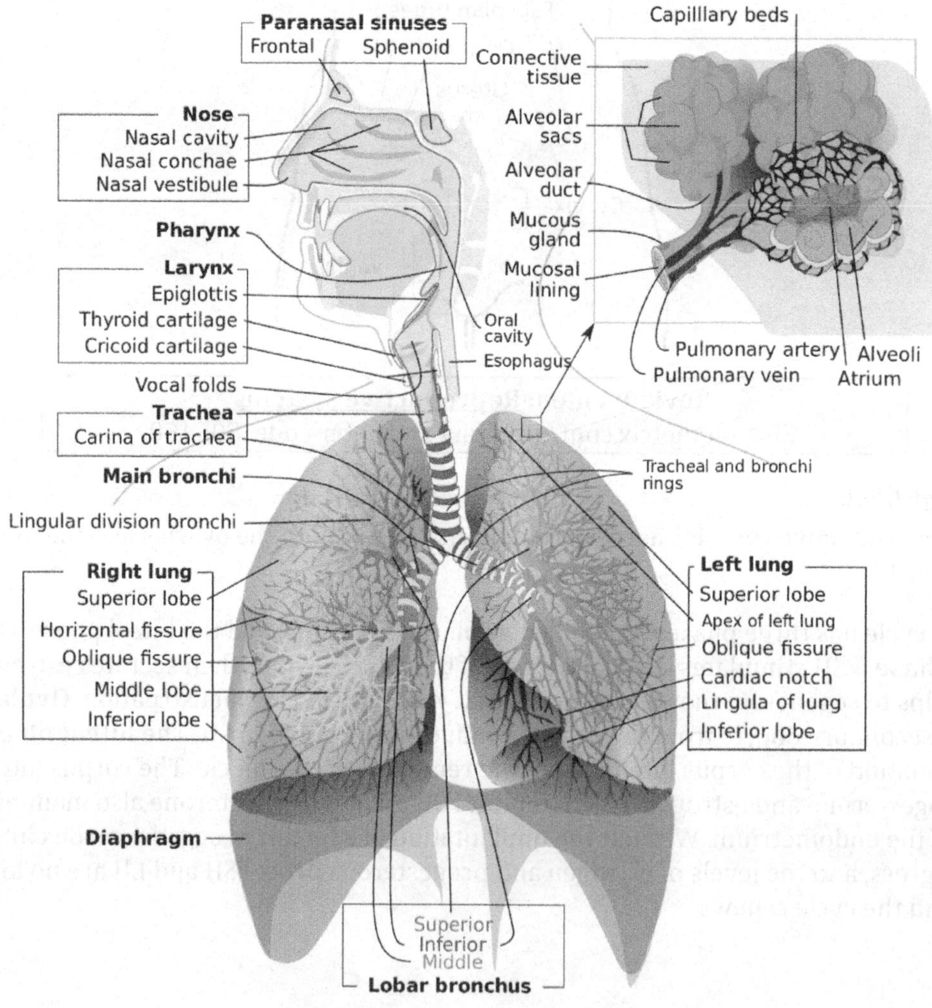

Review Video: Respiratory System
Visit mometrix.com/academy and enter code: 783075

Control of Respiration

Respiratory neurons in the medulla, pons, and brainstem control the speed and depth of respiration and are responsible for maintaining its normal rhythm. The normal respiration rate in adults is 12-20 breaths per minute. Infants breathe faster; the newborn rate is 44 breaths per minute. The respiratory neurons stimulate motor neurons in the spinal cord to cause the contraction of the muscular diaphragm and intercostal muscles. The respiratory neurons also receive information from receptors about the levels of carbon dioxide (CO_2), oxygen (O_2), and hydrogen (H) in the body, as well as the degree of stretch present in the lungs and chest. Chemoreceptors in the carotid arteries inform the respiratory neurons when the concentration of oxygen falls; chemoreceptors located in the medulla, carotid arteries, and aorta keep track of the levels of carbon dioxide and hydrogen. Breathing can be controlled consciously to a certain extent but is basically an autonomic function.

Mechanics of Respiration

Respiration occurs when the air pressure within the alveoli differs from the air pressure external to the body. The air pressure in the lungs is altered by changes in the size of the thoracic cavity, which occur as a result of the contraction and relaxation of the muscular diaphragm and intercostal muscles. The muscular diaphragm is primarily responsible for allowing respiration. Inhalation is brought about by two actions that increase the size of the thoracic cavity. The contraction of the diaphragm causes it to flatten, lengthening the thoracic cavity, and the contraction of the intercostal muscles pulls the rib cage upward, widening it. With the enlargement of the thoracic cavity, the pressure within decreases and air enters the lungs. Air is then pushed out of the lungs as the muscular diaphragm and intercostal muscles relax and the volume of the thoracic cavity decreases.

Internal and External Respiration

Internal respiration refers to the exchange of oxygen, carbon dioxide, and trace gases at the cellular level. **External respiration** refers to the exchange of oxygen, carbon dioxide, and other gases between the lungs and blood, commonly known as breathing. The passage of gases through the respiratory system can be traced as follows:

1. **Inspiratory neurons** in the respiratory center of the medulla oblongata (brain stem) tell the body to inhale.
2. **Nostrils** and **mouth** warm inhaled air by moving it over nasal conchae and sinuses.
3. Air passes through the **pharynx** to the **larynx** (voice box).
4. The **epiglottis** flips to cover the esophagus.
5. Air passes into the **trachea** (windpipe).
6. **Diaphragm** contracts and flattens to raise the ribs as breathing occurs.
7. **Intercostal muscles** between the ribs pull the ribs up enabling the chest to expand and air to pull inward.
8. Trachea splits into the left and right **bronchi** that connect to the **lungs**. The bronchi split into fine branches called **bronchioles**.
9. Bronchioles end in thin-walled, grape-like **alveoli** where the red blood cells absorb oxygen (O_2) from the inhaled air and give off carbon dioxide (CO_2).
10. **Expiratory neurons** in the brain stem tell the diaphragm and ribs to relax and exhale carbon dioxide into the atmosphere.

Review Video: Pulmonary Circuit
Visit mometrix.com/academy and enter code: 955608

Nasal Cavity

The inside of the nose is the nasal cavity. The external nares (nostrils) are its outside openings; the internal nares (conchae) are its posterior openings; and the vestibule refers to the front (anterior) portion. Air is taken in through the external nares, warmed, humidified, and filtered by the conchae. The posterior part of the septum is made of bone, and the anterior part is cartilage. The nasal cavity is divided into left and right halves by the nasal septum (vomer). The hard palate forms the cavity floor. The nasal cavity is lined with mucous membrane. The goblet cells of the mucous membrane secrete mucus to trap particles of dust and debris. Ciliated cells wave hairs to stop large particles from advancing any further into the respiratory tract.

Pharynx

The internal nares lead to the pharynx. Mucous is swept back in the nasal cavity to the pharynx, where it is swallowed and excreted through the digestive tract. Air is humidified and warmed in the nasal cavity before passing into the pharynx to prevent damage to the lining of the deeper respiratory passages. The pharynx is the common opening from the nasal cavity to the rest of the respiratory tract, as well as the digestive tract. It is split into three regions: the nasopharynx, oropharynx, and laryngopharynx. The nasopharynx is the upper (superior) part of the pharynx; it extends from the internal nares down to the uvula and contains the pharyngeal tonsil. The oropharynx runs between the uvula and epiglottis. The laryngopharynx lies below the upper edge of the epiglottis and opens to the esophagus.

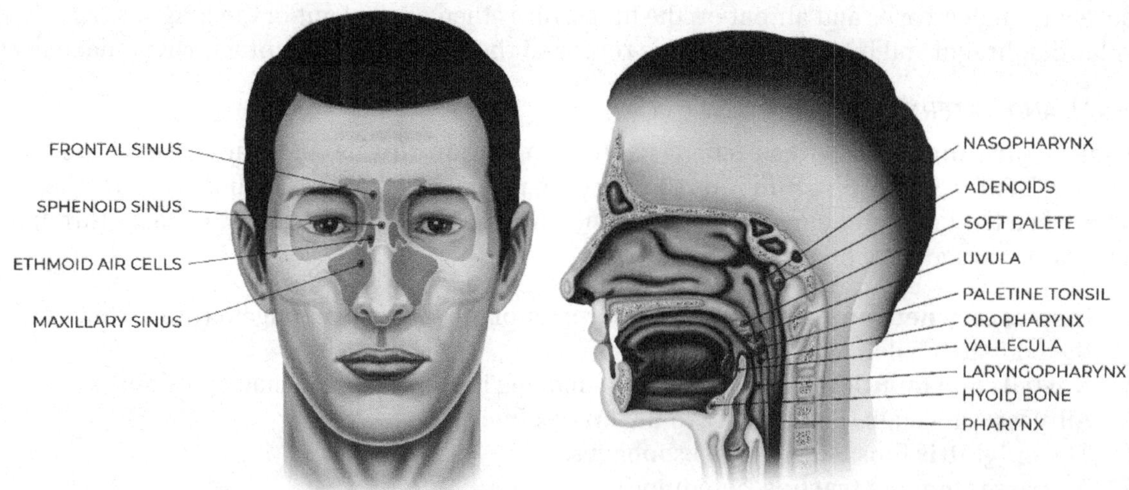

LARYNX

The larynx is comprised of a cartilaginous skeleton, muscles, ligaments, and mucosal lining. The cartilages making up the larynx are the thyroid, cricoid, and arytenoid. The largest and most superior of these is the thyroid cartilage, or Adam's apple. The cricoid cartilage is the most inferior of the cartilages. If the patient's airway is closed by trauma, foreign body obstruction, or edema from anaphylaxis, the cricoid can be punctured to permit breathing (cricothyrotomy). The arytenoid cartilage lies between the cricoid and thyroid cartilages. The thyroid cartilage is attached to the epiglottis. It covers the opening of the larynx during swallowing to prevent food and fluid from entering the larynx. The vallecula is a depression that lies anterior to the epiglottis. The larynx contains the vocal folds (vocal cords) for speech and provides an entrance to the lower respiratory passages. The movement of the intrinsic muscles of the larynx alters the shape and tension of the vocal cords, adjusting voice pitch.

TRACHEA

Also called the windpipe, the trachea is a tube comprised of connective tissue, cartilage, and smooth muscle. Its lateral sides are made of cartilage, which protects the trachea and keeps the structure open for the passage of air. The posterior position of the trachea consists of ligamentous membrane and smooth muscle. The smooth muscle can alter the trachea's shape. The esophagus is positioned posterior to the trachea's back wall. Cilia in the trachea push mucus and particles of foreign matter toward the larynx. Their movement allows the mucus and foreign matter to enter the esophagus, where it can be swallowed. The trachea splits into the right and left mainstream bronchi at the carina.

PRIMARY BRONCHI

The primary bronchi (extrapulmonary bronchi) are large passageways that conduct air into the lungs; no gas exchange takes place. They form where the trachea splits at the carina and run from the mediastinum down into the lungs. The two primary bronchi are different shapes. The right bronchus is shorter, wider, and positioned more vertically than the left bronchus. If a patient has an obstructed bronchus, it is more likely the right one. The primary bronchi are supported by C-shaped cartilage rings and split into the secondary bronchi as they enter the lungs. This site, where the bronchi, vessels, and nerves enter the lungs, is called the hilus.

BRONCHIAL TREE

The primary bronchi split to form the **secondary bronchi**, and the secondary bronchi divide to form the **tertiary bronchi**. The tertiary bronchi reach into the lobules of the lungs and continue to branch into the bronchioles. The bronchioles divide many times to form the terminal bronchioles, which split into respiratory bronchioles. Each individual respiratory bronchiole also divides and becomes an alveolar duct. The alveolar ducts terminate in the alveoli, clusters of air sacs that resemble clusters of grapes. A single alveolus is 0.1-0.2 mm in diameter. Each one is surrounded by capillaries. It is here in the alveoli where the exchange of respiratory gases (oxygen for carbon dioxide) occurs.

Lungs

The lungs (pulmones) are the main organs of respiration. They are light enough to float in water, elastic, smooth, shiny, and spongy. When touched, the tiny, grape-like alveoli crackle. The lungs are covered in a double-walled sac called the pleura. The base of each lung rests on the diaphragm, which raises and lowers the lungs. The right lung is the larger of the two lungs, comprised of three lobes, versus two lobes in the left lung. The lung's lobes are separated by fissures on the surface of the organs. Each lobe of the lung is split into lobules that are separated by connective tissue. Major blood vessels and bronchi do not pass through the connective tissue, so surgeons can remove diseased lobules fairly easily. The right lung contains 10 lobules, and the left lung holds nine. As the primary bronchi enter the lungs, they split into secondary bronchi.

Review Video: Lung Sounds
Visit mometrix.com/academy and enter code: 765616

Pleura

The pleura is the thin membrane that protects the lungs. The parietal pleura lines the inside of the chest cavity; the visceral pleura covers the lungs. The space between the two is called the pleural space. The visceral pleura lubricates the surfaces of the lungs by secreting small amounts of fluid. The lungs expand and contract during respiration, and pleural fluid allows the different lung surfaces to glide smoothly across each other. Pleurisy is a painful condition in which the pleura become inflamed as a result of fluid collecting in the pleural space (wet pleurisy) or the two membranes rubbing together (dry pleurisy). A pleural rub may be audible with a stethoscope (auscultation) if the patient has pleurisy, pleural effusion, pneumonia, pulmonary infarction, neoplasm, lupus, or asbestosis.

Dyspnea, Hyperpnea, Bradypnea, and Orthopnea

Dyspnea is characterized by difficulty breathing, such as shortness of breath (SOB) or painful breathing. **Hyperpnea** is rapid breathing. **Bradypnea** is abnormally slow breathing. **Orthopnea** causes difficulty breathing unless the patient is sitting upright or standing, as in congestive heart failure (CHF).

Regulating the Acid-Base Balance

The lungs control blood pH by releasing **carbon dioxide**, a slightly acidic waste product of oxygen metabolism. The carbon dioxide is excreted by cells into the blood, carried into the lungs by red blood cells, and exhaled. As the level of carbon dioxide builds up in the blood, the blood pH decreases. The amount of carbon dioxide exhaled is controlled by the respiration rate. The normal respiration rate for seated adults is 12-20 breaths per minute. As the rate increases and breathing becomes deeper, the amount of carbon dioxide exhaled increases. As a consequence, the pH of the blood also increases. To decrease pH, the brain slows the speed and depth of breathing.

Respiratory Alkalosis

Respiratory alkalosis is characterized by lower-than-normal levels of carbon dioxide in the blood, causing an increase in blood pH. Respiratory alkalosis disrupts the acid-base balance, with a decrease in PCO_2 (hypocapnia). Respiratory alkalosis can result from any heart or lung disease that causes fever, anxiety, shortness of breath, or hyperventilation from exhaling too much carbon dioxide. Drugs like progesterone, nicotine, salicylates, catecholamines, and methylxanthines can cause hypocapnia. Pregnant women have naturally increased progesterone and so are prone to this condition. If the patient rebreathes through a paper bag, it may help. However, patients with brain and spinal cord problems, who already have a low pH in their cerebrospinal fluid (CSF), may become worse if they use a paper bag. Signs and symptoms of respiratory alkalosis include agitation; dizziness; numbness in the hands, feet, and around the mouth; fainting (syncope); and in extremely rare cases, seizures. Respiratory alkalosis is rarely life threatening.

Respiratory Acidosis

Respiratory acidosis is a disturbance of the body's acid-base balance, which occurs when the lungs are unable to get rid of all their carbon dioxide. Respiratory acidosis decreases blood pH, and the body becomes too acidic. $PaCO_2$ increases (hypercapnia). Any disease, which makes the body less efficient at expelling carbon dioxide, weakens the chest muscles, or interferes with the nerve signals that inflate and deflate the lungs, can cause respiratory acidosis. Asthma, COPD, myasthenia gravis, Lou Gehrig's disease, Pickwickian syndrome of obesity, muscular dystrophy, and Guillain-Barré syndrome all cause respiratory acidosis. Signs and symptoms of respiratory acidosis include confusion, lethargy, sleepiness, fatigue, disturbed organ function, respiratory failure, and shock. Severe respiratory acidosis constitutes a medical emergency.

Additional Respiratory Diseases and Infections

Common respiratory diseases and infections include the following:

Asthma	Condition characterized by recurrent attacks of severe wheezing, coughing, and shortness of breath because of spasms and contraction of the bronchi, limiting airflow. May be triggered by allergies, temperature variations, or exercise.
Bronchitis	Bacterial or viral infection of one or both bronchi resulting in severe cough, shortness of breath, and thick usually purulent sputum production. Bronchitis may be acute or chronic (recurrent).
Pneumonia	Bacterial, viral, or fungal infection of air sacs in the lungs, resulting in cough, fever, chills, malaise, difficulty breathing, and chest pain.
Diphtheria	Contagious bacterial (*Corynebacterium diphtheria*) infection of the mucous membranes of the nose and throat resulting in difficulty speaking, swallowing, and breathing. Most people in US are vaccinated against diphtheria.
Tuberculosis	Contagious bacterial (*Mycobacterium tuberculosis*) infection of the lungs resulting in weakness, weight loss, cough, fever, night sweats, chest pain, and bloody sputum.
Measles	Highly contagious viral infection that results in generalized rash, cough, high fever, sore throat, and runny nose. Usually resolves in 1–2 weeks but some may develop pneumonia or encephalitis. Prevention is through vaccination.

URINARY SYSTEM

The urinary system is comprised of two kidneys (which are located in the right and left flank areas), which filter the blood of toxins and excess fluid, creating urine. Ureters carry the urine to the bladder, and a urethra carries the urine to the external meatus (opening) during urination. The urethra of the female is about 0.5-1.5 cm long, and the male urethra is about 15-29 cm long, so the female is more at risk for ascending infections.

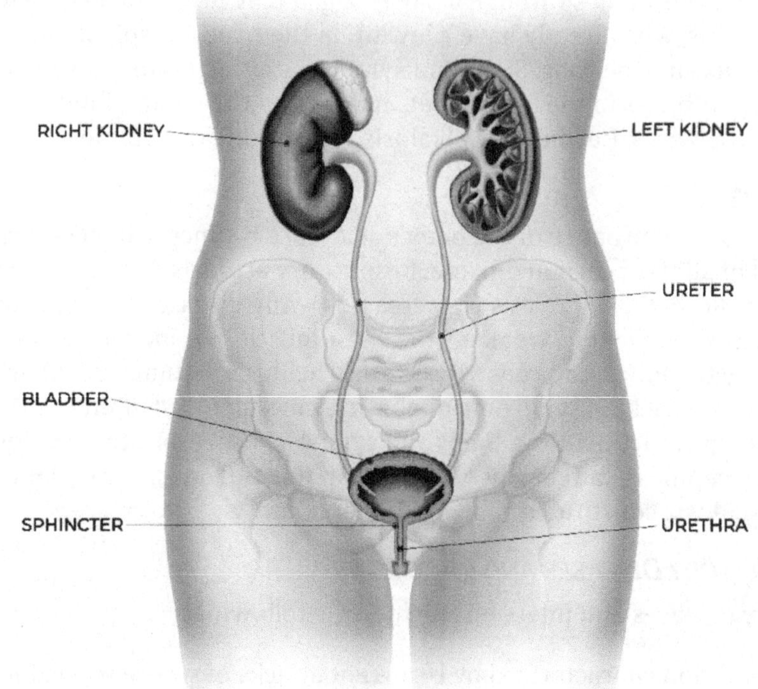

Review Video: Urinary System
Visit mometrix.com/academy and enter code: 601053

KIDNEYS

Two kidneys are located in the retroperitoneal space, in the posterior abdomen, one on each side of the spinal column. They are bean-shaped and concave on their medial aspects. The concave area contains an opening called the hilum, the point of entrance for the renal artery, renal vein, nerves, and ureter. The kidney controls blood pressure through the renal artery with the hormone renin.

The kidney is surrounded by a capsule of fibrous and connective tissue. The renal cortex is the outer part of the organ, lying underneath this capsule. Inside the cortex is the renal medulla, split into 10–20 renal pyramids. A renal pyramid and the overlying cortex associated with it form a renal lobe. The tip of a renal pyramid is called a papilla. Each papilla drains into a minor calyx. A number of minor calyces act together to drain into a major calyx. The major calyces, in turn, drain into the renal pelvis, from which urine then drains from through the ureter into the urinary bladder.

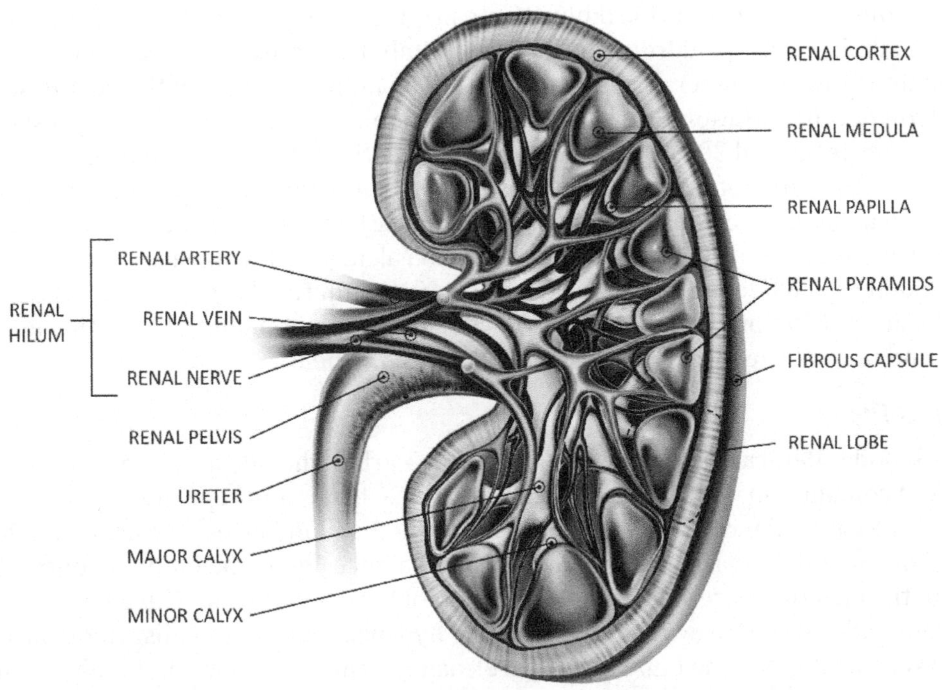

Path of Blood and Urine

The path of blood through the kidney and the subsequent path of urine is as follows:

1. Unfiltered blood enters the **nephron** through the afferent arteriole and flows into the **renal corpuscle.**
2. Minerals and some fluid filter out of the blood in the **glomerulus**, a tuft of blood vessels.
3. Filtrate enters **Bowman's capsule**, a shell around the glomerulus, where the majority of filtration takes place.
4. Blood leaves the glomerulus through the efferent tubule and enters the **peritubular network**.
5. Water and salt get reabsorbed in the **proximal convoluted tubule** (PCT), and return to the bloodstream.
6. Filtrate flows into the **descending loop of Henle**.
7. Blood continues through the peritubular network and out of the nephron through a venule.
8. Filtrate flows into the **ascending loop of Henle**, and into the **distal convoluted tubule (DCT)** in the cortex.
9. Hormones fine tune the filtrate to reabsorb only what amino acids, glucose, and salts the body needs.
10. **Filtrate** is now urine, and flows into the **collecting duct**, where ADH controls its concentration.
11. Urine passes from the kidney to the **ureters, bladder, urethra, and meatus** for micturition (urination).

Kidney Function

The kidneys produce 2-3 liters of urine daily. Waste products excreted in the urine include urea from protein catabolism, uric acid from nucleic acid metabolism, creatinine, excess water, and some drugs and toxins. Necessary minerals are reabsorbed. The kidneys maintain the acid-base balance, regulate electrolyte concentrations, control the volume of blood, and govern blood pressure. The entire blood supply is filtered 20-25 times per day through the 1.4 million nephrons of a healthy kidney cortex. If the number of nephrons decreases to 700,000, the patient develops hypertension. The kidneys help maintain the body's homeostasis (balance) by communicating with other organs using three hormones: erythropoietin (EPO), renin, and calcitriol. EPO signals the bone marrow to produce red blood cells while the lack of it causes anemia, renin regulates blood pressure, and calcitriol is the active form of Vitamin D. Calcitriol aids in the maintenance of calcium, needed for bones, teeth, and normal chemical balance, particularly in the heart.

Regulation of PH

The pH of the blood is determined by the blood levels of carbon dioxide and bicarbonate. The kidneys work in conjunction with the lungs to modify these levels and regulate acid-base homeostasis. Acid-base balance is achieved by controlling the blood levels of carbon dioxide and bicarbonate. The lungs help to regulate carbon dioxide balance, while the kidneys control the levels of bicarbonate through the secretion and reabsorption of bicarbonate and hydrogen ions. The kidneys prevent and respond to acidosis by secreting hydrogen ions and reabsorbing bicarbonate ions. They correct alkalosis in the opposite way, releasing bicarbonate ions and reabsorbing hydrogen ions. Because the body normally contains 20 times more bicarbonate than carbonic acid, it is better able to correct acidosis than alkalosis.

RAS

The **renin-angiotensin system** (RAS), also referred as the renin-angiotensin-aldosterone system (RAAS), regulates blood pressure. Renin in the distal convoluted tubule reacts to sodium depletion (e.g., through sweating) and blood pressure drops (e.g., due to blood loss) by converting angiotensinogen, a blood protein, to angiotensin I. Angiotensin I is converted into angiotensin II in the lung capillaries via the angiotensin-converting enzyme (ACE). Angiotensin II stimulates the adrenal cortex to secrete aldosterone, which acts on the renal tubules. Aldosterone balances salt and water levels by increasing the reabsorption of sodium ions in the distal convoluted tubules and water in the loop of Henle. Retaining water and salt causes blood volume to increase, which raises blood pressure.

Urinary Tract Infections

Urinary tract infections include the following:

- **Cystitis** (bladder infection): Cystitis is especially common in females. It causes burning, frequency, urgency, pelvic pain, and discolored urine and is treated with oral antibiotics.
- **Urethritis** (urethral infection): Urethritis is caused by bacteria from fecal residue infect the urethra or from sexually-transmitted infection. It causes pain and swelling and can be treated with oral antibiotics.
- **Pyelonephritis**: Pyelonephritis is an infection that spreads from the bladder upward to infect the body of the kidney and the collecting tubules. It causes flank or back pain, nausea, vomiting, fever, chills, painful urination, and dark foul-smelling urine. Pyelonephritis can be treated with IV and oral antibiotics.

The Eyes

The main **parts of the eye** and their functions are as follows:

- **Aqueous humor** is watery fluid that maintains eye pressure.
- The **bony orbit** is the socket protecting the eye.
- **Cranial nerves** that help with the function of the eye such as movement or vision include:
    - the optic nerve (cranial nerve II)
    - oculomotor (III)
    - trochlear (IV)
    - trigeminal (V)
    - abducens (VI)
    - vagus (X) nerves
- **Eyelashes and lids** protect the eye and sweep out particles.
- **Extrinsic muscles** focus the eye.
- The **lacrimal glands** are tear ducts to moisten the eye.
- The **lens** refracts light.
- The **optic disc** is the blind spot.
- The **pupil** regulates light entry.
- The **retina** has rods for black and white imaging and cones for color imaging, and helps trigger the optic nerve to send impulses to the brain.
- The **macula** is at the retinal center that is very sensitive to light. The black spot in the center is called the fovea which provides the sharpest vision.
- The **choroid** is a black layer behind the retina that absorbs light and nourishes the retina.
- The **cornea** is the window at the front of the eye that helps with focus.
- The **iris** regulates light entry.
- The **sclera** is tough, white fibrous connective tissue holding nerves and vessels that acts as protection for the eye.
- The **suspensory ligament** connects the lens to the ciliary muscles of the iris.
- The **vitreous humor** is jelly that maintains the eye's shape and refracts images.

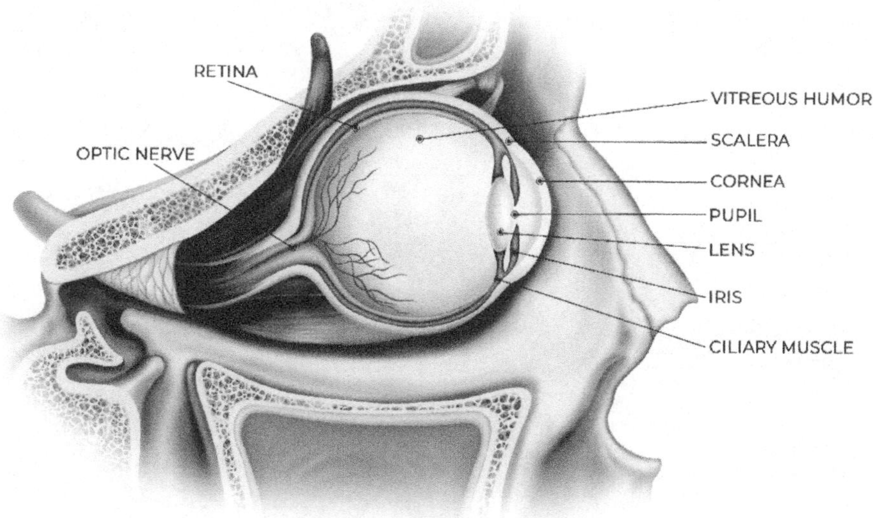

Eye Diseases

The following eye diseases are common:

- **Astigmatism** results from faulty curvature and focusing errors, also called refractive error. Normal eyes are spheres, but eyes with astigmatism are football- or spoon-shaped. Patients with astigmatism require corrective eyeglasses to prevent headaches, blurred vision, and eye fatigue.
- **Cataracts** are clouded lenses, a problem common among the aged, diabetics, steroid users, head-injured patients, and workers exposed to radiation.
- **Conjunctivitis** is a red, inflamed conjunctiva due to chemicals or infection.
- **Glaucoma** sufferers have blocked aqueous humor between the lens and iris, which can cause blindness. Open-angle glaucoma is chronic; closed-angle glaucoma is acute. The condition affects people with a family history and is most prevalent in African Americans.
- **Hyperopia** results in farsightedness.
- **Myopia** is nearsightedness.
- **Presbyopia** is the inability to focus due to an aged, inelastic lens and requires reading glasses.
- **Strabismus** patients are cross-eyed.

Instrument Sterilization

Sanitization, Disinfection, and Sterilization

Sanitization is the decontamination process that is intended to reduce the number of pathogenic organisms to a number that is no longer considered harmful, although some viruses and spores are resistant to sanitization. Sanitizing agents include sodium hypochlorite, chlorine gas, and calcium hypochlorite.

Disinfection is a decontamination process that is intended to greatly reduce pathogenic microorganisms from inanimate objects, including surfaces, most often through the use of chemical disinfectants, such as hydrogen peroxide, peroxyacetic acid, and isopropanol.

Sterilization is a process that is intended to kill or deactivate all microorganisms, including viruses, bacteria, fungi, spores and unicellular eukaryotic organisms, rendering the items sterile. Methods of sterilizations include heat (dry, steam incineration), irradiation (non-ionizing, ionizing), filtration, and high pressure as well as the application of chemicals (ethylene oxide, glutaraldehyde, formaldehyde, peracetic acid).

Spalding Classification System of Disinfection

Earle H. Spalding developed a 3-category classification system for different levels of **sterilization/disinfection** based on the type of item (instrument and/or equipment) and its use. While not applicable in all situations, this system is often used for reference:

- **Critical items** are items or pieces of equipment entering the vascular system or sterile tissue, including breaching the mucosal barrier. These include surgical instruments, probes, and urinary catheters and must be sterilized before use. Many of these items are purchased as already sterilized; others are sterilized with steam sterilization or high-level chemical sterilants, such as 7.5% stabilized hydrogen peroxide.
- **Semicritical items** are those items that contact mucous membranes or non-intact skin, including respiratory and anesthesia equipment and manometry probes and catheters. These devices require high-level disinfectants, such as glutaraldehyde and hydrogen peroxide, in accordance with FDA guidelines.
- **Noncritical items** are those items that come in contact with skin that is intact, such as bedpans and blood pressure cuffs. These devices require low-level disinfectants, such as alcohol or diluted bleach.

Sanitization of Equipment, Exam Room Surfaces, and Instruments

Sanitization of equipment, surfaces in the exam room, and instruments should first begin with cleaning to remove all organic and other residue so that the sanitization process can make direct contact. Guidelines vary depending on the sanitizing agent utilized, but manufacturing guidelines should be carefully followed in order to achieve reduction of 99.9% of microorganisms within 30 seconds of application:

- **Equipment**: Must be cleaned according to manufacturer's guidelines with special attention to any knobs or switches.
- **Surfaces**: High-touch surfaces, such as doorknobs, handles, light switches, and telephones, must be cleaned frequently following manufacturer's guidelines and regulations (government, CDC, OSHA). Other surfaces (floors, walls) require periodic sanitization.
- **Instruments**: Should be cleaned thoroughly with soap and water before sterilization, and cleaning must take place in a special "dirty" area. The process for sanitation depends on the classification of the instrument.

Care and Handling of Local Anesthetic Setup

When sanitizing the **local anesthetic setup**, sanitize the harpoon of a stainless-steel reusable aspirating syringe after each use, and then autoclave the entire syringe. From time to time, lubricate parts or the harpoon may require replacement. Discard plastic syringes in a biohazard container. Discard the cannula into a sharps container after normal use if there is any evidence of a broken seal or if tissue penetration occurs more than four times. Anesthetic cartridges come in sterilized, sealed blister packs and should be stored at room temperature in a dark area. Inspect the cartridge before use. Discard a cartridge that has expired or has large bubbles, rust, corrosion, or extruded stoppers. Dispose of a used cartridge in a tamper-proof container approved by the pharmacist. Be aware that addicts scavenge garbage for residual drugs.

Gas and Chemical Sterilization Methods

Gas sterilization methods have been developed because many of the synthetic materials in use are not heat tolerant; however, many gases are highly toxic.

- **Ethylene oxide** is an effective sterilizer but is toxic and combustible, so specialized equipment is necessary to ensure safety.
- **Hydrogen peroxide plasma gas** provides low temperature, low moisture sterilization of medical devices. Because there is no heat involved in the process, the items can be removed as soon as the process completes.

Chemical sterilization may be used for heat sensitive critical and semi-critical items that can be immersed in a liquid. The duration of time required varies. In some cases, the difference between chemical sterilization and disinfection relates to the length of time the process takes. For example, many chemicals require 10–20 minutes (and some up to 12 hours) for effectiveness. Chemical sterilants include glutaraldehyde, hydrogen peroxide, and peracetic acid, sometimes in combination.

Preparing a Tray for the Autoclave

An **autoclave oven** sterilizes instruments. The medical assistant cleans instruments promptly after use by immersion in an ultrasonic bath or instrument washer. Instruments that cannot be cleaned immediately are presoaked in disinfectant temporarily. Use a scrub brush for stubborn debris. Separate the blades of all instruments. Ultrasonic solution should cover all the instrument parts. Instruments that have hinges (e.g., scissors and forceps) should be sanitized first and later sterilized in the open position. Remove instruments from the ultrasonic bath, hold them under running water, dry, and then wrap them for the autoclave. Seal the pack with pressure-sensitive striped tape, which turns color when the correct temperature has been reached. Set the autoclave thermostat to:

- Dry heat at 170 °C (340 °F) for 1 hour for powders and swabs that deteriorate when wet
- Steam at 121 °C (250 °F) and 15 psi for 30 minutes for most metal and glass

Dry the instruments well prior to storage. If the doctor requests an instrument that is not on the autoclaved tray prepared, then use a flash pre-vacuum sterilizer at 134 °C (275 °F) for 4 minutes to sterilize the instrument.

Records of Sterilized Instruments

Records of sterilized instruments must be kept in case there is a recall that requires the items to be traced, retrieved, and re-sterilized. All sterilization records must include the following:

- Date, sterilizer number, and load number
- Lot number and general contents of load
- Exposure time, temperature, and pressure
- Operator's name or initials
- Chemical indicator results
- Biological indicator results
- Bowie-Dick test results for steam vacuums

A record of every sterilizer's performance must also be kept for accreditation. It should show the model and serial number, service dates, reason for the service request, services performed by the technician, and parts replaced.

Laboratory Procedures and Specimen Collection

Venipuncture

Equipment

Routine adult venipuncture equipment includes the following:

- Completed requisition with a physician's signature and billing information
- Soap, water, and towels for hand washing
- Sufficient evacuated blood tubes with the right color stopper
- One 21- or 22-gauge cannula, 1.5" length
- Plastic vacutainer holder with a Luer lock hub
- Isopropyl alcohol or povidone-iodine swab
- Clean, dry cotton balls
- Band-aid or Micropore tape, if the patient is allergic to adhesive
- Tourniquet (rubber Penrose catheter or blood pressure cuff)
- Kidney basin or tray to hold the specimen during collection
- Latex or vinyl gloves
- Pen with indelible ink
- Plastic biohazard bag with outer pouch for the requisition
- Well-buttoned lab coat to protect clothing
- Reclining chair or bed to support the patient
- Certain tests require chemical additives, ice, or a hot water bath
- Sharps disposal container
- Garbage can

Patient Identification and Consent Procedures

Patient identification and consent procedures include the following:

1. If the patient requires an interpreter, provide one.
2. Identify oneself to the patient.
3. Tell the patient which doctor requested the blood sample.
4. Explain in general terms of what is going to be done.
5. Check the patient's armband or health card to confirm identity.
6. Verify the correct spelling of the patient's name and date of birth.
7. If there is any discrepancy between the patient's written identification and the requisition, STOP. Get a doctor or nurse who knows the patient to confirm the identity, and note this on the requisition.
8. A conscious, adult patient has the right to refuse treatment. If the medical assistant proceeds with collection after the patient has refused it, they can be charged with battery. Mark "PATIENT REFUSED" with initials, the date and time on the requisition, return it to the patient's chart, and inform the charge nurse at once. If the patient is unconscious, the law considers the medical assistant to have been given implied consent.

PREPARATION

Preparation for a venipuncture is as follows:

1. Check the expiration dates on all tubes, cannulae and swabs. Get fresh products if any have expired.
2. Wash, dry, and glove the hands.
3. Place the equipment in the kidney basin on an easily accessible table, not on the bed where they can break if the patient rolls over.
4. Select the patient's arm that has no intravenous fluid drip or injury.
5. Tie the tourniquet around the patient's bicep, or inflate a blood pressure cuff to 20 mmHg.
6. Ask the patient to clench a fist. Palpate the veins in the ante cubital fossa.
7. If the arm turns blue, or if the patient complains the tourniquet is too tight, loosen it immediately. Wait until the arm returns to a normal color before reapplying. Prolonged or repeated use of the tourniquet or blood pressure cuff can result in artificially high calcium levels in the specimen.

DRAWING BLOOD

Procedures for drawing blood include the following:

1. Position the patient's arm on a pillow so blood flows downwards. Tell the patient to remain still.
2. Apply tourniquet and cleanse the planned needle insertion site with an alcohol pad, allowing the alcohol to air dry.
3. Retract the skin from the site by anchoring the vein using the non-dominant hand below the insertion site.
4. Uncap the 21- or 22-gauge cannula. Rest the first tube inside the holder. Do not push it onto the hub.
5. Insert the cannula, bevel up, into the vein at a 30° angle until flash of blood is visualized.
6. Grasp the holder with one hand. Push the tube onto the hub with the other. Blood flows automatically into the evacuated tube when the stopper is pierced and stops when its vacuum is depleted.
7. Detach the filled tube from the hub and invert the tube several times to mix the anticoagulant and blood.
8. Place the filled tube in the kidney basin.
9. Release the tourniquet. The tourniquet should not be applied for longer than one minute to prevent hemoconcentration.
10. Rest cotton over the puncture site.
11. Remove the cannula while still on the end of its holder, without unscrewing it. Apply steady pressure to the wound for 4-6 minutes to stop bleeding—longer if the patient is taking anticoagulant drugs like aspirin or coumadin.
12. Ask the alert patient to continue applying pressure after the first minute and dispose of the used equipment in appropriate containers. Elevate the puncture slightly to help slow bleeding, but do not bend the arm. Apply a band-aid.

Blood Collection by Capillary Puncture

Capillary puncture is suitable when a very small quantity of blood is required and the patient has difficult veins. Examples of when capillary puncture is appropriate include:

- Newborn PKU
- Diabetic glucose via glucometer
- Anemic hemoglobin via hemoglobinometer
- Bleeding time before surgery

Capillary puncture is inappropriate for blood cultures or large quantities because the site clots quickly.

Perform newborn capillary puncture with a short point lancet on the lateral or medial plantar heel surface to avoid nicking the calcaneus (heel bone) and causing osteomyelitis. The infant may require a foot amputation if the site becomes gangrenous. Older infants can have the plantar surface of their big toes pricked with a short point lancet. Children and adults have the distal phalanx palmar surface pricked with a long point lancet.

Procedure

Wash the puncture site with warm water to dilate capillaries. If the site remains cold, apply a chemical warming pack. Wrap the pack in a cloth so it does not directly contact the infant's thin skin. Swab the site with alcohol. Puncture the skin quickly with a lancet. Draw blood into the Microtainer tube by capillary action and GENTLE squeezing in the following order:

Color	Additive	Order of Draw	# of Inversions
Lavender	EDTA	First	Mix 20 times
Dark Green	Lithium Heparin	Second	Mix 10 times
Mint Green	PST	Third	Mix 10 times
Gold and Amber	SST	Fourth	Do not mix
Red	None	Last	Do not mix

The order of draw is different than that used for venipuncture because capillary blood is more likely to clot or hemolyze during collection.

Wiping the puncture with alcohol to encourage bleeding when the wound has already clotted will dilute the specimen. Vigorous squeezing can cause interstitial fluid to leak into the specimen and dilute it, or hemolysis of red blood cells, giving a false result.

Culture and Susceptibility Testing

Sensitivity testing is also called **culture and susceptibility testing** (C&S). Wash hands. Don gloves and a lab coat. Sterilize a loop. Streak body fluid (stool, urine, blood, sputum, or wound drainage) across an agar plate with the loop. Rotate the loop and streak again so the bacteria are evenly distributed across the agar. Tissue may also be placed directly on media by the RMA. Incubate at body temperature (37 °C) for 24-48 hours.

If growth occurs, the lab distinguishes normal flora from pathogens by chemical and enzyme tests. A lab tech inoculates pathogens with antimicrobials to see if they can be killed (susceptible), or cannot be killed (resistant). If the antimicrobial that works best requires high doses (intermediate), it is likely to be toxic to the patient. The doctor initially prescribes the antimicrobial to which the pathogen is susceptible, except if the patient is allergic to it. The doctor consults with a pharmacist and microbiologist to choose the least toxic alternative, but the intermediate dose may need to be given over a long time and the patient may suffer side-effects. If the pathogen is resistant to many antimicrobials, then expensive intravenous combination therapy may be the only effective treatment.

Hematocrit Test

A hematocrit (Hct) test separates the blood cells from the plasma in a centrifuge as part of a complete blood count (CBC). Hct indirectly measures red blood cell (RBC) mass, so if the RBCs are of normal size, then the Hct should confirm the RBC count. Patients with macrocytic, microcytic, or iron deficiency anemia with small RBCs will not have parallel Hct and RBC counts. Report results as Packed Cell Volume (PCV), meaning the percentage by volume of packed red blood cells in whole blood. Normal values for venous blood are: Males 42-52%; females 36-48%. Microhematocrit readings from capillary tubes are a little higher. Infants have higher hematocrits than adults because they have more macrocytic RBC's. An abnormal hematocrit suggests follow-up tests must be done for a firm diagnosis. Low hematocrit readings (less than 30%) may indicate many diseases, including adrenal insufficiency, anemia, burns, Hodgkin's disease, leukemia, or poisoning. High hematocrit can be from erythrocytosis, polycythemia vera, or shock.

ESR

An erythrocyte sedimentation rate (**ESR** or **sed rate**) measures how far blood cells with anticoagulant (EDTA or sodium citrate) will fall in a clump (aggregate) in a Westergren or Wintrobe tube in one hour, due to changes in plasma proteins (Rouleaux formation). Normal RBC's do not form Rouleaux, and they settle slowly. Normal values are as follows:

- Males <50 years of age: 0-15 mm/hr
- Males >50 years of age: 0-20 mm/hr
- Females <50 years of age: 0-20 mm/hr
- Females >50 years of age: 0-30 mm/hr
- Children: 0-10 mm/hr

If RBC's settle quickly, the Rouleaux indicates some type of inflammation, necrosis, or parasites are present and further tests are required, but a sed rate does not definitively diagnose a disease. A high ESR can indicate many diseases: Anemia, arthritis, cancer, heart attack, lupus, pelvic inflammatory disease, kidney disease, pneumonia, poisoning with heavy metals, syphilis, thyroid disease, toxemia, and tuberculosis. A low sed rate can result from heavy blood loss.

C-Reactive Protein

C-reactive protein (CRP) is a globulin required to resist bacterial infections and inflammation. CRP binds to dying cells to activate the complement system, triggering it to fight infection and disease. Young people normally have a CRP less than 10 mg/L. Pregnant women, the elderly, and patients with mild viral infections or inflammation have a slightly elevated CRP of 10-40 mg/L. However, CRP rises in 6 hours after a severe infection or inflammation occurs, up to 200 mg/L, and peaks in 48 hours. People with massive burns or overwhelming bacterial infections have CRP levels over 200 mg/L. CRP is elevated in patients with rheumatic fever, heart disease, colon cancer, pneumonia, tuberculosis, lupus, diabetes, vasculitis, rheumatoid arthritis, septic arthritis, and osteomyelitis. Athletes who train excessively decrease their CRP and become more susceptible to infections as a result. To perform a CRP test, draw 10 mL of blood in a red stoppered tube. The immunohistochemistry lab performs an ELISA latex agglutination test to measure the C-reactive protein level. A positive result indicates only inflammation somewhere in the body.

Pregnancy Testing

Beta Human Chorionic Gonadotropin (beta-hCG) is the substance the lab tests urine or blood for to confirm female pregnancy or gestational tumors, or testicular tumors in males. It is performed preoperatively as a precaution for women of childbearing age.

Qualitative hCG just confirms the pregnancy, as it is detectable one week after conception. Tell the patient to collect the first morning urine sample, if possible, because it is the most concentrated at that time. Avoid taking diuretics or the antihistamine promethazine, because it could create a false-negative result. The patient should tell the doctor if they take drugs to control epilepsy or Parkinson's disease, or tranquilizers or hypnotics to induce sleep, because they can cause false-positive results. At least 50 mL is required in a clean jar. The specimen must not be contaminated with stool, menstrual blood, semen, or prostate extractions.

Quantitative hCG helps diagnose ectopic or failing pregnancy, ovarian or testicular tumors, or monitors a woman after a miscarriage. Draw a red stoppered tube of blood for the lab. High levels of beta-hCG in blood indicate tumor progression. Low levels indicate effective cancer treatment.

Monitoring RBC, WBC, and Platelets

The medical assistant performs a quality control test on the Coulter counter every 8 hours by manually comparing RBC, WBC, and platelet counts on a smear against the machine's reading for the same patient. The patient's blood may be normal, but the machine could report an incorrect result if the quality of the stain used was poor (too acidic or alkaline), the specimen was diluted incorrectly, or the machine's calculation was inaccurate.

Test	Normal Values
RBC count	Infants: 3-5 million cells per microliter of blood (cells/mcL)—varies greatly from newborn to toddler Adult males: 4.35-5.65 million cells/mcL Adult females: 3.92-5.13 million cells/mcL, but lower in pregnancy
WBC count	3,400-10,000 WBCs per microliter (cells/mcL) Differential: 1% basophils, 1-3% eosinophils, 50-70% neutrophils, 15-40% lymphocytes, and 2-8% monocytes
Platelets	Infants: 200,000-475,000 per mcL Adults: 150,000-450,000 per mcL

Monitoring Patients on Anticoagulation

The three tests used to monitor patients who take the blood thinner (anticoagulant) coumadin are **INR**, **PT**, and **PTT**. Note that PT and PTT are being phased out in favor of INR.

INR (international normalized ratio) checks clotting Factor VII to I. It standardizes different tissue factors (thromboplastin) used worldwide for testing. Normal INR is 0.9-1.2. If a patient has an INR under 0.8, there is little bleeding (due to rapid clotting). If a patient has an INR of 3.0-4.5, there is heavy bleeding (hemorrhage). Most patients on anticoagulant therapy (coumadin, heparin, and warfarin) are kept with an INR of 2.0-3.0, depending on their condition. If the patient is very likely to develop blood clots, the doctor may push the INR to 3.5. Therapeutic INR is checked every 4-6 weeks. Prolonged INR may be due to bile deficiency, cirrhosis of the liver, lack of Vitamin K, or small intestine disease.

Normal PT (prothrombin time) is 10-12 seconds. Therapeutic value for patients on coumadin is 13-18 seconds. PT checks Factor VII to I.

Normal PTT (partial thromboplastin time) is 25-38 seconds. Therapeutic value for patients on coumadin is 38-76 seconds. PTT checks Factor XII to I.

Blood Sugar Monitoring

The following tests monitor blood sugar for suspected or confirmed diabetes:

- **Fasting blood sugar**: Instruct the patient to fast for 8 hours before collection. Do not drink excessive water, as it dilutes the blood (and therefore the sugar level). Normal fasting blood sugar is less than 100 mg/dL. Use a grey stoppered tube because the oxalate preservative stops the blood cells from eating sugar.
- **2 hr. p.c.**: Two hours post cibum (after eating). After the fasting blood collection, the patient takes a normal meal and returns for a second collection exactly 2 hours after it was finished. Blood sugar should peak two hours after eating (postprandial), and then drop precipitously.
- **HbA1c**: A test for glucose bound to hemoglobin in red blood cells over their 120-day lifespan. It is a snapshot of blood glucose control for the past three months and can help to evaluate the effectiveness of strategies being used to control diabetes such as medication or diet.
- **GTT**: A 3- or 5-hour glucose tolerance test diagnoses hyperglycemia (high blood sugar) that is a precursor to diabetes. Collect blood and urine fasting, 30 minutes after a glucose drink was finished, and at 1 hour, 2 hours, and 3 hours. Occasionally it is ordered at 4 and 5 hours.

Liver Function Tests

ALP (Alkaline Phosphatase) normally ranges from 40-129 IU/L in adults and up to 300 in children with growing bones. Doctors use ALP to differentiate between bone and liver diseases. ALP increases in bone fractures and Paget's disease, liver cancer, hyperparathyroidism, hyperphosphatasia, infarcted bowel, and rheumatoid arthritis. ALP decreases in pernicious anemia, celiac disease, hypothyroidism, low serum phosphorous (hypophosphatemia), and malnutrition.

ALT (Serum Alanine Aminotransferase) normally ranges from 7-55 IU/L. ALT increases in liver disease. AST:ALT ratio should be 1:1. If it is greater than 1:1, this can indicate cirrhosis, congestion, or tumors of the liver. If the ratio is less than 1:1, suspect hepatitis or mononucleosis.

AST (Serum Aspartate Aminotransferase) normally ranges from 8-48 IU/L. AST increases in conditions that affect the heart such as congestive heart failure, liver such as chronic alcohol or drug abuse or cirrhosis, muscles such as muscular dystrophy, or pancreatitis.

Bilirubin normally ranges from 0.1-1.2 mg/dL (0.3-1.0 mg/dL for individuals under 18 years of age). It is a reddish-yellow bile pigment created when the liver breaks down old red blood cells, and is stored in the gall bladder. Excess bilirubin causes jaundice. The medical assistant can artificially lower bilirubin by leaving a specimen tube exposed to light at room temperature for one hour, shaking the specimen, or allowing air bubbles in it.

Lipid Profile

A lipid profile tests for hyperlipidemia, elevated fats and oils in the blood which clog blood vessels and result in heart attack, stroke, and ischemia. Routinely screen men over 35, women over 45, and younger patients with risk factors or a significant family history of cardiovascular disease.

Lipid	Normal Value
LDL cholesterol (bad cholesterol)	High: >160 mg/dL Borderline high: 130-159 mg/dL Near optimal: 100-129 mg/dL Optimal: <100 mg/dL
HDL cholesterol (good cholesterol)	Male: >40 mg/dL Female: >50 mg/dL
Total cholesterol	Desirable: <200 mg/dL Borderline high risk: 200-239 mg/dL High risk: ≥240 mg/dL
LDL/HDL ratio	<4
Triglycerides	Normal: <150 mg/dL Borderline high: 150-200 mg/dL High: >200 mg/dL

Instruct the patient to fast for 12-14 hours before testing. Random lipids are inaccurate because fatty meals spike them. Treatment is diet modification, exercise, weight loss, niacin supplements, statins for cholesterol (Lipitor, Mevacor), and fibrates for triglyceride (Lopid, Tricor).

Urine Collection Procedures

Routine Urinalysis

Below are the common urine dipstick tests in routine urinalysis. Normal values are bracketed:

1. **Blood** (negative): Intact or hemolyzed red blood cells indicate bleeding due to infection, menstruation, paroxysmal hemoglobinuria, or trauma.
2. **Glucose** (negative): Uncontrolled diabetes and women with gestational diabetes spill sugar into their urine when their renal threshold is exceeded.
3. **Ketones** (negative): Uncontrolled diabetes, extreme dieters, and starving people produce ketones in urine when their bodies burn fat instead of sugar.
4. **Leukocytes** (negative): White blood cells indicate infection.
5. **pH** (5-9): Acidic urine helps the bladder resist infection. Alkaline urine encourages bacterial growth.
6. **Protein** (up to 8 mg/dL): Albumin is shed from the kidneys if the nephrons are damaged. Trace protein can be from genitals or feces.
7. **Nitrites** (negative): Some bacteria, like E-coli, produce nitrites after eating nitrates, so this is an indicator of infection.

If kidney stones, infection, or damage is suspected, then a microscopic urinalysis is performed with the routine urinalysis for casts, crystals, and cells.

Microscopic Urine Examination

On microscopic urinalysis, assess for:

1. **Red blood cells (RBC)**: Up to two RBC at low-power field are normal. Five or more indicate tumor, infection, glomerulonephritis, or trauma; this is recorded as microscopic hematuria.
2. **White blood cells (WBC)**: Up to four WBC at low-power field are normal. Five or more indicate a urinary tract infection.
3. **Casts**: Negative or occasional hyaline casts are normal. Record many hyaline casts as proteinuria. The cast types and diseases they indicate are WBC, pyelonephritis; RBC, glomerulonephritis; waxy and granular, non-specific; broad casts, chronic renal failure; and fat casts, nephritic syndrome.
4. **Crystals**: None are normal. Urate crystals indicate gout. Phosphate and calcium oxalate crystals appear in hyperparathyroidism and malabsorption conditions. "Coffin lid" struvite casts occur with urea-splitting bacteria. Tyrosine or cystine indicates metabolic disease or poisoning.
5. **Bacteria**: Normal urine is sterile, with no bacteria. Many indicate a urinary tract infection (UTI).
6. **Artifacts**: Squamous cells from the vagina, cotton fibers from clothes, and starch granules from baby powder are all examples of extraneous artifacts.

Random and Midstream Urine Collections

Random urine is used at any time of day for a routine checkup, in any clean container. It does not require a sterile container nor does it require a lid if it will be tested immediately, only if it will be transported or stored. Urine is generally tested in the chemistry department. Routine checkup tests include blood, protein, glucose, ketones, and pH. Hands should be clean and free of contaminants that could affect the results.

Midstream urine can also be collected at any time of day but requires a sterile, lidded container. It is used for bacteriology studies to diagnose bladder and kidney infections. The patient cleans the urinary opening (meatus), voids a little urine, collects the midstream of urine, and voids the remainder in the toilet. If hands touch the inside of the container, the specimen may be contaminated and produce a false positive.

Plating a Midstream Urine Sample

The procedure for plating a midstream urine sample for culture and sensitivity testing (MSU for C&S) is described below:

1. Touch the outside of the MSU container only.
2. Open an agar plate; do not touch the inner surface or lid.
3. Dip a sterile swab or loop in the urine.
4. Press the swab or loop lightly across the surface of the agar to plant the possible bacterial infection for culture.
5. Close the plate tightly. Label it with the patient's name, date and time, physician's name, and test ("urine for C&S").
6. If the specimen will be sent to an outside lab, refrigerate it until pickup. If testing it onsite, place it in an incubator for 24-48 hours so the microbiologist can make a determination about the infection.

7. If growth occurs, a microbiologist places several small circles of paper impregnated with different antibiotics on the plate.
8. If the bacteria are sensitive to the medication, a small area surrounding the paper circle will have no apparent growth.
9. If bacteria are resistant, growth is uninhibited.

KIDNEY (RENAL) FUNCTION TESTS

The following are kidney (renal) function tests and their normal values:

- **BUN**: Blood urea nitrogen (BUN) is a nitrogenous waste byproduct of amino acid metabolism. Urea is the end product. BUN is normally excreted by the kidneys at 7-20 mg/dL. Patients with end-stage renal disease (ESRD) have BUN levels between 60-100 mg/dL and are monitored monthly.
- **Creatinine**: Creatinine is the end-product of muscle metabolism and is normally removed by the kidneys at 0.7-1.5 mg/dL. High creatinine (over 1.5 mg/dL) and BUN (over 20 mg/dL) means the patient has a kidney disease (e.g., glomerulonephritis, pyelonephritis, stones, tubular necrosis, or tumors).
- **Protein**: A normal serum protein test includes total protein 6-8 g/dL, albumin 3.5-5.0 g/dL, and globulin 2.5-3.0 g/dL. Albumin deficiency causes swelling (edema) and can be from protein malnutrition, kidney or liver, and disease. Low globulin indicates severe burns, malnutrition, or kidney or liver disease.
- **Urea**: Carbamide, a nitrogenous waste product of protein metabolism made by the liver from ammonia and aspartic acid (an amino acid). Healthy kidneys eliminate about 10 g of urea daily. Purified urea is used as a diuretic, pressure reducer, and antiseptic.

24-HOUR CREATININE CLEARANCE TEST

The 24-hour creatinine clearance test determines if kidneys are damaged by measuring their output of creatinine against the blood level. If the kidneys do not filter properly, creatinine output in the urine decreases and blood levels increase. In a normal male, creatinine clearance results fall between 110 and 150 mL/min; in normal females, they are between 95 and 125 mL/min. A BUN-to-creatinine ratio between 15:1 and 20:1 is a normal finding.

Patients should be instructed to prepare for the test in the following way: Two days before and during the test, do NOT eat more than 8 ounces of red meat, take Vitamin C, drink caffeine, or exercise strenuously. Discard the first morning urine in the toilet. Note the start time. Collect all urine in the jug up to and including the same time the next morning. Keep the jug on a bucket of ice or in the refrigerator. Note the time of the last collection. Return to the lab the next morning to have a blood creatinine level drawn for comparison.

Drugs that affect the test include diuretics, vitamin C, levodopa, Tagamet, Mefoxin, Dilantin, Garamycin, quinine, procainamide, amphotericin B, and tetracycline.

STOOL COLLECTION PROCEDURES

O&P AND PINWORM

Stool for ova and parasites (O&P) is a test that assesses for worms (helminths) and protozoa that can cause anemia in feces samples, such as tapeworm and round worms. Give the patient a clean jar containing an ounce of formalin. Tell the patient to use a popsicle stick to mix a teaspoon of stool with the preservative and return it, tightly capped and labeled, to the lab.

Pinworms are white, thread-like parasites usually contracted by children from sand boxes in which infected cats and dogs have defecated. The child often scratches his/her itchy bottom and grinds the teeth while sleeping. Give the parent a stool container containing a pinworm paddle, or tell the parent to use a jar with clear tape. When the child sleeps, use a flashlight to visualize the anus. Female tapeworms leave the bowel to lay eggs around the anus at night. Gently touch the paddle or tape to the anus and place it in the jar. Cap tightly. Wash hands well. Return the labeled jar to the lab.

Occult Blood and Guaiac

Patients who use aspirin regularly or have ulcers may lose microscopic amounts of blood in their feces. The lab examines stool smears on a mail-in card for **occult blood**. Provide the patient with an occult blood kit. Instruct the patient to follow the enclosed diet for three days before collection, as foods that cause bleeding must be avoided (e.g., cantaloupe, turnip, broccoli, and horseradish). Tell the patient to place plastic wrap under the toilet seat and defecate. Use the enclosed popsicle sticks to smear thin samples of stool from three consecutive bowel movements on the three windows in the card. The patient mails the card back to the lab in the envelope provided.

Guaiac also detects occult blood, but is collected by the doctor in the office during a rectal examination with a gloved finger. The doctor wipes the soiled glove across a window that contains guaiac resin on a card and adds two drops of peroxide. If the sample oxidizes (turns blue) in 2 seconds or less, the patient is losing blood.

These two tests are not reliable tests for bowel cancer.

Sputum Culture

Sputum is phlegm (mucous) and other matter expelled from the lungs and trachea. It should contain as little saliva from the mouth as possible. Sputum can be cultured (C&S) to identify an infection, such as pneumonia. Sputum can be examined microscopically to identify cancer or a disease-causing agent, such as asbestos fibers. If the doctor orders sputum for AFB (acid fast bacilli stain), then the lab searches for bacteria that cause tuberculosis. Drink fluids the night before specimen collection, to encourage secretions. Collect the specimen upon arising, because sputum collects in the air passageways during sleep. Tap on the chest. Cough deeply. If unable to produce any sputum, try inhaling steaming salt water. If any sputum arises, spit it into a sterile cup. Cap it tightly and label it. Bring the sputum to the lab immediately for testing. If unable to transport it immediately, refrigerate it up to 3 days. The doctor may order specimen collection on 3 consecutive days.

Manual Hemoglobin Test for Hemodialysis Patient

When performing a manual hemoglobin test for a hemodialysis patient, test the hemoglobinometer with known controls first. Polish a clean hemocytometer slide with lens paper. Fill a blue-ringed, unheparinized capillary tube with blood. Place one drop of blood on the hemocytometer slide. Roll the heparinized, wooden hemolysis stick over the blood drop until the blood is hemolyzed and transparent (about 30 seconds). Place the cover slip over the slide. Slide them together into the hemoglobinometer. Look through the viewer. Adjust the light until the two fields are exactly the same color. (Most hemoglobinometers use green and black.) Read the scale (usually on the side of the meter) and record the hemoglobin level. Normal values are 12-16 g/dL for women, and 14-16 g/dL: for men. Disassemble the slide and cover slip. Sanitize, disinfect, polish, and case them. Wipe the test area and outside of the hemoglobinometer with disinfectant. Hemoglobinometer readings with capillary blood show about 10% false-positives for anemia, as compared to venous Coulter Counter readings. Hemoglobinometers are for point-of-care testing for "ballpark" estimates.

Tests for Mononucleosis

Epstein-Barr virus (EBV) causes mononucleosis. The **Monospot** heterophile antibodies test confirms the patient is in the early stage of mononucleosis (2-9 weeks). To perform a Monospot, drop capillary or venous blood on a glass slide. Mix with guinea pig kidney antigen to absorb Forssmann antibodies. Mix with beef red blood stroma to absorb non-Forssman antibodies. Mix with horse blood. Guinea pig agglutination means the patient has early mononucleosis. Beef should not agglutinate. Monospot can be false-negative on children under 10, or before two weeks of infection. False-positives are caused by adenovirus, Burkitt's and Hodgkin's lymphomas, cytomegalovirus, hepatitis, HIV, leukemia, lupus, pregnancy, rheumatoid arthritis, rubella, and toxoplasmosis. Monospot may not detect an infection that is older than six months.

If the patient has late-stage mono, the doctor orders EBV antibody titer, CBC, and throat swab. To perform a titer, serially dilute blood serum or other body fluids with saline. Negative is less than 1:40 EBV and no IgM antibodies are present. Positive is greater than 1:40 and antibodies are present. IgM indicates the active phase of mono. IgG antibodies mean the patient is recovering from mononucleosis.

Test for Strep Throat

Often, acute pharyngitis results from group A streptococci. **Strep throat** especially affects children 5-15 years old in the winter and spring. Strep throat can develop into rheumatic fever when it travels through the bloodstream to destroy the heart, joints, and kidneys. "Super Strep" strains are resistant to antibiotics. To perform a Quidel QuickVue rapid strep test:

- Swab the patient's tonsils and pharynx for no more than five seconds with the swab in the kit. Use a tongue depressor to avoid swabbing the cheeks and tongue. The patient will gag briefly.
- Place the swab in the test cassette chamber.
- Crush the extraction reagent delivery device.
- Mix the extraction solutions until they turn green.
- Add the solution to the top rim of the swab chamber.
- Stand the swab upright in the chamber so capillary action draws the solution up to the rabbit reagent pad.
- Read the window at five minutes. A red stripe on the reagent strip indicates strep infection. The control is the blue line next to the letter C, and it should always appear. The absence of a red line indicates no strep infection. A positive result means the patient requires antibiotic treatment to avoid rheumatic fever.

Test for Tuberculosis

The tests that identify tuberculosis (TB) are a positive **Mantoux skin test** or **QFT-G blood test**. Both must be confirmed by chest x-ray and sputum culture to determine whether the TB is active or latent. 10% of exposed persons with positive Mantoux tests develop active TB infection. Employers offer prophylaxis with Isoniazid (INH) if a medical assistant is exposed to an active TB case.

To perform the two-step Mantoux skin test:

- Week 1: The medical assistant injects 0.1 mL of 5 units of tuberculin intradermally in the patient's forearm.
- 2-3 days later: The patient returns to have the test read. A negative test has no redness or swelling.
- Week 2 or 3: The medical assistant repeats the test again to prevent identification of a booster reaction as a positive TB result.

Patients with AIDS, lupus, renal failure, or kidney transplant have false-negative reactions to Mantoux. The patient who received BCG vaccine against TB will have a false-positive reaction. Ask the registered nurse to perform the QFT-G blood test for these patients, instead of Mantoux.

Vaginal Swab for Maternal Strep B

The procedure to collect a vaginal swab for maternal strep B is described below:

1. Wash and glove hands.
2. The patient should be informed that two swabs will be collected to ensure there is no danger to her newborn.
3. Tell the patient to remove her trousers and panties, but she may retain a skirt.
4. Cover the patient with a clean drape for modesty.
5. Position her face up on the exam table and move her buttocks to the bottom edge.
6. The patient must spread her legs widely, so if she has difficulty, place her feet in the stirrups.
7. Do not use lubricant.
8. Gently open her labia with one hand.
9. Clean mucous away from the mother's cervix with a clean, dry vaginal swab. Discard the swab.
10. Apply a Strep B swab to her cervix for 10 seconds to collect a sample.
11. Place it in the media container.
12. Snap off the end of the stick so the lid fits tightly.
13. Label the vial with the patient's name and date.
14. Give the patient a disposable wipe to clean herself before departing.

Collecting a Wound Culture

To obtain a wound culture, first gather a biohazard waste bag, a microbiology requisition, a cleansing pack, and a sterile dressing. Use a red-stoppered swab for MRSA testing and a charcoal swab for all other tests.

1. Wash and glove hands and don personal protective equipment (PPE).
2. Create a sterile field with drapes; examine the wound.
3. Note in the patient's chart the presence of pus; foul odor; discharge; cellulitis; discoloration; delayed healing; friable, granulated tissue; increased pain to touch; pocketing; or wound enlargement.
4. Wet the swab with sterile saline and rotate it 360° across the wound in a zigzag.
5. Place the swab in the media and cap tightly.
6. Clean the wound with disinfectant (e.g., Betadine) and dress it.
7. Discard soiled articles and doff PPE.
8. If the patient is taking antibiotics, note it on the requisition.
9. Do not refrigerate the swab; transport it to the lab immediately.

Specimen Labeling and Common Preservation Methods

Appropriate specimen labeling and preservation is critical in obtaining accurate results and readings:

- **Specimen labeling**: Before collecting a specimen, the patient's identity should be confirmed with two identifiers (name and birthdate). Every specimen container must have a label directly attached at the time and point of collection. The following information must be on each specimen: Patient's first and last name, medical record number, date of birth, date and time of collection, and initials of person collecting the sample. Infant samples also require the mother's first name, infant's gender, and infant's ID band number. Some labels may contain a barcode and/or the physician's name as well.
- **Preservation**: Some specimens may be stored in the refrigerator, including urine and stool specimens, after being properly labeled. Fresh tissue specimens should be inserted into a container holding the fixative already with volume 20:1 in comparison with specimen. The container should be gently agitated for a few minutes after the specimen is inserted to ensure penetration.

Tools and Methods of Specimen Preparation and Examination

Tools and methods of specimen preparation and examination include the following:

Incubator	Equipment used to store cell and tissue cultures in a temperature-controlled environment for optimal growth. Shaking incubators provide a shaking platform and agitation to promote cell growth.
Centrifuge	Equipment used to spin and separate components of a specimen, such as blood, placed inside in a vial.
Microscope	Used to examine slides of tissue to note microscopic elements, such as abnormal cells, and wet mounts to identify microscopic organisms.
Culture inoculation	Procedure by which a specimen is applied to an agar plate or injected into a liquid medium for a bacterial culture.
Microbiologic slides (wet mount)	A sample, such as vaginal discharge, is placed on a slide and a drop of water or NS placed on top of the specimen before the top slide is carefully put in place. This method is especially useful for viewing and identifying motile (moving) microscopic organisms.

Gram-Positive and Gram-Negative Bacteria

Bacteria are either gram-negative or gram-positive. Identifying this quality is important in planning treatment:

- **Gram-negative**: Thin-walled bacteria that turns **RED** when Gram stained from absorbing crystal violet, pink safranin, and fuchsin. Lipopolysaccharide in their walls repels blue stain. Lipid-A is the endotoxin found outside the cell wall. Parts include: flagellum (motility), pilus (adherence, conjugation), capsule (protection), peptidoglycan wall (support, shape), cytoplasmic membrane, and periplasmic space (holds enzymes and proteins). Examples: *Escherichia coli, Klebsiella pneumoniae, Pseudomonas aeruginosa, Haemophilus influenzae, Enterobacter aerogenes.*
- **Gram-positive:** Thick-walled bacteria that turns **VIOLET-BLUE** when Gram stained. Walls contain teichoic acid and a membrane that increase virulence. Examples: group B streptococcus, *Staphylococcus aureus* and *epidermidis,* and *Listeria monocytogenes.* Most bone infections (osteomyelitis) are caused by Gram-positive bacteria.

Laboratory Standards and Regulations

Occupational Safety and Health Administration (OSHA)

OSHA stands for Occupational Safety and Health Administration. It is an organization designed to assure the safety and health of workers by setting and enforcing standards; providing training, outreach, and education; establishing partnerships; and encouraging continual improvement in workplace safety and health.

SDS (formerly MSDS) stands for **Safety Data Sheets**. These sheets are the result of the "Right to Know" Law also known as the OSHA's Hazard Communication Standard (HCS). This law requires chemical manufacturers to supply SDS sheets on any products that have a hazardous warning label. These sheets contain information on precautionary as well as emergency information about the product.

OSHA Regulations Regarding Laboratory Services

The Occupational Safety and Health Administration (OSHA) requires that facilities provide safe medical equipment and devices. OSHA also regulates workplace safety, including disposal methods for sharps, such as needles, and blood disposition. OSHA requires that standard precautions be used at all times and that staff be trained to use precautions. OSHA requires procedures for post-exposure evaluation and treatment and availability of hepatitis B vaccine for healthcare workers. OSHA defines occupational exposure to infections, establishes standards to prevent the spread of bloodborne pathogens, and regulates the fitting and use of respirators. OSHA requires the use of needleless blood transfer devices as a means of decreasing the risk of needlestick injuries and infection as part of OSHA's Bloodborne Pathogen Standard. Sharps used for blood draw should have sharps injury protection devices whenever possible. Needles without this protection should never be recapped as this increases risk of needlestick. States may have their own OSHA-approved programs but must meet the minimum standards developed by OSHA.

Laboratory Standards and Integrity Assessment

Laboratory standards are established by a number of agencies, including OSHA, which establishes safety standards; the EPA, which established good laboratory practices; CLSI, which provides global laboratory standards; and ISO-9000, which establishes standards for quality management. Laboratory standards are norms or requirements stablished for the profession. **Integrity assessment** is carried out to determine if a laboratory is meeting standards or has engaged in fraud or misconduct (as opposed to accidents or errors), such as through:

- Failure to properly carry out procedures
- Falsification of records or measurements, incomplete documentation, manipulation of data
- Violation of standards or rules of conduct, violations of codes of ethics
- Misrepresentation of quality assurance results
- Failure to adequately calibrate equipment
- Failure to retain samples for the required time
- Improper storage of reagents, samples, and supplies
- Failure to follow standard operating procedures
- Alterations of log book
- Employment of personnel without appropriate license or certification

Integrity assessment may include reviewing data, comparing manual logs with computer logs, conducting an audit trail, carrying out unannounced audits, and encouraging and supporting whistleblowers.

Governmental and Nongovernmental Regulatory Entities

The **Clinical and Laboratory Standards Institute (CLSI)** provides standards for a wide range of performance and testing and covers all types of laboratory functions and microbiology. These standards are used as a basis for quality control procedures. Standards include: labeling, security/information technology, toxicology/drug testing, statistical quality control, and performance standards for various types of antimicrobial susceptibility testing.

In the United States, all laboratory testing, except for research, is regulated by the CMS (Centers for Medicare and Medicaid) through **Clinical Laboratory Improvement Amendments (CLIA)**. CLIA is implemented through the Division of Laboratory Services and serves approximately 244,000 laboratories. Laboratories receiving reimbursement from CMS must meet CLIA standards, which ensure that laboratory testing will be accurate and procedures followed properly.

The **Centers for Disease Control and Prevention (CDC)** is a federal agency that supports health promotion, prevention, and health preparedness. The CDC partners with CMS and the FDA in supporting CLIA programs.

The **National Accrediting Agency for Clinical Laboratory Sciences** is responsible for approving and accrediting clinical laboratory science and similar healthcare professional education programs.

The **College of American Pathologists** is the primary organization for board-certified pathologists serving to represent the interests of the public, as well as pathologists and their patients by fostering excellence in the pathology and laboratory medicine practice.

The **Joint Commission** is a large organization that aims to improve the quality of care provided to patients through implementing healthcare accreditation standards and other supportive services aimed at improving the performance of healthcare organizations.

SOP for Laboratories

Each laboratory should draw up a **standard operating procedure (SOP) document** that outlines all the processes and procedures associated with the reception of a sample and processing, including:

- **Specimen collection processes**: PPE, patient identification, collection tubes, collecting procedures, need for special handling, labeling, transporting specimens, criteria for rejecting inadequate sample, protocols for adverse reactions
- **Chain of custody**: Labeling, storing, packing, and transporting
- **Sample reception**: Specimen identification, logging, specimen condition, specimen accountability, retention times
- **Rejection criteria**: Incorrect collection tube, leaking tube, incorrect labeling, incorrect sample for test, volume inadequate, order unverified, mismatch between order and labeling
- **Delivery** (from reception to processing): Process for delivery to correct department, specimen retention policies
- **Processing**: Procedures for testing, accountability standards, storage, and retention policies
- **Reporting**: Methods of reporting and timeframes

Principles of Pharmacology

Six Rights of Medication Administration

Six rights of medication administration include the following:

- **Right patient**: The medication should be prescribed specifically for the patient and the medical assistant should check two identifiers before giving medications.
- **Right medication**: The medication should be the correct choice for patient's condition and should match the prescription. Always verify that the medication is correct. Check the medication label when obtaining the medication, when preparing it, and before administering it.
- **Right route**: Administration should be the route that is appropriate for patient's condition and the type of medications (oral, sub-lingual, rectal, injection [IV, IM, or SC], etc.).
- **Right dose**: The dose must be as prescribed and appropriate for age, weight, and condition. If the medication is provided in a different dose from that prescribed, check calculations with a nurse.
- **Right time**: Medication should not be expired (always check date) and must be administered at the time ordered, such as "stat" (immediately) or "every 5 minutes times three."
- **Right documentation**: Documentation should be done immediately after administration and recorded in the correct format.

Actions Required If Patient Brings Their Own Medications for Self-Administration

A patient may **bring his or her own medications** into the facility for self-administration, for example, an Epi-pen, asthma inhaler, insulin, pain pump, or nitroglycerin. This means that the patient gets instant treatment, but it also represents a liability to the facility. The drugs could be improperly stored, shared, stolen, or mistakenly administered to another patient. The syringes used to administer the medication may be disposed of incorrectly in the regular garbage, instead of a sharps container, and present a hazard to cleaning staff.

The medical assistant may assist the patient with self-administration to the extent of:

- Checking the label and dosage to ensure it is taken as directed
- Opening the case and placing the medication in the patient's hand
- Ensuring safe disposal of sharps (e.g., broken ampoules, needles)

However, the medical assistant may not actually inject or otherwise administer the medication without the doctor's expressed instructions. The medical assistant's liability is greatest for medications marked "as needed" (prn). Most states require caregivers to take a 4-hour training course with a pharmacist or registered nurse before allowing medication assistance.

Common Drug Types

Drug	Function	Examples
Analgesics	Acts as a minor pain reliever.	Aspirin, Tylenol, Advil, or Aleve
Anesthetic	Produces loss of sensation for painful procedures.	Local anesthetics: Procaine and lidocaine General anesthetics: Halothane, and methohexital
Antibiotics	There are 7 classes of antibiotics, all targeting different types of bacteria. The mode of action varies; some kill bacteria by impairing the cell membrane, others interfere with cell metabolism, leading to death of the cell.	Common classes: Penicillins, cephalosporins, aminoglycosides, carbapenems, fluoroquinolones, glycopeptides, macrolides, sulfonamides, and tetracyclines
Beta Blockers	Lower blood pressure by blocking adrenaline and slowing the heart	Inderal, Lopressor, and Tenormin
Cathartics	Encourages bowel movements (defecation) before x-rays of the colon or to treat poisoning	Sorbitol and senna
Diuretics	Increases the formation of urine to relieve edema (swelling) or high blood pressure	Hydrochlorothiazide, Furosemide (Lasix), and Triamterene
Expectorants	Helps expel mucous from the lungs through coughing by breaking down and mobilizing the secretions	Guaifenesin
Hypoglycemics (diabetic)	Oral medications help the body metabolize carbohydrates, decrease production of glucose (sugar) by the liver, or stimulate the pancreas to produce more insulin. Insulins (given by injection) replace natural insulin the pancreas can no longer produce to metabolize carbohydrates.	Oral: Sulfonylureas (glipizide), biguanides (Metformin) Insulin injection: Rapid-acting, Regular (short-acting), Intermediate-acting, Long-Acting, Ultra-long-acting
Sedatives	Makes insomniacs drowsy, relieves seizures, or calms anxious patients	Nembutal, Seconal, Ativan, Xanax, and Valium
SSRIs	Increase the level of serotonin (a neurotransmitter) to decrease depression	Prozac
Statins	Inhibit production of cholesterol in the liver and lower blood cholesterol levels	Atorvastatin (Lipitor), Simvastatin (Zocor)
Vaccines	Builds the patient's active immunity against a specific disease.	DPTP (diphtheria, polio, tetanus, and pertussis) and MMR (measles, mumps, and rubella)
Vasodilators	Relaxes smooth muscles in blood vessels to allow them to expand, decreases BP	ACE inhibitors, Hydralazine, and Minoxidil

Controlled Substances

Controlled substances are categorized under the *Controlled Substances Act of 1970*. There are five groups of controlled substances, categorized from Schedule I to Schedule V.

- **Schedule I substances** have a high potential for abuse and dependence and have NO accepted medical use in the United States. These drugs are not considered safe to use even under medical supervision. Schedule I substances are for research and instructional purposes only. Schedule I drugs include Ecstasy, Heroin, and LSD.
- **Schedule II substances** have a high potential for abuse, but have an accepted medical use. Use is severely restricted because severe psychological and/or physical dependence may develop. Schedule II drugs include PCP, Methamphetamine, Ritalin, and most narcotics.
- **Schedule III substances** have less potential for abuse than Schedule I and II substances, and have an accepted medical use in the United States. Abuse of these substances may lead to moderate or low physical dependence and/or high psychological dependence. Schedule III drugs include anabolic steroids for body building, like Winstrol, narcotics with less than 90 mg of codeine per dose, and buprenorphine (Suboxone).
- **Schedule IV drugs** have a low potential for abuse compared to substances in Schedule III. Schedule IV substances have an accepted medical use in the United States. Abuse of substances in this category may lead to limited physical and/or psychological dependence. Examples of Schedule IV drugs are Xanax, Librium, Valium, and the date rape drug Rohypnol.
- **Schedule V** substances have a low potential for abuse compared to Schedule IV drugs. Schedule V substances have an accepted medical use in the United States. Abuse of Schedule V drugs may lead to limited physical and/or psychological dependence compared to Schedule IV substances. Examples of Schedule V drugs are Robitussin A-C, Lomotil, and Pediacof.

Complications in Medication Administration and Use

Various complications can arise from drug administration and the medical assistant must be aware of these risks for each specific drug type:

- **Side-effect**: An unwanted effect of a therapeutic dose of a drug. A side-effect may or may not cause the patient harm. An example is drowsiness for cold medications.
- **Adverse event (AE)**: A minor side-effect that may or may not be expected. For example, a patient may develop indigestion after using Aspirin for a headache.
- **Sentinel event (SE)**: An unexpected outcome causing serious physical or psychological harm, or even death. For example, a child may develop brain damage from Reyes Syndrome after taking Aspirin for influenza.
- **Substance abuse**: Excessive use of any substance, but usually drugs or alcohol, which impairs or distresses a patient for 12 months or more. Substance abuse is characterized by failure at school, work, or home due to frequent absences, neglect, or bizarre behavior. Substance abuse produces legal problems, such as arrests for disorderly conduct or driving while impaired. The abuser continues to crave the substance despite its physical hazards and social problems.

Resources

Physicians' Desk Reference (PDR)

The *Physicians' Desk Reference (PDR),* which is issued each year, contains a wealth of information about drugs, and is an invaluable resource for information about adverse effects, correct dosage, and administration. The PDR contains reference lists of telephone numbers for the FDA (such as medical product reporting programs), for poison control centers, and for drug information centers. The product information guide provides colored pictures of medications in actual size to help to identify unlabeled medications. Manufacturers provide information about the drugs that matches the package inserts, which are required by the FDA to provide indications, effects, dosages, routes, methods, frequency and duration of administration and any warning, hazards, contraindications, side effects, and precautions. The PDR is available in a print edition and also an online version (PDR.net) and includes a mobile version with safety alerts.

Drug Reference Manuals

Common drug manuals for the medical office are the *American Drug Index, Compendium of Pharmaceuticals and Specialties,* Lippincott's *Nursing Drug Guide*, and Stoklosa and Ansel's *Pharmaceutical Calculations*. The definitive online drug reference is the *United States Pharmacopeia–National Formulary (USP–NF)*. When in doubt about a drug, always contact a pharmacist.

Medication Administration, Dosage, and Storage

Routes of Drug Administration

The route of administration is the manner by which a drug is introduced into the body. The routes of administration include the following:

- **Enteral** (oral, rectal, or by feeding tube)
- **Topical** (on the skin, in the eyes or nose, vaginal, or inhaled)
- **Parenteral** (IV, subcutaneous, intramuscular, intracardiac, intraosseous, intradermal, intrathecal, intraperitoneal, transdermal, transmucosal, intravitreal, and epidural)

The route of administration affects the way the medication is absorbed, distributed, and eliminated. The effect of a medication is local or systemic. There are many variations on these three basic routes of administration. The FDA acknowledges over 100 different routes of administration. When deciding on the route of administration, the doctor and pharmacist consider:

- How **fast** the patient requires the drug
- How **effective** it will be by a given route
- The likelihood of **toxicity**
- The **discomfort** it will cause
- How likely the patient is to **comply** with the route
- How likely the route is to play into the patient's **addictive habits**

Syringe Parts

The syringe is used to inject medications, to irrigate wounds, and to obtain specimens. The barrel holds the medication or solution and the rubber stop keeps the fluid from leaking out. The plunger is inserted to inject the fluid, and the flanges allow the fingers to grasp the syringe. The needle is interchangeable so that different sizes can be attached to the tip by being inserted into the hub. A Luer lock or slip about the hub helps to secure the needle so that it doesn't inadvertently come loose.

Injections

Forms of Injections

Common forms of injection include the following:

- **Subcutaneous Injection**: Delivers the drug under the skin using a 0.5" long, 24- or 25-gauge needle held at a 45° angle to reach the fat. The upper arm, abdomen, thigh, or lower back can be used as the site. The maximum volume of administration for a subcutaneous medication is 0.5 mL. An example is insulin for a patient with diabetes.
- **Intramuscular Injection**: Delivers the drug into the muscle with a 1" long, 20-gauge needle held at a 90° angle perpendicular to the muscle, to reach the deep tissue. For obese patients, use a 2" needle. In adults, intramuscular injection sites include the vastus lateralis (thigh) in volumes of 0.5-3.0 mL, the ventrogluteal region (hip) in volumes of 0.5-3.0 mL, the deltoid (upper arm) in volumes of 0.5-2.0 mL, or the dorsogluteal region (buttocks) in volumes of 1-3 mL.
- **Intravenous Injection:** Delivers the drug into a vein of the arm, hand, leg, foot, scalp, or neck with an Angiocath, butterfly, or Insyte Autoguard needle. The medication is infused via venous catheter by syringe or pump. The nurse sets the drip rate per minute by adjusting the clamp and monitoring the drip chamber. An example is Zoledronate that is given yearly to prevent bone fractures for individuals with osteoporosis.

Two less frequently used forms of injection are: Intradermal (into the skin) for Mantoux TB test, and intraosseous access (IO) into the bone, which an Emergency Response team uses for emergency cases when intravenous access is not available.

Needle Gauge and Length

The route, needle length and gauge, angle, site, and volume administered depends on the contents of the injection. On the syringe package, the first number indicates the **gauge** and the second number the **length** (e.g., 28-gauge, ½"). Gauge refers to the size of the borehole in the cannula (needle). The higher the gauge number, the thinner the needle and the smaller the borehole. Therefore, a 28-gauge cannula is thinner than a 25-gauge cannula. Thinner needles should be used for children and frequent injections.

Z-Track Method of Medication Administration

The Z-track method of medication administration is used to administer deep IM injections of substances that are irritating to the subcutaneous tissue. The procedure is as follows:

1. Draw up medication into syringe and then change the needle so no drug residue adheres to the needle.
2. Use a circular method with an alcohol wipe to cleanse the tissue of the dorsogluteal injection site.
3. Holding the syringe vertically with needle upward, draw 0.2-0.5 mL of air into the syringe.
4. With the fingers, pull the skin of the injection site 2-3 inches to the left and hold in place.
5. Rapidly insert the needle at a 90-degree angle to the skin and up to the hub (to ensure the aspirated air clears the needle), aspirate slightly, and (if no blood appears) inject slowly to prevent tissue damage. (If blood appears, remove needle.)
6. Rapidly remove needle and release the tissue so that it moves back into place and seals the drug into place.
7. Apply pressure to site with alcohol wipe but do not massage tissue.

Options of Medication Availability

Medication availability comes in the various options. Aseptic technique should be utilized when drawing up and administering medication regardless of its availability.

- **Single dose vials (SDV)**: Provides a single dose of a medication and is used only once within one hour after removal. Any remaining medication is discarded, as using leftover medication has proven to cause infection in patients.
- **Multiple-dose vials (MDV)**: Provide multiple doses but should be used for only one patient. Expires according to manufacturer's date or 28 days after first use. These vials are identified as multiple-use with an FDA label and contain preservatives to prevent the possibility of bacteria growth.
- **Ampules**: Glass ampules contains 1-10 mL of a single dose of medication. A gauze pad should be wrapped about the neck before breaking open. The medication is aspirated into a syringe using a special filter needle in case of glass residue. The needle must be replaced with a regular needle before injecting the medication.
- **Pre-filled cartridge-needle units**: Some cartridge-needle units are placed in special injection devices, for injection and contain a single dose of medication. Other prefilled cartridge-needle units are complete and do not require an injection device. Multi-dose cartridges (such as for insulin) require that a new needle be attached for each use.

Hazard Prevention with Parenteral Medications

Hazard prevention with parenteral medications includes preparing medications in a designated clean area; using appropriate and aseptic techniques when accessing drugs, such as in vials, ampules, and cartridges; and following the manufacturer's guidelines regarding safety. When withdrawing medications from a vial, only sterile needles should be utilized. Medications should not be prepared near a source of running water because the danger of water droplets contaminating the medication. Medications should be prepared immediately before use. Directions must be carefully followed when reconstituting powdered medications or diluting liquid medications to ensure that the appropriate dosage is prepared. Once a medication is reconstituted, the dosage must be carefully calculated to avoid overdose or underdose. The mode of administration (IM, SQ, ID, IV) should be verified to ensure adequate absorption and avoid tissue damage and the correct syringe, needle, and angle of injection utilized.

Completing Prescriptions and Authorization of Medical Refills

Requests for **prescriptions and refills** are often per telephone. In some cases, the physician may need to handle prescriptions and refills personally, but if these tasks are delegated to the medical assistant, the medical assistant should follow established protocol and should determine the identity of the caller (using their name, birthdate, or other identifier) and the telephone number. If the pharmacy is calling, the medical assistant may take a message that includes the name of the patient and the medication, and advise when the physician will respond or ask the pharmacy representative to hold while the patient's record is checked. If a patient/caregiver is calling, the medical assistant should ask the name of the medication and the pharmacy, and then check the patient's record. If the physician authorizes prescriptions/refills, the medical assistant should provide the record to the physician to review. If the medical assistant has been delegated to order refills, the medical assistant should check the original order to make sure that the physician has authorized refills.

Calculating Drug Dosage

The medical assistant must weigh the patient accurately because the drug dosages are calculated by milligrams of medication per kilogram of patient's body weight. For example, if the drug reference manual states the general dosage is 20 mg/kg and the child patient weighs 25 kg (55 lb), then the patient receives 500 mg.

However, in pediatric medicine, some drugs have a maximum dosage that must not be exceeded within 24 hours, regardless of the patient's weight. Divide the maximum dosage by the general dosage to find out if a child gets an adult dose. For example, the maximum dose is 600 mg and the general dosage is 20 mg/kg. The child who weighs 31 kg (68 lb) gets an adult dose but the child who weighs 25 kg (55 lb) gets a pediatric dose.

Sometimes the doctor's prescription is different from the available dosage. For example, the pharmacist has 250 mg capsules of ampicillin in stock but the doctor's prescription calls for a dose of 500 mg. Divide the required dose by the available dose. This patient gets two 250 mg capsules to equal 500 mg.

Storage

Storing Drugs

Correct storage maintains a drug's efficacy and safety. Store most drugs at room temperature (22-25 °C). Protect drugs from insects, dust, light, and humidity. Patients and visitors should not be able to see the automated dispensing cabinet or drug cupboard. Keep all drugs out of the reach of children, known drug addicts, and patients who may be suicidal. Some biologicals, especially ointments, hormones, and vaccines, require refrigeration.

Improper storage causes the drug to degrade before its expiration date. Most drugs last 2-5 years from their date of manufacture, provided they are kept in ideal conditions. However, some specialty preparations, such as eye drops, may only last a few hours, days, or weeks.

Controlled drugs are supervised by the Drug Enforcement Administration (DEA) and include human anesthetics, analgesics, sedatives, and drugs used to euthanize animals. Controlled drugs must be double locked in a wall cabinet and the key must not be kept nearby. Record use in a log. When the drug expires or the bottle is empty, return the log and bottle to Pharmacy.

Storing Vaccines

Vaccinations have various storage recommendations due to the delicate nature of their contents:

- **Flu, DTaP, Hib, HepB, PCV7, PPV23, and EIPV**: Protect vaccines from light. Never store a vaccine on the refrigerator door. Always keep open vials of vaccine on a tray in the main refrigerator compartment. Keep a liquid or mercury thermometer on the same shelf as the vaccine tray. Check and record the thermometer reading twice per day, when the shift starts and before leaving, and record it in a log. The refrigerator *should* be at 5 °C (41 °F), but *must* be 2-8 °C (36-46 °F).
- **Varicella and MMR** must be frozen, ideally at -18 °C (0 °F), but the freezer must be -15 °C (5 °F) or colder.
- Use a plug guard on the refrigerator and post a sign on it that reads "Biologicals" with a biohazard sign.
- NEVER store food or specimens in the same refrigerator as vaccines.
- Rotate stock weekly, so the oldest vaccine is used first. A vaccine marked only with month and year is viable until the last day of the month. Never use an expired vaccine.
- Never pre-draw a vaccine or leave it out of the refrigerator between uses.
- During transport, keep refrigerated vaccines in an insulated container on a cold gel pack and use dry ice for frozen vaccines.
- Report all accidents to the safety officer, and do not use compromised vaccines.
- If an unusual vaccine is encountered, read the product insert, refer to *The Red Book* if the insert is missing, or phone the manufacturer.

Immunizations

Immunization vs. Vaccination

Immunization refers to the body's buildup of defenses (antibodies) against specific diseases. It has an important role in preventing the spread of infection. Immunization prevents the individual from contracting a disease or lessens the severity of the disease, and can also prevent the complications (encephalitis, hearing loss, paralysis) associated with the infectious diseases. **Vaccination** is one method of creating immunity through the introduction of a small amount of the virus's or bacteria's antigen to the body, which then stimulates the body's creation of antibodies against that disease. Vaccination prevents the spread of infection to infants who are too young to have developed immunity and to those who are immunocompromised (cancer patients, transplantation recipients). Herd immunity results from a majority of the population being immune to a disease, therefore minimizing transmission. It is defined in terms of the percentage of the population that must be immunized in order to prevent outbreaks. This percentage may range from 80-85% for some disorders, but those that are highly contagious, such as measles, may require a herd immunity of 93-95%. Herd immunity can be obtained via widespread vaccination or widespread infection, though it is not recommended that individuals avoid immunization and rely on herd immunity for protection, as rates of immunization vary from one community to another.

Types of Vaccines

There are a number of different types of vaccines:

- **Conjugated forms**: An organism is altered and then joined (conjugated) with another substance, such as a protein, to potentiate immune response (such as conjugated Hib).
- **Killed virus vaccines**: The virus has been killed but can still cause an immune response (such as inactivated poliovirus).
- **Live virus vaccines**: The virus is live but in a weakened (attenuated) form so that it doesn't cause the disease but confers immunity (such as measles vaccine).
- **Recombinant forms**: The organism is genetically altered and, for example, may use proteins rather than the whole cell to stimulate immunity (such as Hepatitis B and acellular pertussis vaccine).
- **Toxoid**: A toxin (antigen) that has been weakened by the use of heat or chemicals so it is too weak to cause disease but stimulates antibodies.

Some vaccines are given shortly after birth; others begin at 2 months, 12 months, or 2 years and some later in childhood.

DTaP and Tdap Vaccines

Diphtheria and pertussis (whooping cough) are highly contagious bacterial diseases of the upper respiratory tract. Cases of diphtheria are now rare in the United States, although they still occur in some developing countries. There have, however, been recent outbreaks of pertussis in the United States. Tetanus is a bacterial infection contracted through cuts, wounds, and scratches. The **diphtheria, tetanus, and pertussis (DTaP) vaccine** is recommended for all children. DTaP is a newer and safer version of the older DTP vaccine, which is no longer used in the United States. **Tdap** is the DTaP booster shot meant to continue immunity to these diseases through adulthood, given every 10 years starting at age 11.

DTaP requires 5 doses:

- 2 months
- 4 months
- 6 months
- 5-18 months
- 4-6 years (or at 11-12 years if booster missed between 4-6)

According to recent ACIP recommendations, DTaP may now also be administered to children ages 7-9 as part of a catch-up series, but children will then require their routine Tdap dose at age 11-12. If DTaP is administered to children ages 10-18 it can be counted as their adolescent Tdap booster. Adverse reactions can occur, but they are usually mild soreness, fever, and/or nausea. About 1 in 100 children will have high fever (>105 °F) and may develop seizures. Severe allergic responses can occur.

HPV Vaccine

Human papillomavirus (HPV) comprises >100 viruses. About 40 are sexually transmitted and invade mucosal tissue, causing genital warts, which are low risk for cancer, or changes in the mucosa, which can lead to cervical cancer. Most HPVs cause little or no symptoms, but they are very common, especially in those 15-25. Over 99% of cervical cancers are caused by HPV and 70% are related to HPVs 16 and 18. The HPV vaccine, Gardasil, protects against HPVs 6 and 11 (which cause genital warts), along with 16 and 18, which can cause cancer. Protection is only conveyed if the female has not yet been infected with these strains. The vaccine is currently recommended for females under 26 but studies have determined that those not adequately covered over the age of 26 and up to 45 can benefit. A series of 3 injections is required over a 6-month period:

- Initial dose 11-12 years (but may be given as young as 9 or ≥18)
- 2 months after first dose
- 6 months after first dose

PPV

Pneumococcal polysaccharide-23 vaccine (PPV) (Pneumovax and Pnu-Immune) is a vaccine that has been available since 1977 to protect against 23 types of pneumococcal bacteria. It is given to adults ≥65 and children ≥2 years in high-risk groups that include:

- Children with chronic heart, lung, sickle cell disease, diabetes, cirrhosis, alcoholism, and leaks of cerebrospinal fluid
- Children with lowered immunity from Hodgkin's disease, lymphoma, leukemia, kidney failure, multiple myeloma, nephrotic syndrome, HIV/AIDS, damaged or missing spleen, and organ transplant

Children ≤2 may not respond to this vaccine and should take PCV-7. Administration is as follows:

- One dose is usually all that is required although a second dose may be advised for children with some conditions, such as cancer or organ/bone marrow transplantations.
- If needed, a second dose is given 3 years after the first for children ≤10 and 5 years after the first for those ≥10.

Hepatitis A Vaccine

Hepatitis A is a contagious virus that causes liver disease and can cause serious morbidity and death. It is spread through the feces of a person who is infected and often causes contamination of food and water. The **Hep A vaccine** is now recommended for all children at one year of age. It is not licensed for use in younger infants. Two doses are needed:

- 12 months (12-23 months)
- 18 months (or 6 months after previous dose)

Older children and teenagers may receive the two-injection series if they are considered at risk, depending upon lifestyle, such as young males having sex with other males or those using illegal drugs. It is also recommended if outbreaks occur. Adverse reactions are mild and include soreness, headache, anorexia, and malaise although severe allergic reactions can occur as with all vaccines.

Hepatitis B Vaccine

Hepatitis B is transmitted through blood and body fluids, including during birth; therefore, it is now recommended for all newborns as well as all those <18 and those in high-risk groups >18. Hepatitis B can cause serious liver disease leading to liver cancer. Three injections of **monovalent HepB** are required to confer immunity:

- Birth (within 12 hours)
- At 1-2 months
- ≥24 weeks

Note: If combination vaccines are given after the birth dose, then a dose at 4 months can be given.

If the mother is Hepatitis B positive, the child should be given both the monovalent HepB vaccination as well as HepB immune globulin within 12 hours of birth. Adolescents (11-15) who have not been vaccinated require 2 doses, 4-6 months apart. Adverse reactions include local irritation and fever. Severe allergic reactions can occur to those allergic to baker's yeast.

Rotavirus Vaccine

Rotavirus is a cause of significant morbidity and mortality in children, especially in developing countries. Most children, without vaccination, will suffer from severe diarrhea caused by rotavirus within the first 5 years of life. The new **rotavirus vaccine** is advised for all infants but should not be initiated after 12 weeks or administered after 32 weeks, so there is a narrow window of opportunity. Three doses are required:

- 2 months (between 6 and 12 weeks)
- 4 months
- 6 months

An earlier vaccine was withdrawn from the market because it was associated with an increase in intussusception, a disorder in which part of the intestine telescopes inside another. Rates of intussusception in those receiving the current (RotaTeq) vaccine have been investigated and incidence of intussusception was within the range of normal occurrences with no evidence linking the occurrences to the vaccine.

Inactivated Poliovirus Vaccine

Poliomyelitis is a serious viral infection that can cause paralysis and death. Prior to introduction of a vaccine in 1955, there were >20,000 cases of polio in the United States each year. There have been no cases of polio caused by the poliovirus for >20 years in the United States, but it still occurs in some third world countries, so continuing vaccinations is very important. Oral polio vaccine (OPV) is no longer recommended in the United States because it carries a very slight risk of causing the disease (1:2.4 million). Children require 4 doses of injectable polio vaccine (IPV):

- 2 months
- 4 months
- 6-18 months
- 4-6 years (booster dose)

IPV is contraindicated for those who have had a severe reaction to neomycin, streptomycin, or polymyxin B. Rare allergic reactions can occur, but there are almost no serious problems caused by this vaccine.

Varicella Vaccine

Varicella (chickenpox) is a common infectious childhood disease caused by the varicella zoster virus, resulting in fever, rash, and itching, and it can also cause skin infections, pneumonia, and neurological damage. After infection, the virus retreats to the nerves by the spinal cord and can reactivate years later, causing herpes zoster (shingles), a significant cause of morbidity in adults. Infection with varicella conveys immunity, but because of associated problems, it is recommended that all children receive varicella vaccine. Two doses are needed:

- 12-15 months
- 4-6 years (or at least 3 months after first dose)

Children ≥13 years and adults who have never had chickenpox or previously received the vaccine should receive 2 doses at least 28 days apart. Children should not receive the vaccine if they have had a serious allergic reaction to gelatin or neomycin. Most reactions are mild and include soreness, fever, and rash. About 1:1000 may experience febrile seizures. Pneumonia is a very rare reaction.

MMR Vaccine

Measles is a viral disease characterized by fever and rash but can cause pneumonia, seizures, severe neurological damage, and death. Mumps is a viral disease that causes fever and swollen glands but can cause deafness, meningitis, and swelling of the testicles. Rubella, also known as German measles) is also a viral disease that can cause rash, fever, and arthritis, but the biggest danger is that it can cause a woman who is pregnant to miscarry or deliver a child with serious birth defects. The **measles, mumps, and rubella (MMR) vaccine** is given in 2 doses:

- 12-15 months
- 4-6 years

Children can get the injections at any age if they have missed them, but there must be at least 28 days between injections. Children with severe allergic reactions to gelatin or neomycin should not get the injection. Severe adverse reactions are rare, but fever and mild rash are common. Teenagers may have pain and stiffness in joints. Occasional seizures (1:3000) and thrombocytopenia (1:30,000) occur.

PCV-7

Heptavalent pneumococcal conjugate vaccine (PCV-7) (Prevnar) was released for use in the United States in 2001 for treatment of children under 2 years old. It provides immunity to 7 serotypes of *Streptococcus pneumoniae* to protect against invasive pneumococcal disease, such as pneumonia, otitis media, bacteremia, and meningitis. Because children are most at risk ≤1, vaccinations begin early:

Administration is in 4 doses:

- 6-8 weeks
- 4 months
- 6 months
- 12-18 months

Although less effective for older children, PCV-7 has been approved for children between 2 and 5 years of age who are at high risk because of the following conditions:

- Chronic diseases: sickle cell disease, heart disease, lung disease, liver disease
- Damaged or missing spleen
- Immunosuppressive disorders: diabetes, cancer
- Drug therapy: chemotherapy, steroids

PCV-7 may also be considered for all children ≤ 5, especially those ≤3 and in group day care and in some ethnic groups (Native American, Alaska Natives, and African Americans).

Meningococcal Vaccine

Meningitis is severe bacterial meningitis that can result in severe neurological compromise or death. A number of different serotypes of *meningococci* can cause meningitis and current vaccines protect against 4 types although not against subtype B, which causes about 65% of meningitis cases in children. However, the vaccines provide 85-100% protection against sub-types A, C, Y, and W-135. There are 2 types of vaccine:

- **Meningococcal polysaccharide vaccine (MPSV4)** is made from the outer capsule of the bacteria and is used for children 2-10.
    - One dose is given at 2 years, although those at high risk may receive 2 doses, 3 months apart.
    - Under special circumstances, children 3-24 months may receive 2 doses, 3 months apart.
- **Meningococcal conjugate vaccine (MCV4)** is used for children ≥11 (who have not received MPSV4). One dose is required:
    - Ages 11-12, all children should receive the vaccine.
    - If not previously vaccinated, high school and college freshmen should be vaccinated.
- Side effects are usually only local tenderness.

Hib Vaccine

***Haemophilus influenzae* type b (Hib) vaccine** (HibTITER and PedvaxHIB) protects against infection with *Haemophilus influenzae,* which can cause serious respiratory infections, pneumonia, meningitis, bacteremia, and pericarditis in children ≤5 years old. *Administration* is as follows:

- 2 months
- 4 months
- 6 months (may be required, depending upon the brand of vaccine)
- 12-15 months (this booster dose must be given at least 2 months after the earlier doses for those who start at a later age than 2 months)

Children over age 6 usually do not require Hib, but it is recommended for older children and adults. Here are some conditions that place them at risk:

- Sickle cell disease
- HIV/AIDS
- Bone marrow transplant
- Chemotherapy for cancer
- Damaged or missing spleen

Some chemotherapy drugs, corticosteroids, and other immunosuppressive drugs may interact with the vaccine.

Infant Immunization Schedule Summary

The recommended schedule for immunizations for the infant is summarized below:

- All newborns receive **ophthalmic drops or ointment**, to prevent blindness from possible gonorrhea infection, and an injection of vitamin K to prevent hemorrhagic disease.
- Before discharge, newborns are tested for **phenylketonuria** and **hypothyroidism**, and will possibly have their **hematocrit** and **hemoglobin** checked.
- **Hepatitis B vaccine** is given at birth, 1-2 months, and 6-18 months.
- **Diphtheria/tetanus/pertussis vaccine** is administered at 2 months, 4 months, 6 months, and 15-18 months.
- **Hib (Haemophilus influenza type b) vaccine** is given at 2 months, 4 months, and 12 months or later.
- **Poliovirus vaccine** is given at 2 months, 4 months, and 6-18 months.
- **MMR vaccine** is given at 12-18 months.
- **Varicella (chickenpox) vaccine** can be given at 12 months.

Required Immunization History for Children up to 6 Years of Age

According to the Centers for Disease Control and Prevention, by 6 years of age, children in the United States should receive a three-part series of hepatitis B, three doses of rotavirus prevention; four injections protecting against diphtheria, tetanus, and pertussis; four doses of *Haemophilus influenzae* type b; four doses of pneumococcal vaccine; four doses of polio vaccine; two injections that protect against measles, mumps, and rubella; two varicella vaccinations; one hepatitis A vaccination; and a yearly influenza prevention injection.

Vaccination of Children with Uncertain Immunization Histories

Children who have uncertain immunization histories may need vaccinations to meet guidelines. The number of vaccinations needed depends on the child's history. For children who are not up-to-date on immunizations, the necessary injections must be determined. These vaccinations can then be given on a schedule so that the child can catch up. For children with no immunization history or uncertain status, such as refugees or internationally adopted children, restarting the immunization series may be necessary to ensure adequate coverage with all vaccines, particularly measles, mumps, and rubella; varicella; hepatitis B; *Haemophilus influenzae* type b; and polio.

Possible Side Effects

Immunization reactions can be minimized and the child made more comfortable by giving acetaminophen prior to the immunizations. Common reactions to immunizations include irritability, decrease in appetite, fever less than 102 °F, and swelling, redness and tenderness at injection site. These may last for the first 1-2 days and can be treated with acetaminophen every 4-6 hours for the first day. If more severe reactions occur, such as fever greater than 102 °F, severe prolonged irritability, or high-pitched crying, or the symptoms last more than 2 days, the parents should call the healthcare provider immediately.

Important Considerations When Giving Immunizations

Every time a child comes into contact with the healthcare system, his **immunization status** should be assessed. Children are required, by all states, to be immunized before entering a licensed school or day care. Specific requirements will vary from state to state. Vaccines must be handled and stored according the manufacturers guidelines. Immunizations must be documented according to specific guidelines and parents must sign a consent form every time a vaccine is administered. Common illnesses such as colds, ear infections and diarrhea will not usually preclude giving vaccines. The MMR and varicella vaccines should not be given during pregnancy. There are two situations in which immunizations are contraindicated: a previous severe allergic reaction to a vaccine or one of its components and encephalopathy occurring within 7 days of giving a DTP or DTaP vaccine.

The Anti-Vaccination Movement

While **opposition to vaccination** is not a new concept, it is a movement that has gained momentum with the power of information sharing via social media. Opposers to vaccination, often referred to as "Anti-Vaxxers," believe that vaccinations can cause complications such as autism and SIDS, especially when administered in infancy and early childhood, and believe that these risks far outweigh the benefits. There are also those who oppose such medical interventions due to religious beliefs.

While the therapeutic effects of vaccinations have been supported by evidence for both individuals and communities, it is important that healthcare professionals be equipped to respectfully inform and care for those that oppose vaccinations. Individuals should be educated regarding the evidence supporting vaccinations and the vaccinations required by law. The CDC offers a wealth of resources for healthcare workers and for individuals regarding vaccinations. The most notable resource is the CDC's Vaccine Information Statement, a living document that outlines the benefits and risks of vaccines, that healthcare workers can use to inform individuals and parents. If, despite efforts to educate, the individual or caregiver still refuses vaccination, there are ICD codes that providers are required to use to document this refusal (for example, ICD-10-CM: Z28.82: Immunization not carried out because of caregiver refusal). The healthcare worker must also document that preventive medical counseling was provided.

Vaccinations Programs

Vaccination programs seek to promote health by preventing large-scale outbreaks of preventable disease. Public health has the responsibility of weighing the benefits and risks of a vaccine before recommending widespread vaccination for any given disease. Vaccines consist of an **antigen** in solution designed to stimulate the immune system of an individual to produce **antibodies** against the antigen to prevent disease from future exposure. The antigen may be alive or dead. The CDC periodically updates recommendations for all ages and has information concerning each vaccine's composition, contraindications, dosage, administration, and storage. Vaccines are recommended for adults who travel, have occupational risks of exposure, have chronic disease, or are immunocompromised. Some individuals may not receive certain vaccines due to allergies or the presence of certain diseases. Vaccines that are currently recommended for adults include tetanus, diphtheria, pneumococcal, Hepatitis A and B, measles, mumps, rubella, varicella, influenza, and meningococcal.

Chapter Quiz

Ready to see how well you retained what you just read? Scan the QR code to go directly to the chapter quiz interface for this study guide. If you're using a computer, simply visit the bonus page at **mometrix.com/bonus948/certmedasst** and click the Chapter Quizzes link.

General

Transform passive reading into active learning! After immersing yourself in this chapter, put your comprehension to the test by taking a quiz. The insights you gained will stay with you longer this way. Scan the QR code to go directly to the chapter quiz interface for this study guide. If you're using a computer, simply visit the bonus page at **mometrix.com/bonus948/certmedasst** and click the Chapter Quizzes link.

Medical Laws/Regulatory Guidelines and Medical Ethics

OSHA AND THE FDA

The US Department of Labor's **Occupational Safety and Health Administration (OSHA)** sets standards for:

- Proper hand washing
- Wearing gloves and other personal protective equipment (PPE)
- Bagging specimens in biohazard bags
- Disposing of needles and lancets in a sharps container
- Cleaning up spills to prevent spread of bloodborne pathogens
- Harmful chemical control
- Safe equipment use
- Adequate work space

Check for updates regularly at OSHA's website at http://www.osha.gov. These updates are required to be adopted as part of the facility's standards of practice.

The US **Food & Drug Administration (FDA)**:

- Assigns the official (generic) name for drugs when it approves them
- Reports recalls and adverse events through *MedWatch*
- Publishes a free, downloadable *Orange Book* of approved drugs
- Divides drugs into five schedules, based on their potential for abuse, numbered Schedule I (generally illegal) to Schedule V (generally benign)
- Sets the temperature regulations for dish sanitization

HIPAA

HIPAA stands for **Health Insurance Portability and Accountability Act** of 1996. HIPAA's Title I regulates healthcare accessibility, especially in the cases of job change and loss; Title II regulates patient privacy rights. HIPAA requires the following:

- Every patient's medical record must bear a unique identifier to prevent misidentification
- Patients must be given access to their protected health information (medical records) at any time, upon request
- Only relevant health information can be disclosed to authorized parties
- A record must be kept of every disclosure
- Every patient or the parents/guardian must receive a *Notice of Privacy Practices*, outlining how the protected health information will be used

- Physical access to protected health information must be limited (including electronic files via password protection or swipe cards, firewall, and SSL encryption)
- Retired electronic equipment must have all data records wiped clean

Review Video: What is HIPAA?
Visit mometrix.com/academy and enter code: 412009

ADA

Americans with Disabilities Act (ADA) of 1990 provides the following protections for individuals with disabilities:

- Prevention of discrimination in employment
- Access to public services, accommodations, and goods
- Sophisticated telecommunication services to facilitate the hearing and speech impaired
- Requires medical offices to have ramps, entryways, and at least one treatment room that provides access and accommodates the needs of the disabled
- Applies to facilities with more than 15 employees, but all medical offices should strive to comply with ADA

DEA

DEA stands for **Drug Enforcement Agency**. Medical offices are targeted by drug addicts for syringes and narcotics, so the assistant may need to contact the DEA and local police. Medical assistants must be familiar with government sites that list drugs, so they can stay up-to-date with the industry, and spell and classify drugs correctly.

- US Drug Enforcement Agency Drug Scheduling: https://www.dea.gov/drug-scheduling
- FDA Electronic Orange Book: http://www.fda.gov/cder/ob/default.htm
- FDA National Drug Code Directory: https://www.fda.gov/drugs/drug-approvals-and-databases/national-drug-code-directory
- US National Library of Medicine (Medline): http://www.nlm.nih.gov/medlineplus/druginformation.html
- US Pharmacopeia: http://www.usp.org/aboutUSP/

HITECH Act

The American Recovery and Reinvestment Act (2009) (ARRA) included the **Health Information Technology for Economic and Clinical Health Act (HITECH),** which provided incentives for healthcare providers to switch to electronic health records and allowed patients greater access to their electronic health records. Security provisions include:

- Individuals and HHS must be notified of breach in security of personal health information.
- Business partners must meet security regulations or face penalties.
- The sale/marketing of personal health information is restricted.
- Individuals must have electronic access to electronic health information, although the law doesn't specify the form that the disclosed information must take (email, CD, web portal). Copies must be in a format that is readable if the individual requests it, and the healthcare provider may charge a fee.
- Individuals must be informed of disclosures of personal health information.
- Individual can direct healthcare providers to transmit a copy of their health records to individuals or entities of their choosing.

Public Health Statutes Related to Public Health and Welfare Disclosure

Public health statutes related to public health and welfare disclosure include:

- **Communicable diseases**: Title 42 (The Public Health and Welfare) and each state's regulations control reporting requirements for communicable diseases and for quarantine. Diseases that must be reported to the CDC include cholera, giardiasis, hepatitis, salmonellosis, shigellosis, cryptosporidiosis, and COVID-19. State requirements vary, but generally include influenza and measles.
- **Vital statistics**: Each state has a department of vital statistics that compiles birth and death records.
- **Abuse/neglect against children or older adults**: All states have laws regarding abuse/neglect, and all healthcare providers are mandatory reporters. Reporting agencies may differ from one state to another.
- **Wounds of violence**: All states have laws regarding which types of wounds of violence (usually knife and gunshot wounds) must be reported to the police.

Subpoena Duces Tecum

Subpoena duces tecum literally means "bring [it] with you under penalty of punishment." It is a court order for a witness to produce documents. The judge must carefully consider if *subpoena duces tecum* transgresses the patient's HIPAA rights.

The physician and other health professionals must report to authorities:

- Gunshot wounds
- Possible terrorist incidents, especially if they involve the spread of disease
- Known or suspected abuse of a child, senior, or disabled person
- Sexual assault of a juvenile or disabled person
- Poisoning
- Wounds intentionally caused by knives and sharp objects
- Criminal violence, including domestic violence
- Client-specific information for the central cancer registry
- Specific contagious diseases determined by each state

The medical assistant must keep a written record of the patient's information that was disclosed to authorities.

Good Samaritan Act

There are two kinds of Good Samaritan Acts:

- A first aider who provides unpaid assistance to the injured in an emergency and acts as "a reasonable man" up to his or her level of training is protected by state law from unfair prosecution for death, disability, or disfigurement. A judge would dismiss assault and battery charges.
- A living donor who offers a non-directed donation of an organ to the transplant center is a Good Samaritan. The following organs can be donated by a living donor: kidneys, liver lobes, lung lobes, pancreas segments, and small bowel segments. Non-direct donors do not have anyone particular in mind whom they would like to receive their donated organ. The donation is usually anonymous and the Good Samaritan is blameless for complications the recipient suffers.

Anatomical Gift

The ***Uniform Anatomical Gift Act*** of 1968 facilitates organ transplantation under one standard, which is important when organs are transported across state lines. The Act was revised in 1987 and 2006 to cover transplants from cadavers and fetuses only through the national Organ Procurement and Transplantation Network (OPTN). Organ donations from living donors have many ethical and legal pitfalls, and are addressed in separate laws by each state.

American Association of Medical Assistants

The professional organization that certifies medical assistants is the **American Association of Medical Assistants.** Candidates must complete an accredited medical assistant training program and write an exam. Topics covered include anatomy, physiology, terminology, law, medical records, finance, diagnostics, medication, nutrition, and communication. The test consultant for the medical assistant national certification exam is the National Board of Medical Examiners, which examines physicians. Therefore, employers consider the certification results reliable and valid.

Advance Directive, Code Blue, and DNR Order

An **advance directive** is a legal document in which the patient communicates to his or her family and physician what kind of medical intervention he or she desires. A **living will** is a type of advance directive that terminally ill patients often make. Specific laws regarding advance directives vary by state, but the patient must always be competent.

A **"do not resuscitate" order** is a type of advance directive. A DNR order must be written in the patient's chart by the attending physician in order to be valid. All discussions with the patient and the family should be clearly documented in the chart. In the absence of a written DNR order, call a full Code Blue and proceed with resuscitation.

Code blue is a distress call that indicates a patient is in cardiac arrest. Call the resuscitation team immediately. Some patient rooms have code blue buttons that can be pushed to activate the code blue. Additional codes exist for respiratory distress, patient/family violence, elopement, or the abduction of a newborn or child.

Informed Consent

Informed consent protects patients by ensuring that they or those legally responsible for them are fully educated about tests, treatments, and procedures. The patient has the legal right to know about his or her own condition. The exceptions are life-threatening emergencies and legal incompetence. Informed consent protects healthcare professionals from battery lawsuits. Informed consent is obtained when the patient is given written information in regards to the treatment plan, risks, benefits, and alternative treatment options, the provider truthfully answers any questions, and the patient/parent/guardian comprehends the discussion. The patient or legal guardian then voluntarily signs the consent form, without duress or coercion. The medical assistant must obtain signed consent from the patient/guardian before treatment commences. Moreover, it is advisable to obtain the minor patient's assent prior to the procedure. Always keep the original informed consent form in the patient's chart. Assent should also be recorded in the medical record.

Medical Jurisprudence, Civil Laws, and Criminal Laws

Jurisprudence is the legal system set up and enforced at various governmental levels. Civil and criminal laws that pertain to medical situations are referred to as **medical jurisprudence.** Medical jurisprudence also involves applying the science of medicine to legal issues such as forensics or paternity testing.

Civil laws are more often invoked in the medical setting, as they pertain to either contracts or torts.

- A **contract** is an enforceable covenant between two or more competent individuals. An agreement between a doctor and his or her patient is a contract. It can be an expressed contract, with written or verbal terms, or it can be an implied contract, where actions create the contract.
- **Tort law** governs the other branch of civil law. Torts relate to standards of care and wrongful actions that cause injury to a patient.

Criminal laws speak to crimes that endanger society in general. There are occasions when criminal law may apply to medicine, usually resulting in fines, incarceration, and discipline by the state medical board.

Contract Law

There is an expressed or an implied contract between the doctor and patient. The medical assistant and other personnel are the doctor's agents. The doctor is ultimately responsible for breach of contract under the *Doctrine of Respondeat Superior. Respondeat Superior* is Latin for "let the master answer." The *Doctrine of Respondeat Superior* means if a medical assistant is involved in a legal action resulting from work, then the doctor is ultimately responsible for the medical assistant's actions or losses incurred. However, the medical assistant employee is also held accountable for due diligence.

Breach of contract is failure to fulfill and complete the terms of the contract. There are four situations where a contract can be legally abandoned:

- The patient releases the doctor by failure to return for treatment. Ideally, the patient sends the doctor a certified letter of discharge, but this is not required.
- The patient/guardian does not comply with specific instructions from the doctor regarding care.
- The patient no longer requires treatment.
- The doctor formally withdraws from the case by sending a certified letter to the patient explaining the situation, to preclude any charges of patient abandonment.

Terminating Patient's Care

Regardless of the medical assistant's personal opinion, it is his or her responsibility as a healthcare professional to support and respect the choices made by the patient and family. If the family's choices conflict with the medical assistant's strong personal opinions related to care, then the medical assistant must **terminate care**, after giving adequate written notice to the patient and physician to avoid charges of patient abandonment. The medical assistant is legally required to wait until relieved by another member of the healthcare team who has equal or greater training. Examples of common conflicts that arise are:

- Parents refuse blood transfusions, pain relief, and treatments for minors
- Safety hazards (e.g., a dangerous dog, sexual harassment, or threats)
- Patient will not or cannot pay bills because of insurance problems
- Patient is unruly and obnoxious

Reportable Incidents

A reportable incident is a dangerous event that must be reported to the supervisor or Safety Officer within a specific time frame, usually 24 hours to 5 days. Reportable incidents include:

- Medication errors
- Failure to assess and treat a patient according to state protocols, especially if it results in serious injury or death
- Injuries or death while in care (e.g., attempted suicide)
- Inappropriate use of a device or drug that results in death or injury
- Motor vehicle accident resulting in death or injury
- Suspicion of drug or alcohol abuse by a healthcare provider
- Acts or omissions that threaten public safety or result in poor patient outcome

Important Legal Terms

Important legal terms for the medical assistant to understand include the following:

- **Consent to treatment**: Required for all treatment, unless the patient is unconscious or an unaccompanied minor in an emergency. Patient agrees to receive basic, routine services, diagnostic procedures, and medical care.
- **Consent to release information**: Patient's signature authorizes release of health information between provider and other entities, such as third-party payers. Design of this form should be carefully considered, and may include language translation (verbal and/or written).
- **Subpoena**: A legal writ (order) requiring a person to come to court, to testify in court, and/or to produce documents or evidence. Failure to do so may result in fine or jailing.
- **Res ipsa loquitur ("the thing speaks for itself")**: The principle of law that allows the use of circumstantial evidence as proof.
- **Locum tenens ("to substitute for")**: Allows one medical professional to serve temporarily in place of another. For example, a physician's practice may be covered by another physician usually for a few days up to 6 months when the first goes on vacation or takes leave. Companies specialize in providing *locum* physicians to work on a contract basis.
- **Deposition**: This is a sworn out-of-court witness statement taken under oath, usually in an attorney's office prior to a court case to document what the witness knows and to preserve the statements for use in court.
- **Statute of limitations**: A law defining the maximum period the complainant or appellant can wait before filing a lawsuit. The limitation date varies according to the type of case and if it falls within state or federal jurisdiction. Usually, the limitation is 1-6 years. Homicide has no limitation. If the complainant misses the deadline, then the right to sue is "stats barred" (dead). Rarely, a judge will "toll" (extend) the deadline if the injury was discovered late or a trusted person hid misuse of funds or failure to pay. Minors' rights to bring negligence charges are tolled until the age of 18.
- **Assumption of risk**: (A.) A defense against an accusation of negligence. The defendant states the situation was obviously hazardous, so the complainant should have realized injury could result. (B.) An insurance company takes the risk of extending coverage, realizing the policyholder might make a claim, but it is statistically more likely to make a profit from the premiums.
- **Arbitration agreement**: The patient agrees to give up the right to sue the doctor. An arbiter (arbitrator) awards damages if injury results. Settlement is faster for the patient, and the doctor gets a malpractice insurance discount. Both parties save on legal fees.

- **Negligence**: Taking an unreasonable, careless action that could foreseeably cause harm. Failing to exercise due care for others that a prudent, reasonable person would do. Negligence is accidental. Negligence is not an intentional tort, such as trespass or assault. Business errors, miscalculations, and failure to act can be negligent.
- **Contributory negligence**: If a person is injured partially because of his or her own negligence—even if it is slight—then the person who caused the accident does not pay any damages (money) to the injured person. Forty-four states recognize that applying the rule of contributory negligence could lead to unfair acquittal of genuinely negligent defendants, so they now use a comparative negligence test as a more balanced approach. In the 6 states that still have contributory negligence rules, juries tend to ignore it as unfair.
- **Comparative negligence**: A rule used in accident cases to calculate the percentage of responsibility of each person (joint tortfeasors) directly involved in the accident. Damages (money compensation) are awarded based on a complex formula.

Core Ethical Principles for Medical Assistant Practice

Core ethical principles include:

- **Beneficence**: Performing actions that are for the purpose of benefitting another person. In the care of a patient, any procedure or treatment should be done with the ultimate goal of benefitting the patient.
- **Nonmaleficence**: Providing care in a manner that does not cause direct intentional harm to the patient. Care must be intended only for good effect, and good effects must have more benefit than bad effects that result.
- **Autonomy**: The right of the individual to make decisions about his or her own care. In the case of children, the child cannot make autonomous decisions, so the parents serve as the legal decision maker.
- **Justice**: Relates to the distribution of the limited resources of healthcare benefits to the members of society. Resources must be distributed fairly and decisions made according to what is most just.
- **Privacy/confidentiality**: Protecting information (conversations, assessments) and body (close door, pull curtains, use drapes to avoid exposing patient) and protecting personal information about a patient and the patient's health condition.

Patients' Rights

The Advisory Commission on Consumer Protection and Quality on Health Care Industry, an initiative under President Clinton, outlined eight **rights and responsibilities of American patients** as follows:

- The right to information
- The right to choose
- The right to access emergency services
- The right to fully participate in decisions regarding one's own health care
- The right to care without discrimination
- The right to privacy
- The right to speedy complaint resolution
- The responsibility for maintaining one's health to retain those rights

The American Hospital Association replaced its *Patients' Bill of Rights* in 2008 with a brochure called *The Patient Care Partnership*, which is available in many languages on the AHA website. Information about how HIPAA protects patients' rights can be found on the HHS website.

Therapeutic Communication

Communication Cycle

The communication process, which includes the **sender-receiver feedback loop**, is based on Claude Shannon's information theory (1948) in which he described three necessary steps:

1. Encoding a message
2. Transmitting the message through a channel
3. Decoding the message

The resultant communication process begins with the sender, who serves as the encoder and determines the content of the message. The medium is the form the message takes (digital, written, audiovisual), and the channel is the method of delivery (mail, radio, TV, phone). The recipient (receiver) who acts as the decoder determines the meaning from the message. Feedback helps to determine whether or not the communication is successful and the message understood as intended. This process is referred to as the send-receiver feedback loop. Context is the environment (physical and psychological) in which the communication occurs, and interference is any factor that impacts the communication process. Interference may be external (such as environmental noise) or internal (such as emotional distress or anxiety).

Therapeutic Communication

Communication Techniques in Therapeutic Relationships

The following are appropriate communication techniques to encourage therapeutic relationships:

- **Use active listening**: Paraphrase and repeat back information transmitted by the patient. Ask for clarification when the message is confusing. Summarize what was agreed to at the end of the conversation.
- **Watch for nonverbal cues**: Nonverbal cues are gestures, grimaces, posturing, appearance, and eye movements that comprise 85% of all communication. Nonverbal cues can denote pain, fear, lying, depression, or subterfuge by a caregiver. Gently ask the patient to clarify when verbal and nonverbal cues do not match. Children and psychiatric patients may develop tic disorders (involuntary gestures and movements). If which movements are truly cues and which are tics cannot be deciphered, ask the doctor.
- **Ask open-ended questions**: Encourage the patient to explain their thoughts/feelings/understanding by asking open-ended questions rather than asking questions that require only a yes or no answer (close-ended questions).
- **Consider influences**: Put communication in the context of the patient's developmental age, emotions, values, ethics, health, education, culture, environment, social and familial status, and drug levels.

Non-Therapeutic Communication

The following are non-therapeutic communications techniques that must be avoided:

- **Ask leading questions**: Never shape the patient's answers to questions, or try to change the patient's interpretation of the situation by "putting words into the patient's mouth."
- **Demand an explanation**: Do not ask "why" questions in an accusing tone.
- **Give advice**: The physician advises and the medical assistant supports.
- **Demand an immediate response**: Allow the patient sufficient time for silent reflection before responding.
- **Disinterested body language**: Do not appear distracted or make the patient feel inconsequential with impatient motions, bored posture, or rolling eyes.
- **Minimize the patient's feelings**: Do not compare feelings and experiences.
- **Negatively empower**: Do not help the patient to manipulate another person.
- **Make false promises**: Never promise the patient that the doctor will definitely cure the condition, or make other promises that cannot be kept.
- **Play into stereotypes**: Racist, sexist, and religious prejudice must not influence the treatment of the patient.
- **Deliberately mislead**: Always disclose upcoming treatments, tests, or procedures.

Examples of Non-Therapeutic Communication

Examples of non-therapeutic communication include the following:

- **Making negative judgments**: "You should stop arguing with the nurses."
- **Devaluing patient's feelings**: "Everyone gets upset at times."
- **Disagreeing directly**: "That can't be true," or "I think you are wrong."
- **Defending against criticism**: "The doctor is not being rude; he's just very busy today."
- **Subject-changing** to avoid dealing with uncomfortable topics:
  - Patient: "I'm never going to get well."
  - Medical Assistant: "Your parents will be here in just a few minutes."
- **Making inappropriate literal responses**, even as a joke, especially if the patient is at all confused or having difficulty expressing ideas:
  - Patient: "There are bugs crawling under my skin."
  - Medical Assistant: "I'll get some bug spray."
- **Challenging to establish reality**, which often just increases confusion and frustration: "If you were dying, you wouldn't be able to yell and kick!"

Importance of Nonverbal Communication

Any type of message transmitted between two people that does not involve words is considered **nonverbal communication**. As much as 85% of successful communication depends on nonverbal cues. Remember that the patient is likely apprehensive and English may not be his or her first language. The patient may have difficulty speaking due to injury, drugs, age, deformity, developmental disability, or the instruments used during a procedure. Watch the patient's facial expressions, gestures, posture, and position. Tight posture and/or crossed arms and legs suggest resistance. Conversely, relaxed posture and uncrossed appendages suggest openness. Additionally, one's own posture affects the patient. Sit closely beside the patient, rather than towering directly over him or her in an intimidating manner. Explain what is going to be done. A patient feels more comfortable when he or she is well informed beforehand. Maintain the proper social distancing (territoriality) between oneself and the patient during discussions (about 3 feet apart).

Proper Therapeutic Responses with Certain Populations

Therapeutic responses for specific populations include the following:

- **Pediatric/Adolescent**: Use vocabulary appropriate to age and encourage adolescents to make decisions whenever possible ("Which arm should I use?"). Avoid approaching young children too abruptly and chat with the child and caregiver to ease the child's fear. Explain in advance any actions to be taken, such as temperature or BP, and allow the child to see and hold the equipment when possible.
- **Geriatric**: Treat patients with respect, address them by their names ("Mrs. Jones") and avoid terms like *honey* and *dear*. Be alert for barriers to communication, such as hearing deficits, and encourage patients to ask questions and discuss concerns. Avoid rushing and interrupting and utilize active listening skills.
- **Terminally ill**: Avoid being excessively sympathetic ("You poor thing"), but remain patient and empathetic. Utilize active listening and allow the patient time to express feelings or concerns. Understand that patients may be in pain, weak, frightened, nauseated, and/or depressed and may, for that reason, overreact or underreact.

Serving Multicultural Patients' Needs

Respect and tolerate **multicultural beliefs and values**, even if the patient is nonverbal. Most patients and their families willingly share their beliefs, so do not be embarrassed to ask about their preferences. Ask the supervisor for multicultural sensitivity training. Obtain a guide from The Association of Multicultural Counseling and Development. Keep a list of translators' phone numbers. Speak slowly while facing the patient, and do not address the translator first. Order translations of patient guides and forms. Post pictorial direction signs. Allow multicultural families as much latitude as possible, without causing undue stress for other patients. If there is the possibility that a ritual will be noisy or alarming for other patients, respectfully guide the family to the Quiet Room. Realize some cultures have beliefs about specific food having healing or soothing qualities. Stay alert for symptoms of poisoning from traditional Chinese, Indian, Pacific Islander, and Mexican herbal medicines, which often contain mercury.

Communicating with Disabled Patients and Coworkers

The *Americans with Disabilities Act* of 1990 affects hiring, promotion, pay, and reasonable accommodations. It is enforced at business and service providers with more than 15 workers, on public transit, and with telecommunications.

The US Department of Labor suggests the following techniques when communicating with individuals with disabilities:

- Gain the person's attention before speaking by gently tapping the shoulder or arm.
- State clearly who you are. Speak in a normal tone of voice.
- Wait until one's offer of assistance is accepted. Then listen to or ask for instructions.
- Treat adults as adults. Address people who have disabilities by their first names only when extending the same familiarity to all others.
- Do not lead the person without first asking; allow the person to hold your arm and control her or his own movements.
- Be prepared to repeat what you say, orally or in writing.
- Use positive phrases, such as *person with a developmental disability*, rather than negative phrases, such as *mentally defective*.

Communication Techniques with the Hearing Impaired

Hearing impaired patients may have some hearing and may use hearing aids while deaf patients typically have little or no hearing. Some patients are able to use lip reading to various degrees, so the medical assistant should always face the patient (at 3-6 feet) and speak slowly and clearly, using gestures (not excessively) to augment speech:

- **Hearing impaired**: Assistive devices (hearing aids, writing material) should be available and used during communication. Use a normal tone of voice and speak in short sentences. Minimize environmental noises.
- **Deaf**: If patients are deaf, sign language interpreters should be used for important communication (face the patient, not the interpreter). Assistive devices, such as writing materials, TDD phone/relay service, should be available for use. Always announce presence on entering a room by waving, clapping, tapping the foot (whatever works best for the patient). Ensure alarms have visual feedback (lights). Do not chew, smoke, or eat while speaking to the patient.

Communication Techniques with the Vision Impaired

Visual impairment is unrelated to intelligence or hearing, so the medical assistant should speak with age-appropriate vocabulary in a normal tone of voice, facing the patient so the medical assistant can observe their facial expression. Depending on the degree of visual impairment the patient may not be able to see gestures or materials, so alternate forms of materials (braille handouts or enlarged text) or manipulatives must be considered. The field of vision may be impaired so that the patient sees shapes or has better vision in some areas than others, and the medical assistant should try to position herself or himself for the patient's advantage. The medical assistant should also announce his or her presence, explain actions and movement ("I'm putting your dressing supplies on the counter"), announce position ("I'm at your right side") and always tell the patient if intending to touch the patient ("I'm going to take your blood pressure on your right arm").

Communication with the Intellectually Disabled and Illiterate

Communicating with patients who are **intellectually disabled** can be challenging, and patients may have very different and individual responses, so observation of the patient must serve as a guide. Patients may be apprehensive and frightened, so the medical assistant should maintain a friendly, normal tone of voice and should speak with the patient often to establish rapport, even if the response is not clear. The medical assistant should always ask the patient before touching his or her things. Initiating communication by talking about familiar things (family, pictures, the past) may be comforting for the patient. If responses are unclear or inappropriate, the medical assistant can say, "I'm sorry, I didn't understand that," but should not laugh or indicate frustration.

Communicating with patients who are **illiterate** is not different than with most patients because the patients may be quite intelligent, but the medical assistant should take care to explain procedures and provide oral rather than written instructions.

Communication Techniques When Assessing Understanding

Communication techniques used when assessing patient's understanding include the following:

- **Reflection**: Referring to both the meaning of the patient's words and the emotions. If a patient states, "I understand how to monitor my blood pressure," a reflecting question might be, "You feel confident that you know how to take your blood pressure and when to notify the physician?"
- **Restatement**: Restating or paraphrasing something a patient said, such as, "I've been having dizzy spells for two weeks." Restatement might be, "You've been having dizzy spells for two weeks."
- **Clarification**: Asking for more information. If a patient states, "I haven't been feeling well," a clarifying question might be, "What exactly do you mean when you say you haven't been feeling well?"
- **Feedback**: Responding to something a patient has said or done, letting them know that the message/information was received. For example, "You have kept very accurate records of your blood pressure and pulse."

Modes of Questioning When Collecting Data

The three modes of questioning used when collecting data include:

- **Exploratory**: Exploratory questions are often used as a beginning point when collecting data because it may provide a wide range of information. For example, "Are there any problems in the office that you think should be addressed?" Based on responses, more specific questions may be developed.
- **Open-ended**: Open-ended questions are intended to be answered with whole sentences rather than a simple "yes" or "no," so the response is not limited. Open-ended questions typically start with Wh- or H- words, such as who, which, whom, whose, what, why, when, where, how, how many, how old, and how much: "What do you think about the new equipment?" The data obtained with open-ended questions can be hard to evaluate, but is critical in collecting the full perspective and history of the patient.
- **Closed-ended**: Closed-ended questions are those that require a short or brief answer, often "yes," or "no" and leave no room for discussion: "Do you like the new equipment?" The data obtained can be easily counted, for instance, 20 yes, and 16 no.

Internal and External Distractions That Disrupt Communication Cycle

Distractions (interference) that disrupt the communication cycle include:

- **Internal**: The communicator's or recipient's emotional status, such as increased anxiety or anger, can negatively impact communication. Biases, prejudices, and belief systems may also interfere with a person's ability to attend to the ideas of another person. Pain and hunger can be so distracting that the person is unable to focus on communication. When under stress, the brain may process information differently, interfering with comprehension.
- **External**: Noise in the environment (conversation, traffic, alarms, air conditioning) can make it hard for some people to hear clearly, especially those with hearing impairment, and may make concentration difficult. Additionally, people may find noise very stressful to the point that they have difficulty thinking. Other environmental factors, such as extremes of heat or cold, may cause physical discomfort that interferes with the ability to communicate.

Professional Behavior in Therapeutic Relationships

Maintaining Professional Behavior in Therapeutic Relationships

The patient shares confidential information with the medical assistant, which makes the patient vulnerable. At the beginning of a therapeutic relationship, the medical assistant is responsible for establishing:

- Trust
- Clear, identifiable boundaries
- Mutual expectations
- Confidentiality ground rules

Respond to the patient's needs, but pursue the treatment objectives established by the doctor foremost. Demonstrate acceptance, humor, and compassion to the patient, but keep an appropriate emotional and physical distance. Limit patient contact to assisting with medical procedures, bookings, and casual conversation. It is unprofessional conduct to date or befriend patients, or give them insider information. Remember, the primary purpose of the interaction is to be therapeutic to the patient. Stay alert for:

- Inappropriate emotions imposed on another person (transference and countertransference)
- Conflict of interest (using the relationship for personal gain)

At the end of a therapeutic relationship, arrange a monitoring schedule, so that the patient is not lost to follow-up.

Role as Patient Advocate

A patient advocate speaks on the patient's behalf to obtain services and information, and protect rights. If an institution works on the case management system, it will appoint an advocate for each patient, who is usually an RN or social worker. The medical assistant often spends more time with the patient than the case manager. Therefore, the patient will sometimes feel more comfortable with the medical assistant because of this. Relate the hopes, wishes, fears, and concerns of the patient to the healthcare team. Do not become embroiled in emotional family dynamics by revealing confidences. However, expressing the patient's desires through the healthcare team is an appropriate avenue to ensure the patient's voice is heard.

Interpersonal Skills

The medical assistant must interact with colleagues, patients, families, insurance personnel, and salespeople, among others, so **interpersonal skills** (qualities and behaviors one utilizes when interacting with others) are essential. The medical assistant serves as a liaison among different parties (such as the physician and patient) and must appear friendly, cooperative, and empathetic, being especially sensitive to the needs of patients and family members, who are often anxious. The medical assistant should utilize active listening, paying attention to not only the spoken words, but also nonverbal communication and should ensure that personal nonverbal communication is appropriate. The medical assistant should understand conflict resolution and should avoid passing judgement without understanding all aspects of a problem. The medical assistant should value teamwork and model collaboration, showing respect for the opinions of others and providing positive feedback. The medical assistant should also model a positive attitude toward work, colleagues, and patients/families.

Grief and Loss

Grief

Grief is an emotional response to a **loss** that begins at the time a loss is anticipated and continues on an individual timetable. While there are identifiable stages or tasks, it is not an orderly and predictable process. It involves overcoming anger, disbelief, guilt, and a myriad of related emotions. The grieving individual may move back and forth between stages or experience several emotions at any given time. Each person's grief response is unique to their own coping patterns, stress levels, age, gender, belief system, and previous experiences with loss.

Kubler-Ross's Five Stages of Grief

Kubler-Ross taught the medical community that the dying patient and family welcomes open, honest discussion of the dying process and felt that there were certain **stages** that patients and family go through. The stages may not occur in order, but may vary or some may be skipped. Stages include:

- **Denial**: The person denies the diagnosis and tries to pretend it isn't true. During this time, the person may seek a second opinion or alternative therapies. They may use denial until they are better able to emotionally cope with the reality of the disease or changes that need to be made. Patients may also wish to save family and friends from pain and worry. Both patients and family may use denial as a coping mechanism when they feel overwhelmed by the reality of the disease and threatened losses.
- **Anger**: The person is angry about the situation and may focus that rage on anyone.
- **Bargaining**: The person attempts to make deals with a higher power to secure a better outcome to their situation.
- **Depression**: The person anticipates the loss and the changes it will bring with a sense of sadness and grief.
- **Acceptance**: The person accepts the impending death and is ready to face it as it approaches. The patient may begin to withdraw from interests and family.

Review Video: Patient Treatment and Grief
Visit mometrix.com/academy and enter code: 648794

Anticipatory Grief

Anticipatory grief is the mental, social, and somatic reactions of an individual as they prepare themselves for a **perceived future loss**. The individual experiences a process of intellectual, emotional, and behavioral responses in order to modify their self-concept, based on their perception of what the potential loss will mean in their life. This process often takes place ahead of the actual loss, from the time the loss is first perceived until it is resolved as a reality for the individual. This process can also blend with past loss experiences. It is associated with the individual's perception of how life will be affected by the particular diagnosis as well as the impending death. Acknowledging this anticipatory grief allows family members to begin looking toward a changed future. Suppressing this anticipatory process may inhibit relationships with the ill individual and contribute to a more difficult grieving process at a later time. However, appropriate anticipatory grieving does not take the place of grief during the actual time of death.

Disenfranchised Grief

Disenfranchised grief occurs when the loss being experienced cannot be openly acknowledged, publicly mourned, or socially supported. Society and culture are partly responsible for an individual's response to a loss. There is a **social context** to grief; if a person incurring the loss will be putting himself or herself at risk if grief is expressed, disenfranchised grief occurs. The risk for disenfranchised grief is greatest among those whose relationship with the individual they lost was not known or regarded as significant. This is also the situation found among bereaved persons who are not recognized by society as capable of grief, such as young children, or needing to mourn, such as an ex-spouse or secret lover.

Grief vs. Depression

Normal grief is preoccupied with self-limiting to the loss itself. Emotional responses will vary and may include open expressions of anger. The individual may experience difficulty sleeping or vivid dreams, a lack of energy, and weight loss. Crying is evident and provides some relief of extreme emotions. The individual remains socially responsive and seeks reassurance from others.

Depression is marked by extensive periods of sadness and preoccupation often extending beyond 2 months. It is not limited to the single event. There is an absence of pleasure or anger and isolation from previous social support systems. The individual can experience extreme lethargy, weight loss, insomnia, or hypersomnia, and has no recollection of dreaming. Crying is absent or persistent and provides no relief of emotions. Professional intervention is required to relieve depression.

Loss

Loss is the blanket term used to denote the absence of a valued object, position, ability, attribute, or individual. The aspect of **loss** as it is associated with the death of an animal or person is a relatively new definition. Loss is an individualized and subjective experience depending on the **perceived attachment** between the individual and the missing aspect. This can range from little or no value of attachment to significant value. Loss also can be represented by the **withdrawal of a valued relationship** one had or would have had in the future. Depending on the unique and individual responses to the perception of loss and its significance, reactions to the loss will vary. Robinson and McKenna summarize the aspects of loss in three main attributes:

- Something has been removed.
- The item removed had value to that person.
- The response is individualized.

Mourning

Mourning is a public grief response for the death of a loved one. The various aspects of the mourning process are partially determined by **personal and cultural belief systems**. Kagawa-Singer defines mourning as "the social customs and cultural practices that follow a death." Durkheim expands this to include the following: "mourning is not a natural movement of private feelings wounded by a cruel loss; it is a duty imposed by the group." Mourning involves participation in religious and culturally appropriate customs and rituals designed to publicly acknowledge the loss. These rituals signify they are adjusting to the change in their relationships created by the loss, as well as mark the beginning of the reorganization and forward movement of their lives.

Bereavement

Bereavement is the emotional and mental state associated with having suffered a **personal loss**. It is the reactions of grief and sadness initiated by the loss of a loved one. Bereavement is a normal process of feeling deprived of something of value. The word bereave comes from the root "reave" meaning to plunder, spoil, or rob. It is recognized that the lost individual had value and a defining role in the surviving individual's life. Bereavement encompasses all the acts and emotions surrounding the feeling of loss for the individual. During this grieving period, there is an increased mortality risk. A **positive bereavement experience** means being able to recognize the significance of the loss while still recognizing the resilience and value of life.

Risk Factors Complicating Bereavement

The caregiver should assess for multiple **life crises** that take energy away from the grieving process. An important factor is the grieving individual's history with past grieving experiences. Assess for other recent, unresolved, or difficult losses that may need to be addressed before the individual can move toward resolution of the current loss. Age, mental health, substance abuse, extreme anger, anxiety, or dependence on the individual facing the end of life can add additional stressors and handicap natural coping mechanisms. Income strains, community support, outside and personal responsibilities, the absence of cultural and religious beliefs, the difficulty of the disease process, and age of the loved one lost can also present additional risk factors.

Counseling and Providing Emotional Support Regarding Grief and Loss to Children

The approach to counseling and providing emotional support regarding grief and loss to children is dependent on the age of the child. When available, children and family should be provided information about **peer support groups** (especially adolescents) and **bereavement art therapy groups** as these may be especially helpful. Healthcare professionals should use appropriate words (death, died) instead of euphemisms (passed on) when talking about the deceased and should encourage the child to ask questions. Children are often reluctant to express feelings directly, so it may be beneficial to encourage them to keep a journal about their feelings or draw pictures to express them. Parents should be encouraged to share their feelings of grief with their children rather than trying to hide their emotions and should be aware that children express grief in different ways and may regress or complain of physical ailments (stomach ache, headache) in response to grief. Children should be prepared for changes in routines or living situations, such as a stay-at-home parent having to take a job, which may occur as a result of a death or serious illness.

Signs of a Child Having Issues Managing Grief

Management of **grief** comes in stages for children as well as for adults. Grief may be complicated for a child who does not understand the significance of the situation, such as in the case of a parent's death, or for someone who does not have the necessary support systems in place, as in the case of a child who has a grieving parent who consequently becomes unavailable. **Signs that a child is not coping well with grief** include extended periods of sadness, lack of interest in regular activities, sleep disturbances, loss of appetite, statements of wishing for death or joining a person who has died, difficulties with concentration, problems taking direction at school, poor school performance, and fear of being alone.

Interventions for Patients and Family Experiencing Loss and Grief

Loss is painful and frightening. Loss can occur through death or loss of health, self-esteem, or relationships. Loss can also occur from threats, such as fire, flood, theft, or severe weather. The severity of the loss, preparation for it, and the maturity, stability, and coping mechanisms of the person all affect the grieving process. Multiple losses and substance abuse can complicate grief and recovery. Previous life experience and cultural and religious beliefs can help in resolution of grief. Many emotions are triggered, and if the loss is not acknowledged, the person may become depressed or develop health problems. **Interventions** for those experiencing grief and loss include:

- Teach patients to recognize symptoms, such as SOB, empty feelings in the chest or abdomen, deep sighing, lethargy, and weakness as signs of grief.
- Assist the patient and family to heal themselves by accepting the loss, recognizing the pain from it, making changes to adapt to and assimilate the loss, and moving toward new relationships and activity.
- Refer to groups or counseling for more intense support if needed.

Supporting Families and Patients as They Receive Bad News

It is often best if the patient can **receive bad news** while being **supported** by family, friends, physicians, nurses, support staff, social workers, and clergy if they so desire. However, the patient may not want family members or others to be present, and this too should be respected.

- Provide privacy and ensure that there will be no interruptions.
- Provide seating for all participants.
- Do not provide too much information at once, as the opening statement may be all that the patient can comprehend at one time.
- Allow time for reactions before providing more information.
- Wait for the patient to signal the need for more information and then provide an honest answer in layman's terms. Information may not be absorbed and may need to be repeated as the patient and family are ready for it later after the initial conference.
- Use techniques of therapeutic communication. People may need others to sit and listen and provide comforting empathy many times before having a conversation about problem solving.

Spirituality

Spirituality provides a connection of the self to a higher power and a way of finding meaning in life experiences. It provides guidance for behavior and can help to clarify one's purpose in life. It can offer hope to those who are ill or facing loss and grief and can give comfort, support, and guidance. **Spirituality** is not always connected to a religion and is highly individualized. A person may lose faith and confidence in his/her spiritual beliefs during trying times:

- Ask patients about their spiritual beliefs.
- Listen attentively and do not offer opinions about their beliefs or share your own unless invited.
- Show respect for their views and offer to obtain spiritual support by calling a spiritual leader or setting up a spiritual ritual that has meaning for them.

This support can help them to regain their beliefs and endure illness by helping them to rise above their suffering and find meaning in this experience.

Palliative and Hospice Care

Palliative care attempts to make the rest of the patient's life as comfortable as possible by treating distressing symptoms to keep them controlled. It does not attempt to cure but only to control discomfort caused by the disease. Palliative care does not require terminal illness/prognosis and can be implemented for any patient with chronic disease and suffering.

Hospice care uses palliative care as it supports the patient and family through the dying process. Hospice teams support the daily needs of the patient and family and provide needed equipment, medical expertise, and medications to control symptoms. They offer spiritual, psychological, and social support to the patient and family as needed and desired. Assistance with end-of-life planning is given to help the patient and family accomplish goals important to them. Bereavement support is also given. The team consists of the attending physician, hospice physician advisor, nurses, social worker, clergy, hospice aides, and volunteers. Hospice care is given in the home when the patient has family who are willing to assume care with the assistance of the hospice team. Hospice care also occurs in hospice facilities, hospitals, and extended care facilities. To qualify for Hospice care, the patient must be deemed terminal and given a 6-month or less life expectancy by two separate physicians. Should the patient survive 6 months in hospice, they can be extended for two 90-day periods, and then an unlimited number of 60-day periods per physician order.

Education Theory

Bandura's Theory of Social Learning

In the 1970s, Bandura proposed the theory of social learning, in which he posited that learning develops from observing, organizing, and rehearsing behavior that has been modeled. Bandura believed that people are more likely to adopt the behavior if they value the outcomes, if the outcomes have functional value, and if the person modeling the behavior is similar to the learner and is admired because of status. Behavior is the result of observation of behavioral, environmental, and cognitive interactions. There are **four conditions** required for modeling:

- **Attention**: The degree of attention paid to modeling can depend on many variables (physical, social, and environmental).
- **Retention**: People's ability to retain models depends on symbolic coding, creating mental images, organizing thoughts, and rehearsing (mentally or physically).
- **Reproduction**: The ability to reproduce a model depends on physical and mental capabilities.
- **Motivation**: Motivation may derive from past performances, rewards, or vicarious modeling.

Transtheoretical Model of Change

The transtheoretical model of change puts forth concepts applicable to the process of educating patients and their family members. The **stages** of the transtheoretical model of change include the following:

1. The first stage is **precontemplation**. At this point, the patient is not aware of any need for a change in the health behavior.
2. In the next stage, **contemplation**, the patient begins to realize why the change may be necessary after recognizing that the health behavior in question is unhealthy and weighing the consequences of continuing this behavior.
3. During the stage of **preparation**, the patient imagines making the change at a future time and starts to formulate a plan to do so.
4. The **action** stage occurs when the patient makes specific modifications in health behavior and begins to note the resulting positive changes.
5. During the **maintenance** stage, the patient is able to implement the change over time by utilizing strategies to prevent a return to previously unhealthy behaviors.
6. **Termination** is the stage at which a patient has incorporated the changed behavior into daily functioning, and the patient will not resume the previous unhealthy behavior.

Kurt Lewin

Force Field Analysis

Force field analysis was designed by Kurt Lewin, a social psychologist, to analyze both the driving forces and the restraining forces for change:

- **Driving forces** instigate and promote change, such as leaders, incentives, and competition.
- **Restraining forces** resist change, such as poor attitudes, hostility, inadequate equipment, or insufficient funds.

The educator can use this force field analysis diagram to discuss variables related to a proposed change in process:

- Write the proposed change in the center column.
- Brainstorm and list driving forces and opposed restraining forces. Score the forces. (When driving and restraining forces are in balance, this is a state of equilibrium or the status quo.)
- Discuss the value of the proposed change.
- Develop a plan to diminish or eliminate restraining forces.

LEWIN'S MODEL OF CHANGE THEORY

Lewin's model of change theory may be used to help some patients make decisions for change. Patients can be educated about the need for change and can be assisted with making alterations in behavior or thoughts in order to better facilitate change; however, only the patient can truly implement the change permanently. Lewin's concept of change theory involves a three-part process:

- **Unfreezing** is the part of the model in which the patient becomes open to change, sees a need for it, and removes the boundaries inhibiting change.
- The patient then makes the **actual change** according to expected outcomes and goals.
- Finally, **refreezing** is the process of maintaining the change so that it becomes a habit, and one that the patient is likely to uphold for a long period of time.

Lewin's theory also involves either driving forces or restraining forces. Driving forces are those outside measures that support the change, while restraining forces inhibit success in implementing the change.

Patient Education

Patient Education Techniques by Age

Age	Learning Issue	Teaching Solution
Infant	Non-verbal	Teach the parents or guardian.
Preschooler	Short attention span	Instruct with visuals (e.g., dolls) and role play. Tell parents to oversee treatment
5-8 yr	Longer attention span and eager for knowledge	Use short videos, visuals, and pictures.
9-12 yr	Good attention span, great curiosity, and some independence; rapid growth issues, such as mixed dentition; desire for group acceptance	Teach pairs or small groups, if confidentiality can be preserved. Use age-appropriate language to indicate respect.
13-15 yr	Peer pressure, interest in personal appearance, poor coordination, and bad eating habits	Give individualized instructions, motivation, and encouragement.
16-19 yr	Question authority, have busy schedules	Act as a friend and mentor. Explain disease process and anatomy.
20-60 yr	Individualized problems	Tailor instruction to the individual circumstances (e.g., pregnancy, depression, drug abuse).
60+ yr	Age-related problems (e.g., eyesight, memory, mobility, multiple prescriptions), fixed income, isolation, dependence on caregiver	Educate caregivers and patient. Emphasize avoiding triggers. Dispense free samples (promotions from suppliers). Register patient with wandering registry, if necessary.

Assessing Readiness to Learn

Reading body language is an important skill the medical assistant can use to assess a patient's stage of readiness. Assume that the patient is open to learning if his or her pupils are slightly dilated, signifying interest, and he or she leans forward and nods his or her head up and down in agreement. Look for direct eye contact, smiling, positive behavior, or a change in position from sitting back to leaning forward. Lowered eyes or looking away can mean fixation on something else or avoidance of the situation in an American-born patient, but in other cultures, direct eye contact is considered rude and challenging. Pursed lips may mean the patient is stressed, angry, or taking psychiatric drugs. Shaking the head from side to side may signal disagreement, while shrugging the shoulders can mean indifference or uncertainty. If the patient hangs his or her head down, this may indicate sadness, anxiety, or lordosis due to a deteriorating spine.

Teaching Points for Health Topics

The following are key teaching points for health topics:

- **Health and wellness**: Weight control, regular exercise, smoking cessation, intervention for substance use/abuse, support groups, resources
- **Nutrition**: Nutrients (fats, proteins, carbohydrates, vitamins, minerals), well-balanced meals, label-reading, and calories
- **Hygiene**: Hand-washing, dental care (brushing, flossing), bathing, and basic skin care
- **Treatment and medications**: Mode of administration, dosage, frequency, duration, and adverse effects
- **Preoperative care**: Any necessary preparation, such as showering, GI cleansing, fasting, and taking/withholding medications
- **Postoperative care**: Mobility, deep-breathing and coughing, wound care, medications, and restrictions on activities
- **Body mechanics**: Lifting, carrying, body alignment, avoidance of muscle strain
- **Personal/Physical safety**: Fall prevention, home safety measures, lighting, and medical ID bracelets

Diabetic Education

Diabetic education should include the following:

- **Glucose monitoring**: Patients should understand how to use the monitor and read and understand the results. The patient should know how frequently to test glucose. The patient should be advised of unsafe lower and higher levels and when to contact the physician or 911.
- **Medications (oral hypoglycemics)**: Patients should know administration, dosage, schedule, and adverse effects.
- **Medications (insulin)**: Patients should know dosage, schedule, and adverse effects as well as sites for injection and site rotation. Patients should practice filling syringes or using prefilled syringes and giving injections under supervision.
- **Ketoacidosis/hypoglycemia**: Patients should be able to describe signs and symptoms of ketoacidosis and hypoglycemia and know what steps to take if these occur.
- **Foot care**: Patients should be advised to avoid going barefoot, to practice good hygiene, and to check feet daily for signs of irritation or infection.
- **Diet**: Patients should understand the prescribed diet and any limitations, such as avoiding sugar and refined carbohydrates. Patients must understand the importance of eating 3 meals daily and staying on the diet.

Patient Education for At-Home Monitoring

Home Anticoagulation Monitoring

Home **INR anticoagulation** monitoring is done with a small device that varies in size from 4.5 ounces to 28 ounces, depending on the manufacturer. The patient must prick a finger with a lancet to obtain a drop of blood, which is placed on a test strip or cuvette. This is inserted into the device for reading. The INR result is displayed in a digital screen. Medicare and most insurances cover the costs of the equipment if used at least one time weekly.

Home Cholesterol Monitoring

Various monitoring systems/devices exist for **at-home monitoring of cholesterol**. One type of device is similar to the anticoagulation monitor, and the procedure is similar: prick the finger with a lancet, place a drop of blood on a test strip, and place into an electronic monitor for results. Some monitoring systems require only a test strip, which changes color according to the cholesterol level. Some monitoring devices provide only total cholesterol while others provide total cholesterol, HDL, LDL, and triglyceride levels.

Patient Instructions for Crutches, Canes, and Walkers

Crutches should be properly fitted before the client attempts ambulation. Correct height is one hand-width below axillae. The handgrips should be adjusted so the client supports the body weight comfortably with elbows slightly flexed rather than locked in place. The client should be cautioned not to bear weight under the axillae as this can cause nerve damage, but to hold the crutches tight against the side of the chest wall. The type of gait used depends on the type of injury.

A **cane** should be held in the opposite hand of the side of injury. When holding the cane in neutral position, the elbow should be bent at about a 15-degree angle and if holding the cane straight down to the side of the body, the top of the cane should be in line with the crease of the wrist.

The same is true of a **walker**, the elbow should be bent at 15 degrees when standing up straight and grasping the handles, and the handle grasps should be in line with to the crease of the wrists. The client should be able to move the walker forward without leaning over.

Patient Instructions for Wheelchairs

Wheelchair instructions should include the following:

- Engage brakes before getting in or out of the wheelchair and ensure the footplates are folded up or swung to the side
- Secure feet on footplates before navigating, but never stand on them
- Check for obstacles before navigating
- Secure safety harness/lap straps as needed
- Use hand rims to navigate forward and backward
- Avoid steep inclines (greater than a one-foot rise per 12-foot distance) and avoid going up or down inclines diagonally
- Bend forward slightly when going up an incline and lean backward slightly when going down
- Avoid rocky, soft, or uneven surfaces and beware of slippery surfaces
- Engage brakes when stopped
- Avoid hanging anything from the chair handles as the weight may lead to imbalance and tipping backward
- Never attempt to navigate stairs or escalators
- Go backward into elevators
- Use a gripper to pick up items and avoid bending forward or reaching down or behind
- Transfer into a seat in a motor vehicle unless it is adapted for wheelchair use and contains a security system

Patient Instructions for Splints and Slings

With both splints and slings, the patient/caregiver should be advised to check circulation by noting the skin color below the injury. The pulse should be palpable. The affected limb below the injury should also be checked for sensation and any feeling of numbness or tingling, which may indicate impaired circulation. The patient should be able to freely move any digits below the injury (toes, fingers).

- **Splints**: Used to limit movement of a limb but are generally removable, so they may be worn during the day and removed at night or while bathing. Commercial splints are often applied and secured with Velcro straps, but some may be formed from casting material that is secured in place by compression bandages.
- **Slings**: Used to elevate the hand or wrist in order to prevent or reduce edema and prevent movement or to immobilize an arm to maintain bone alignment with a broken clavicle (collarbone). If a cast has been applied to an arm, the sling helps to redistribute pressure and reduce strain on the shoulder muscles. Slings are generally applied so that the arm lies bent at the elbow with the lower arm parallel to the floor.

Educational Resources

Obtaining Ready-Made Patient Education Materials

Patients are entitled to **reliable information** about signs, symptoms, safety, and healthy behaviors. Print out information from the National Library of Medicine at http://www.nlm.nih.gov/. Obtain ready-made patient education materials from the drug or device manufacturer, which may include brochures, videos, demonstration models, self-evaluation quizzes, instruction manuals, and free samples. Contact a sales representative or call the supplier's order desk, and be prepared with the doctor's license number. For example:

- If the patient needs education on proper dental care, dispense a free brush, floss, and paste, which are available as a no-cost promotion from many suppliers.
- If the patient has allergies and needs to be taught to avoid triggers, send the patient home with a self-evaluation quiz and instructions to return with it to the next appointment.
- If the patient needs information about maintenance, spare parts, and operating procedures for medical devices, check the facility's computerized maintenance management system (CMMS).

Resource Materials for Parents, Guardians, and Teachers

Parents, guardians, and sometimes teachers and other caregivers are directly responsible for ensuring a patient receives his or her medication(s). Advise them to deal with only one pharmacy, if possible. If consistent compliance is desired, educate the parents about correct drug dosage, timing, administration technique, blood levels, adverse drug interactions, and prohibited foods and herbs. Inform the parents they must first discuss all changes in dose and medication type or drug withdrawal with the attending physician. If the attending physician is unavailable, advise the parents to ask for the doctor on call (locum tenens) and double-check with the pharmacist. Explain that abrupt withdrawal from some drugs can cause severe problems (e.g., neuroleptic malignant syndrome). Give the parents a written list of foods and herbs that could interact badly with the drugs. Parents' and guardians' attitude towards medication and therapeutic regimens highly influence their child. Utilize a translator, if necessary.

Avoiding Prejudice in Patient Resource Materials

The medical assistant often deals with patients who are not of his or her culture, race, religion, ethnicity, or socioeconomic status. **Multicultural skills** are, therefore, a job requirement for medical assistants in the United States. The *Ten Standards of Practice* require medical assistants to exercise compassion and place the welfare of the patient above all else. This means researching the specific cultures, learning their habits, traditions, and preferences. Remember that many immigrants in the United States continue their native practices from their country of origin. Utilize a translator to tailor existing English materials to the target population; do not merely translate material verbatim. Use street language if needed, and avoid medical jargon. To avoid prejudice in resource materials, review the *Patients' Bill of Rights* of 2010.

Appropriate Documentation of Patient Instruction

Documentation of patient instruction should be done as soon as possible, including the date and time, a description of the instruction provided and the method used, the purpose, and the patient response. If a teaching plan is developed, this should be filed in the patient's record as well with a copy or record of any handouts or written instructions provided to the patient. In some cases of standardized instruction (such as wound care after a procedure), a checklist may be utilized to indicate the topics covered, but the checklist should also allow comments so that the medical assistant can indicate the effectiveness of the teaching. One method of assessing effectiveness is to have the person explain his or her understanding or do a return demonstration (such as for wound care). Follow-up should also be documented, such as when the patient returns to determine if the patient has demonstrated understanding or needs further instruction.

Chapter Quiz

Ready to see how well you retained what you just read? Scan the QR code to go directly to the chapter quiz interface for this study guide. If you're using a computer, simply visit the bonus page at **mometrix.com/bonus948/certmedasst** and click the Chapter Quizzes link.

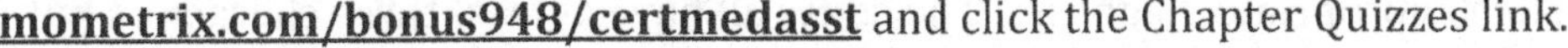

Administrative

Transform passive reading into active learning! After immersing yourself in this chapter, put your comprehension to the test by taking a quiz. The insights you gained will stay with you longer this way. Scan the QR code to go directly to the chapter quiz interface for this study guide. If you're using a computer, simply visit the bonus page at **mometrix.com/bonus948/certmedasst** and click the Chapter Quizzes link.

Coding, Billing, and Third-Party Payments

Coding Systems

The most commonly used coding systems are:

- The International Classification of Diseases, 10th Edition, Clinical Modification (ICD-10-CM)
- Healthcare Common Procedure Coding Systems (HCPCS) Level II
- Current Procedural Terminology 4th Edition (CPT-4)
- Systematized Nomenclature of Medicine (SNOMED CT) by the College of American Pathologists

Some coding systems are classification systems, and some are nomenclatures. Most healthcare organization use multiple coding systems.

ICD-10-CM

International Classification of Diseases, 10th Edition, Clinical Modifications, (ICD-10-CM) is a coding system used to code diagnoses. The ICD-10-CM codes are used for billing purposes to ensure that procedure codes match appropriate diagnoses. The codes all have at least three characters but may have up to four additional sub-categories. Diagnoses are classified by type of disease or system involved. For example, main categories include neoplasms and diseases of the respiratory systems. With ICD-10-CM, injuries are grouped by body part rather than category of injury.

HCPCS Level II

Healthcare Common Procedure Coding Systems (HCPCS) Level II codes are used when filing claims for equipment, supplies and services that are not covered by CPT codes, including durable medical equipment ambulance services, laboratory service, orthotics, and prosthetics:

- D codes: procedures
- E codes: durable medical equipment, such as bedside commodes
- L codes: orthotic and prosthetic procedures and devices, such as orthopedic shoes
- P codes: pathology and laboratory services

CPT Codes

Current Procedural Terminology 4th Edition (CPT-4) codes were developed by the American Medical Association (AMA) and used to define those licensed to provide services and to describe medical and surgical treatments, diagnostics, and procedures. CPT codes specify procedures as well as typical times required for treatment. CPT codes are usually updated each October with revisions (additions, deletions) to coding. The use of CPT codes is mandated by both CMS and HIPAA to provide a uniform language and to aid research. These codes are used primarily for billing purposes for insurances (public and private). Under HIPAA, HHS has designed CPT codes as part of the national standard for electronic healthcare transactions:

- **Category I codes** are used to identify a procedure or service.
- **Category II codes** are used to identify performance measures, including diagnostic procedures.
- **Category III codes** identify temporary codes for technology and data collection.

SNOMED CT

SNOMED CT is the nomenclature system with the most potential to handle the complex data represented in electronic health records (EHRs). **SNOMED** (Systematized Nomenclature of Medicine) offers comprehensive international clinical reference terminology, used worldwide. The CT suffix stands for *clinical terms*. Designed for computers, SNOMED CT offers a consistent language for capturing, sharing, and aggregating health data across specialties and sites of care. SNOMED links synonyms to a single concept. For instance, SNOMED recognizes appendicitis as an inflammatory and GI disease. SNOMED includes domain-specific vocabularies, such as those for nursing. SNOMED maps to interface with other clinical terminologies, such as ICD-10.

Diagnostic-Related Groups (DRGs)

Diagnostic-related groups (DRGs) were instituted in 1982 as a way to classify patients who shared similar diseases and treatments for billing purposes, under the assumption that patients who shared symptoms and/or diseases use the same number of resources and, therefore, should be billed the same amount. There are approximately 500 different DRGs, and patients are placed into specific DRGs using International Classification of Disease (ICD-10-CM) codes, along with specific patient information such as sex, age, and the presence of comorbidities. By placing patients into DRGs, Medicare is able to determine how much the hospital should be reimbursed for patient care. The institution of DRGs has changed the health care system from one that was provider-driven (meaning the individual clinician determined the billable amount) into one that is payer-driven (meaning that Medicare determines reimbursement).

Healthcare Financing Methods

Healthcare financing involves complex options. The payment methods are self-pay (also called direct pay or out-of-pocket payment), which entails the patient paying directly for his or her own health costs, and indirect pay, which involves a third party paying for the health costs. Third-party payers can be the government, insurance companies, managed-care programs, or self-insured companies. A common third-party payer is an insurance company. Insurance providers essentially have a contractual arrangement with individuals and/or companies to cover all or part of health costs incurred for a monthly fee, called a premium. Coinsurance means the insurer is partially responsible for the debt, and the patient is usually responsible for the remainder. Insurance companies generally pay for health costs after they have been incurred through a reimbursement arrangement with the healthcare provider.

Healthcare Reimbursement Arrangements

Healthcare reimbursement is ubiquitous across healthcare providers, in that most healthcare costs are covered by third parties after the costs have been incurred. Often this reimbursement involves several parties, but the general **arrangements** fall into a few key categories called reimbursement formulas or contracted amounts:

- **Retrospective payment systems** encompass several formulas, in which healthcare costs are determined after the healthcare has been provided.
- **Fee-for-service costs** are based on the provider's cost for each service, such as lab tests, and hospitals are paid on a per-diem basis.
- **Usual, customary, and reasonable charges** are based on what is normally charged for physician care or what is reasonable for the service provided.
- **Sliding scale fees** apply in low-income or public health programs, where cost is based on the patient's ability to pay.
- **Capitation** pays a prepaid amount to the provider, based on a predetermined per-person or per-capita amount.

MANAGED CARE

Managed care encompasses various types of plans designed to effectively deliver healthcare by containing costs and use of services, while providing quality healthcare to its subscribers. Managed care organizations (MCOs) contract with employers, unions, individuals, and other purchasers to provide comprehensive healthcare to people who voluntarily enroll in the plan. Providers who participate in managed-care plans may be paid employees or may provide services on a per capita (capitation) arrangement, a fee-for-services arrangement, or other types of payment arrangement. There are many types of managed care programs, but the most common are health maintenance organizations (HMOs) and preferred provider organizations (PPOs). Some models integrate health insurance, delivery, and payment within one organization, and exercise control over utilization. MCOs generate complex information needs, affecting the responsibilities of the medical assistant.

HMO

HMO stands for **Health Maintenance Organization**. An HMO is a collection of doctors, allied healthcare providers, and hospitals that receive fixed monthly payments from the government to care for Medicaid patients or from an employer for its workers, rather than fee-for-service. Cost control is of major importance to the HMO. There are variations of HMOs, called preferred provider organizations (PPO) or point-of-service plans (POS).

Up until the 1980s, most patients had indemnity insurance that was fee-for service. The patient would co-pay for medical care with an insurance company, and had the option of visiting any licensed care provider. Today, more than 50% of Americans deal with HMOs as a cost-saving measure for the government, insurers, and employers. Care at an HMO costs a fraction of that with traditional providers, but the patient can only see providers and get tests that are in-network. Patients do not have to pay up front, fill out claim forms, or wait to be reimbursed at an HMO.

VARIATIONS AND COMPONENTS

PPOs, POS plans, case management, and utilization management are all variations or components of HMOs:

- **Preferred Provider Organization (PPO)**: A network of physicians and/or healthcare organizations that provide healthcare at a discounted rate in return for patient volume. PPOs contract with payers or employers.

- **Point of Service (POS) Plan**: An arrangement in a managed-care organization (MCO) whereby the patient chooses a provider each time a healthcare service is required. A point of enrollment plan refers to one in which the patient chooses a provider at the time of enrollment.
- **Case Management**: The overview and coordination of costs and resources for an MCO. An individual, such as a primary care provider, is designated as a case manager or gatekeeper. Case management is usually employed when a patient is suffering from a chronic, progressive, and/or terminal illness that requires several types of healthcare services.
- **Utilization Management**: The oversight/management of healthcare costs, usually required by the payer. Utilization review is the process of evaluation for healthcare cost/service efficiency.

Federal and/or State Mandated Insurance Options

Medicaid, Tricare, CHAMPVA, and workers' compensation are federal and/or state mandated insurance provided to specific demographics:

- **Medicaid**: The program through which the federal and state governments help low-income individuals by paying for those medical services that are deemed to be absolutely necessary. Medicaid is covered by Social Security Act Title XIX. Medicaid is available to Federal Supplemental Security income recipients, low-income children under 6 years of age, pregnant women, individuals older than 65 with a disability, and individuals deemed categorically needy by their state.
- **TRICARE**: The Department of Defense provides healthcare for active and retired military personnel and their families through the TRICARE program, previously CHAMPUS.
- **CHAMPVA**: Civilian Health and Medical Program of the Department of Veterans Affairs. It is always the secondary payer, after Medicare, to minimize out-of-pocket expenses. CHAMPVA covers the families of veterans who were killed or permanently disabled in the line of duty, who are ineligible for Tricare.
- **Workers' Compensation**: Insurance provided under laws generated by each state, to cover medical expenses and lost income for workers injured on the job, or to their survivors if the injury results in death.

Medicare Part A

Medicare Part A is no-cost hospital insurance for the following individuals:

- Social Security recipients over 65 years old
- Patients receiving disability benefits for a minimum of 24 months
- Patients with renal failure (requiring dialysis or transplant)

Medicare Part A covers care in the following **facilities**:

- Critical access hospitals
- Home care
- Inpatient hospitals
- Hospice
- Skilled nursing facilities

Medicare Part A is financed primarily through payroll tax, and is unavailable to beneficiaries who are ineligible for federal retirement benefits.

Medicare Part B

Medicare Part B insurance covers outpatient treatment for necessary and preventative services including the following:

- Blood transfusion
- Diagnostic tests like glaucoma, Pap smears, mammograms, and prostate exams
- Doctors' office visits
- Durable assistive devices, like beds, oxygen, walkers, and wheelchairs
- Laboratory tests
- One physical exam in the first 6 months
- Outpatient clinics for mental health, occupational therapy, and physiotherapy
- Outpatient surgery
- Vaccines, such as Hepatitis B and Pneumococcus

Part B is financed by federal appropriations with monthly premiums paid by the beneficiary, who also pays some deductibles and copayments.

Medicare C and D

Medicare Part C is also known as **Medicare Advantage**. It is available to beneficiaries enrolled in Parts A and B (hospital and outpatient insurance coverage). Part C offers various managed-care plans, including HMO, POS, and PPO plans. Medicare Part D is a recently added option to be bundled into Medicare Advantage that provides prescription drug coverage. There are several plans available, but the beneficiary always pays a monthly premium and part of the drug cost. Medicare providers are reimbursed through an insurance company contracted by the federal government as a fiscal intermediary. Congress passed the *Tax Equity and Fiscal Responsibility Act* (TERFA) in 1983 to combat spiraling medical costs. TERFA created the Prospective Payment System (PPS), a method whereby reimbursement amounts are predetermined based on the services rendered. CMS annually reviews standardized rates, represented by classifications called Diagnosis-related Groups (DRGs) for inpatient care, and Resource-based Relative Value Scale (RBRVS) for physician services.

Review Video: Medicare and Medicaid
Visit mometrix.com/academy and enter code: 507454

Requesting Third-Party Payer Reimbursement

Third-party payers are insurance companies or employers that use patient care data as the basis for claims processing to pay for healthcare services provided. Many third-party payers encourage the use of ambulatory care by providing financial incentives. It is very time-consuming for the physician to qualify a claim for third-party reimbursement because he or she must specify diagnoses and provide exact details (e.g., a surgical procedure must document the reason for surgery, lesion length, layers of fascia involved, etc.). The medical assistant reduces the time the physician spends on documentation by reviewing the patient's record the day before an appointment and isolating the pertinent information. The patient must authorize disclosure of his or her information to third-party recipients. The third-party payer will probably redisclose the patient's information to the Medical Information Bureau (MIB), which allows access to other potential insurers for up to 7 years. Only drug or alcohol abuse cases are exempt. Third-party payers require a Progress Note for each visit billed.

Sending Information to Third-Party Payers

The medical assistant deals with occasional third-party payers through surface mail, and with regular third-party payers through a virtual private network (VPN), or Extranet. One component of the VPN is a demilitarized zone (DMZ), which sits between the internal network and the VPN. It allows outside access to a third-party portion of the network, while protecting the Intranet, or internal, information.

Enrolling Doctor as Participating Provider

In order for a doctor to be considered a participating provider, they must produce specific documentation to payers to obtain billing privileges, for example:

- A doctor must meet **credentialing standards** established by the National Committee for Quality Assurance (NCQA).
- Individual healthcare providers and business owners must supply the payer with a **tax identification number** for the IRS.

Master Charge Lists

Master charge lists delineate how much can be charged for each service, as identified by a CPT-4 code. These lists are also known as charge master, charge description master (CDM), or fee schedule. Charges are impacted by clinical modifiers, which affect reimbursement. Modifiers are given numeric or alphabetical codes. Either the medical assistant or the HIM manager is responsible for monitoring the accurate and timely coding of all services rendered, and regularly analyzing contracted reimbursement rates and expenses associated with services or product costing.

Financial Bookkeeping

Bookkeeping

The medical assistant should understand the following elements of bookkeeping:

- Petty cash
- Single-entry bookkeeping
- Bank deposits, checking, and reconciliations
- Patient accounts and statements
- Payroll

The medical assistant completes the financial records when the office is not busy. Usually, a certified accountant (CPA) sets up the doctor's accounting records and provides instructions for how the medical assistant is to record transactions. For purchases, the medical assistant records the following:

- Date of purchase
- Reason for payment in the "explanation" column
- Check number used to pay for the purchase
- Amount

The accountant calculates the annual income tax and completes the financial statements through double-entry bookkeeping. The medical assistant is not typically involved with a practice's taxes or financial statements.

Petty Cash Accounts

Petty cash is a small amount of cash (usually no more than $100) that is kept on hand to pay for miscellaneous costs, such as for overdue postage, tips for delivery, parking costs, and supplies, such as coffee or tea, for a break room. Petty cash should be kept in a locked, secure drawer or container. Money placed into petty cash should come from a practice account but never directly from cash payments directly received from a patient. That money should be kept separate. A petty cash record should be maintained and should include a record of any disbursement and replenishment. The date and purpose of disbursements must be recorded along with the signature of the person withdrawing funds. Additionally, petty cash receipts should be filled out each time a person receives money from petty cash, such as when a person withdraws money to purchase breakroom supplies.

Data Entry Procedures

Data entry procedures include posting the following:

- **Charges**: If the physician or nurse practitioner manually checks off services, print out a charge slip from the computer program and later use the information on the form to enter data into the computer application. In the charge posting screen, post the patient's name, identification number, date of service, the service provided (office visit, ECG, injection), the CPT code, the ICD-10-CM diagnostic codes, HCPCS Level II codes, and the charge for the service. The application may require co-payments and payments to be entered as well. Diagnostic codes must match the service provided.

- **Payments**: Access the payment posting screen, which should list the procedure charge history. Then post the correct date, payment type (cash, check, credit card), and amount and check the balance (view ledger).
- **Adjustments**: Discounts, such as for Medicare or insurance, are usually entered in the charge posting screen, but this may vary from one application to another. The adjustment is to the balance owed.

Revenue Cycle, Front-End and Back-End Activities, and Payer Contracts

The **revenue cycle** begins when the patient enters the healthcare system for diagnosis, treatment, and follow-up services. It includes the flow of patient and financial information and ends with reimbursement for services rendered.

Front-end activities take place before a patient receives treatment, such as collection and verification of demographics, billing, and insurance information. **Back-end activities** involve billing and claims processing after admission, and even after discharge, if applicable.

Payer contracts are legally binding documents describing the obligations of both providers and payers. Healthcare billing adheres to industry standards of language and service codes, as noted by the Common Procedure Coding System (HCPCS) of the Healthcare Financing Administration (HCFA). A provider who contracts with a payer is considered a participating provider. If no contract exists, then the provider is considered a non-participating provider. He or she may be reimbursed less by a third-party payer. Non-participating providers usually obtain additional co-payment from the patient. This is especially true of mental healthcare providers, such as counselors and psychologists.

Claims Processing

Claims processing requires accurate, complete information and must meet standard formats. Denials of claims based on incomplete or inaccurate information can be avoided by monitoring for correct patient information and medical codes. Primary and secondary billing is generated for patients covered by multiple insurance plans. Insurance payments are accompanied by either a remittance advice (RA) or explanation of benefits (EOB), indicating the billed amount, allowable amount by insurance coverage, payment amount, patient liability, and the amount disallowed by insurance. Review accounts to ensure that the correct payment was made according to the individual payer's contract, which may be based on a percentage, per unit, DRG rate, or another fee schedule. A case mix analysis results in a "case mix index" or average, which is then multiplied by the number of cases.

IRS

The **Internal Revenue Service (IRS)** is the federal government agency responsible for tax collection and tax law enforcement. Often, the medical assistant is responsible for payroll in a small office and must be familiar with IRS withholding requirements. For example, Medicare A is financed primarily through payroll tax. The medical assistant must learn to prepare paychecks and deduct income tax, pension, unemployment insurance, and healthcare premiums. The medical assistant can obtain IRS forms from the IRS website. The medical assistant enters payroll records on a master sheet, which is a computer file that contains long-term information that changes infrequently, such as employees' names and addresses. The master is updated regularly, and the medical assistant refers to it as the most reliable source of information. The medical assistant must keep the payroll master entirely separate from accounts payable. An IRS auditor may ask to review the payroll master, and the medical assistant is obliged to show it.

Truth in Lending Act

The federal *Truth in Lending Act* (Regulation Z) (1968) is part of the *Consumer Protection Act* and is enforced by the Federal Trade Commission. When a healthcare provider engages in a credit agreement, a truth-in-lending statement must be provided to the patient/guardian/payor at the time the credit agreement is made. The statement must be easily understood by the payor. The credit agreement includes the total amount owed and the payment schedule and amounts that have been agreed upon (usually monthly payments). When applicable, the truth-in-lending statement must include the maximum dollar amount that can be charged to the account, the interest rate, the method used to calculate the interest rate, and the method used to determine the minimum monthly payment. If a party pays in four or fewer installments without a specific agreement, the provisions of the *Truth in Lending Act* do not apply.

Accounts Receivable Aging Reports

The accounts receivable aging report is used to track insurance payments, including those that are past due. The aging of accounts is done by 30-day increments (0-30, 31-60, etc.). Unless a payment agreement has been agreed upon in advance, all payments are considered past due after 30 days. Those that exceed 120 days are usually referred to a collection agency or written off by the practice. In some cases, the practice may send a letter asking for payment and indicating plans to take the matter to small claims court if payment is not received and the amount due is within the small claims court limits.

Collections Process

Identifying Delinquent Accounts

The turn-around time for a claim submitted to an insurance company is usually 30–60 days if submitted on paper and 10–15 days if submitted electronically. Payments received after this time are considered delinquent. If a claim is **delinquent**, then the usual policy is to send a tracer within a few days to determine if there is a problem with the claim or if the insurance company requires more information. The insurance claim register should be checked routinely to ensure that delinquent claims are not overlooked. The tracer form should include:

- Name and address of insurance company
- Patient's and insured's names
- Employer's name (if applicable)
- Date claim was initially submitted and the amount of the claim
- Note indicating excess time has passed with no word from insurance company or request for further information
- Area for the insurance company to explain reason for delay (pending, processing, denied)
- Physician's name, address, and telephone number

Fair Debt Collection Practices Act

The federal *Fair Debt Collection Practices Act* (1977) is intended to protect debtors from third-party collection agencies or others acting on behalf of another (such as an attorney) regarding consumer debts (medical bills) and to ensure debtors are treated fairly. The regulations, however, do not apply to a healthcare provider attempting to collect his or her own debts. Third party agents are prohibited from harassing debtors, making false statements or threats in order to gain payments, or being in any way frightening or verbally abusive. Third parties may not make threats that they cannot legally follow through on, such as threatening to have a debtor arrested. Additionally, third parties are prohibited from calling or contacting debtors before 8 AM or after 8 PM. The debtor must receive appropriate notices, and third parties must identify themselves as debt collectors. If requested to cease communication, they must do so, and they cannot attempt to collect from those who have filed for bankruptcy.

Operating Budget

The operating budget for a facility is a summary of all projected income and expenses for a specific time period. Operating budgets are often constructed on a monthly basis and include projections for the year. Seasonal expenses, such as lawn mowing and snow removal, must be included. Fluctuations in such items as payroll, administrative expenses, prices for materiel and supplies, taxes, insurance, and general costs should be forecast as accurately as possible. The budget should be reviewed monthly by the facility manager and accounting and at least quarterly by a member of upper management. Discrepancies between the budgeted amount of a line item and the actual cost should be investigated and revisions made as necessary.

Formulation of Operating Budget

Senior management and departmental managers negotiate and prepare the operating budget. The **operating budget team** considers both corporate guidelines and forecasts of departmental activity. Each department estimates the demand for its services, but the priorities that must be met are primary care, hospitalizations, surgeries, births, and emergency care. The management team creates forecasts based on market trends, past history, and executive judgment. The team evaluates trends in resource prices and the cost of in-house personnel versus contractors. Purchasing and human resources provide the statistics for these forecasts. The operating budget affects the medical assistant most directly. The capital budget concerns the actual building, and the utilities budget concerns how the building is heated, cooled, and lit.

Financial Mathematics

Financial mathematics related to patient and practice accounts require primarily a basic knowledge of addition and subtraction, but the medical assistant needs to have an understanding of financial documents, such as invoices, which are essentially billing forms that describe a purchase/service and the amount due to pay for the purchase/service. Additionally, the medical assistant should be familiar with single-entry bookkeeping, which is often utilized to record income and expenses:

Date	Description	Income	Expense	Balance
Jan 1	Balance			500.00
Jan 12	Printer cartridges		126.00	374.00
Jan 15	Vitamin supplements		50.00	324.00
Jan 16	Cash deposit	220.00		544.00

Important Terms

Important finance and bookkeeping-related terms for the medical assistant to understand include the following:

- **Relative value studies**: A schedule that assigns a unit value to a medical procedure to compare costs.
- **Resource-based relative value scale (RBRVS)**: The Center for Medicare and Medicaid (CMS) reviews its standardized rates every year. Resource-based Relative Value Scale (RBRVS) are standardized rates the CMS pays providers for physician services.
- **Contracted fees**: The participating provider agrees to accept a list of specific fees from the payer. A fee is the total the provider can charge. This benefit plan prohibits extra billing.
- **Accounts receivable (A/R)**: Money owed to the practice by a patient for services and products the provider sold on credit and for which the patient has been invoiced. Enter A/R as a current asset on the balance sheet.
- **Accounts payable (A/P)**: Unpaid bills the practice owes to suppliers. A/P does not include payroll, rent, taxes, or accrued interest. Enter A/P as current liabilities (short-term) on the balance sheet.
- **Billing cycle**: The period between billing for services and products, which is usually one month in most practices.
- **Aging of accounts**: Classifying the accounts according to risk by the number of days that have elapsed since the due date or billing date. Most practices have an aging schedule of 1-30 days, 31-60 days, 61-90 days, and more than 90 days. The longer an account is unpaid, the greater the risk that the patient will default.
- **Collections**: The medical assistant transfers a delinquent account more than 90 days overdue to the collection department or a private collection agency. It is cheaper for the medical assistant to negotiate with the patient than it is to accept 10% of recovered money from the collection agency or risk that no money will be recovered if the patient files for bankruptcy.
- **Itemization**: The medical assistant prepares a bill for the payer with a detailed list of all procedures performed and products used during one visit for a particular patient. The supplier prepares a bill for the practice listing all products sold in detail (size, shape, quantity, color, material, etc.).
- **Consumer Protection Act**: A legal statute that prohibits deceptive marketing, encourages the seller to give the consumer information, and enforces product safety standards.
- **Ordering**: The medical assistant issues a Purchase Order (PO) Number to the supplier to confirm a request for goods or services. When the medical assistant accepts receipt of the goods or services, the PO becomes a binding legal agreement for the practice to pay the supplier.
- **Invoice**: A bill of sale or contract that identifies the practice and patient, or the seller and buyer. This lists the quantity of products or services sold and describes them. Invoices also show the date of service or shipment, delivery or transport mode, price, and payment terms, including discounts. When the medical assistant or doctor signs the invoice, it becomes a demand for payment. When the patient pays the invoice in full, it becomes a document of title.
- **Tracking**: The monitoring of performance or delivery. As a person or product passes through checkpoints, the medical assistant notes if there is deviation from a benchmark through tracking software.

Scheduling

Schedule Types

Multiple schedule types are used in the medical office setting, including the following:

- **Stream**: The standard booking method, where patients are slotted in 15-minute intervals. A patient with a complex procedure takes two or three slots.
- **Double-booking**: Two patients are booked simultaneously. Staff take the history, vital signs, weight, height, and any standard tests (e.g., visual acuity, urinalysis, PFT). The physician performs a short exam and prescribes medications. Long wait times can result.
- **Wave**: A booking method for dealing with late arrivals. Schedule three patients simultaneously, at the beginning of each half hour. The doctor sees them in the order of their arrival. If one patient is late, it does not affect the other two. The longest wait is 20 minutes.
- **Modified wave**: Two to three patients are scheduled at the top of each hour, and all other call-ins may come in and wait their turns.
- **Open booking**: First-come, first-served. A booking method for dealing with no-shows and emergencies. Give the patient an appointment on the same day he or she calls. Used by walk-in clinics.
- **Clustering**: All patients of one type only are seen in a clinic on predetermined days/parts of days to increase efficiency, such as diabetics, pregnant mothers, or arthritics. Also called **categorization**.

Appointment Matrix

An appointment matrix is the template on which the appointment schedule is recorded (on paper or in the computer). Typically, the matrix lists the physicians and nurse practitioners, and the times of day (usually in 10 minute-increments and the days of the week). The appointment matrix may be quite simple (as below) or complex. Any time that a physician or nurse practitioner is not available, that time slot is blocked out so that no appointments will be made at those times. If the physician or nurse practitioner sets aside certain days or times for extended visits, such as for admission history and physical, these times may be color-coded or otherwise noted. Example:

Dr. Smith	Hr.	May 15	May 16
	8:00	Mrs. Jones—BP check	Staff meeting
	8:10	Mr. Brown—Glucose	" "
	8:20	Miss White—UTI	" "
	8:30	" "	Mr. Smythe - Ulcer exam
	8:40	Telephone calls	" "

* "   " indicates that the schedule block is a continuation of what is mentioned above. This is used for appointments or meetings that run over the 10-minute increment used in this example.

Scheduling Considerations

Depending on the appointment being scheduled, the medical assistant must consider the following elements:

- **Scheduling a first appointment**: Necessary information includes the patient's name, date of birth, address, telephone number or other contact information as well as the purpose of the visit, name of referring physician/healthcare provider, and the patient's insurance company. Insurance information should include primary and secondary insurers as well as ID numbers and group numbers and a contact number necessary for preauthorization or referrals.
- **Scheduling subsequent appointments**: The patient's name and birthdate should be obtained to verify status, and the patient should be asked the purpose of the visit and the physician/nurse practitioner the patient wants to see. Confirm that there have been no changes to insurance since the last appointment.
- **Legal aspects of scheduling**: Patients may be charged for missed appointments only if a protocol is in place that applies to all patients. The patients must be advised at the time the appointment is made of the charge for missing the appointment or failing to notify the office within 24 hours. Medicare and many insurers don't pay for these charges.

Handling No-Shows, Cancellations, Delays, and Emergencies

Remind patients the day before an appointment is scheduled. If a patient misses an appointment, notify a doctor and the referring doctor. If missing an appointment could compromise the patient's care (e.g., a suicidal patient), the medical assistant may be required to follow up. **No-shows and cancellations** that notify the medical office in less than 24 hours before an appointment may be charged a fine to cover the doctor's lost fees.

Always have patients' contact numbers handy in the scheduler. If the doctor is delayed, ensure urgent patients are seen by the *locum tenens* (doctor-on-call). Never leave an urgent case unattended. Rebook routine appointments. If a routine patient shows up anyway: Apologize, explain the absence (e.g., delivering a baby), estimate how long the wait will be, suggest rebooking, and offer hospitality if the patient decides to wait.

Always consider calls with complaints of chest pain, high fever, and earache an emergency. Ignoring or delaying emergency calls can result in legal action against the medical assistant and the doctor. Leave at least 20 minutes per day open on the schedule to handle emergent patients.

Referrals

Completing a Requisition to Refer Patient for Outside Services

After the doctor finishes the consultation with a patient, review the written Physician's Orders in the chart before the patient leaves the office. The medical assistant may be required to book an appointment with a specialist, such as a dietitian, physiotherapist, or psychiatrist. The assistant may be required to arrange outside tests, such as audiology, bloodwork, ultrasound, or allergy screening. Call the outside service to book an appointment on the patient's behalf. Remember that a debilitated patient is unable to tolerate more than one invasive test per day. Obtain the correct requisitions for the tests from the outside services. Complete them by accurately transcribing information from the patient's chart into the requisition form. The medical assistant will find the patient's prescribed drugs on the nursing history chart. Send the requisition with the patient to the appointment. Remind the patient that most hospital operating rooms are booked several months in advance. The doctor may also dictate a referral letter to the specialist, which is typed later, and send it by fax or surface mail so that it arrives well before the appointment.

Receiving Referred Patients

Because referrals are an important source of new patients, patients that are referred are often given priority in scheduling, according to practice policy and depending on the urgency of the referral. If the referral is made directly, as per telephone, then the medical assistant should ask about urgency and obtain as much information as possible, including a request for medical records to save time later. In some cases, the patient calls after being advised to do so by a referring healthcare provider. In that case, medical records should generally be obtained in order to assess urgency before making the appointment. Three **types of referrals** are most common:

- **Consultation**: Usually these patients are referred to a specialist for diagnostic testing, surgery, or additional treatment. Some types of testing and treatment may require preauthorization for insurance companies.
- **Therapy/Treatments**: These may include psychological therapy, physical therapy, occupational therapy, or speech therapy. The therapy may require preauthorization for insurance companies.
- **Community resources**: These include home health agencies, meals programs, and respite care.

Preauthorization Process

Insurance carriers may require preauthorization for diagnostic procedures, hospitalization, and surgical procedures. Managed care programs often also require preauthorization for referrals. For this reason, determining the need for preauthorization should be part of verification of insurance benefits. Insurance cards often list a telephone number, fax number, or other contact information for preauthorization. The medical assistant should gather necessary information before contacting the insurance company and fill out the **preauthorization/referral form** with the following information:

- Patient's name and demographic information
- Healthcare provider's name, provider identification number, address, and telephone number
- Name of the insurance plan, address, and contact information (telephone, fax, secure email)
- Patient's preliminary diagnosis, including diagnostic codes
- Planned procedure/referral, including procedure codes
- Name, address and telephone number or other contact information for referrals
- Amount of patient's copayment and/or deductible
- Hospital benefits (inpatient and outpatient)
- Healthcare providers within the network (if applicable)

The preauthorization/referral form is usually faxed to the insurance company although in emergency situations preauthorization may be obtained by telephone.

Scheduling Hospital Admissions

When scheduling **in-patient hospitalization** for a patient, the medical assistant should first gather all necessary information before calling the admitting department and should obtain preauthorization from insurance companies as needed. In the case of a non-emergent admission, the medical assistant should determine both the patient's and the physician's availability prior to scheduling. Information that the admitting department needs includes the patient's name, address, date of birth, admitting diagnosis, insurance information (primary and secondary), preauthorization number (if appropriate), and purpose of hospitalization. The medical assistant should also inform the admitting department when the admitting physician plans to see the patient, as the patient must be seen by his or her physician within 24 hours. In some cases, care of the patient is assumed by a hospitalist upon admission and not by the patient's personal physician. The patient must be informed of any prehospitalization testing, restrictions, and other special instructions.

Scheduling Diagnostic Tests

To schedule diagnostic procedures, the medical assistant should gather information about the patient, and then determine the diagnostic test to be scheduled and the appropriate time frame within which the test must be conducted. Steps include:

1. Select a diagnostic center/laboratory and verify that services are covered under the patient's insurance plan.
2. Obtain the appropriate preauthorization necessary, or check with the insurance company if unsure of the need for preauthorization.
3. Discuss availability and time/date preferences with patient.
4. Call the diagnostic center/laboratory to schedule appointment.
5. Provide information to the patient regarding the place, date, and time of the diagnostic procedure.
6. Provide any pre- or post-test instructions (such as dietary restrictions or special preparation) to the patient and review with the patient to make sure the patient understands.
7. Record the scheduled procedure in the patient's medical record.
8. Record the scheduled procedure in the diagnostic procedure tracking log.

Scheduling Surgeries

When scheduling surgical procedures, which may be done as an inpatient or in an outpatient surgery center, the medical assistant should first gather all necessary information: The location where the surgery is to be performed, the patient's name, the telephone number, the date of birth, the type of surgery that is to be scheduled, the timeframe, and the name of the surgeon and any assistants as well as the anesthesiologist. Additionally, the medical assistant should contact the insurance company for preauthorization and obtain the preauthorization number that the surgical center will need. If preauthorization testing (PAT), such as CBC, chem-panel, chest x-ray, or ECG, is required, the medical assistant must know who is to perform the testing and may need to schedule the tests as well. Patients must be provided pre-surgical instructions, such as the need to be NPO for a certain number of hours prior to surgery and whether or not to take medications the day of or in the days prior to surgery.

Medical Reception

Comfortable and Safe Medical Reception Area

Considerations regarding situating the medical reception area to provide comfort and safety include the following:

- **Traffic pattern**: The entrance and exit should be clear and layout such that patients can avoid crossing each other's paths.
- **Desk**: The reception desk should be clearly seen on entrance and the focal point of the room. The counter should be low enough to accommodate wheelchairs and chairs should be available for patients who need to sit. If in an open area, an adjacent area should be available for private conversations with patients.
- **Lighting**: Harsh artificial light, such as fluorescent, should be avoided. Windows with natural light are ideal.
- **Furniture/chairs**: Vinyl and manufactured fabrics can be more easily cleaned and usually hold up better than natural fibers. Chairs should be comfortable and large enough to accommodate patients who are obese.

Outfitting a Reception Area

To outfit a reception area optimally, consider the following:

- **Choose colors** to modulate patients' moods. Greens, blues, and pinks are calming and suitable for psychiatric areas. Yellows, oranges, and reds are energizing and suitable for children's areas.
- Keep the area **well ventilated**, regularly vacuumed, well-lit with as much window light as possible, and cool to discourage the growth of pathogens.
- Choose **washable fabrics** and surfaces that are easy to disinfect.
- **Small chairs, tables, and toys for children** help them pass the time easily. Choose large, hard toys with no small parts that can be swallowed and laminated books, which can be wiped with disinfectant every day to prevent the spread of infection.
- **Plants** help to calm and screen patients to give them privacy. Make sure they are not toxic, heavily scented, or parasite carriers.
- **Classical music** and news programs help mask private conversations. Magazines should be current and not contain perfume inserts.
- **Keep absorbent, rubber-backed rugs and boot trays** in the entrance and tile floors in the examining areas.

Maintaining a Medical Office According to Government Asepsis Standards

OSHA requires that medical offices use good aseptic technique to reduce the spread of disease. Disinfection means cleaning objects to eliminate most pathogenic (disease-causing) microorganisms, such as bacteria, viruses, molds, and parasites. Disinfection and sanitization (washing) do not eliminate spores, which are dormant (sleeping) bacteria waiting for more hospitable growing conditions, or the seeds of algae, fungi, plants, and a few protozoans. The only way to kill spores is by autoclave oven. Autoclaving is appropriate for small instruments but not furniture or other large surfaces. To **maintain the office according to OSHA recommendations**:

- Prepare a fresh solution of germicidal detergent daily. Use the detergent to wipe down soiled walls, mattress covers, furniture, and any equipment that is not the responsibility of Central Sterile Supply (CSS). Mop the floors or wet-vacuum them if there is no housekeeping service.
- Post the appropriate signs outside isolation rooms. Keep the necessary isolation equipment outside of the isolation room for staff and visitors to don and doff.
- Keep a pump bottle of 70-80% alcohol cleanser at the entrance to each exam room and at the front desk.

Reception Tasks

The **medical assistant at the reception** desk is responsible for the following:

- Directing outpatient traffic and salespeople
- Accepting drop-off specimens and courier deliveries
- Scheduling appointments
- Collecting insurance information
- Answering the switchboard
- Responding to emergencies

Reputable medical sales representatives sell innovative drugs and equipment that keep doctors current; arrange for the doctor to make additional money as a researcher, lecturer, or demonstrator; and provide important training materials. Representatives book appointments well in advance. Allow only one sales representative on the premises at a time, and do not allow them to touch patients. Ensure a staff member accompanies them to the stockroom and that they do not open sterile supplies or remove a competitor's products. Ask the doctor if staff is allowed to accept gifts or samples from medical companies. When any non-patient visitor is on the premises, do not allow him or her to film or access patient and financial files without a legal search warrant. If a salesperson or reporter arrives unannounced, explain that patient care is paramount, and an appointment is required. Have police wait away from reception, accompanied by staff, until the doctor is available.

Filing Systems

The following are types of filing systems:

- **Alphabetic**: Indexing files from A to Z, in the same sequence as the letters of the alphabet. It is less accurate than numeric filing.
- **Numeric/terminal digit**: Indexing by numbers, especially the last unit. It is more accurate than alphabetical filing.
- **Subject**: Classifying, coding, and storing documents according to their topic, such as *Sales Receipts* or *Surgical Inventory*.
- **Tickler**: Also called a suspense file. Indexing files according to upcoming actions or unconcluded transactions, such as arranging an annual service check by a mechanic before the warranty expires.
- **EDP** (**E**lectronic **D**ata **P**rocessing): Use of a computer to record, classify arrange, summarize, and report information.
- **Cross-reference**: A direction to the reader to check another section for a more complete explanation or related information.
- **Master**: A computer file that contains long-term information, such as a patient database or payroll records. The master is updated regularly and workers refer to it as the most reliable source of information.
- **Color-coded**: Placing colored stickers on files to identify them quickly, usually so they can be purged easily. For example, medical files more than 10 years old can be legally purged; if all 10-year-old files have purple stickers, then the purging job can be safely delegated to a junior clerk.

Office Communication

Correct Comma Use

Commas separate parts of a sentence that need to be emphasized or isolated so that the sentence will make sense. Commas set apart afterthoughts ("You look marvelous, my dear"), interrupting elements ("It makes sense, I think, to go ahead with the plan"), transitional phrases ("Roger, on the other hand, was prepared for action"), or descriptive expressions ("My new book, *Feeling Young Again*, is available in paperback"). Commas set the year apart in a representation of the date, and set apart all of the abbreviations and titles that follow a person's name.

Do not use a comma to set a verb apart from its object or complement. Do not use a comma to separate adjectives from their succeeding nouns or to separate a noun from the prepositional phrase that follows it. Commas can be used to divide two independent clauses in a sentence when the clauses are connected by *and, but, or*, or *nor*. Commas can divide three or more items in a series or more than one adjective that is being used to modify the same noun.

Correct Semicolon Use

Semicolons are meant to be used between independent clauses in a sentence whenever there is not conjunction such as *and* or *but*. Use a semicolon between clauses whenever one of the clauses has several commas, and the addition of another comma separating the two clauses has the potential to make the sentence unclear. Semicolons should be used to separate the independent clauses in a sentence any time the conjunction between the two sentences is *besides, consequently, nevertheless, however*, or *therefore*. It is also appropriate to use semicolons to separate the items in a list when the items in that list contain commas; for instance, a list of dates that includes the years should be separated by semicolons.

Correct Colon Use

Colons are used before the beginning of a list and to separate two independent clauses when the second cause elaborates on the first clause and there is no transitional expression or coordinating conjunction. Use a colon to set apart hours and minutes in a description of the time, as in 8:20. Use a colon to divide the units in a ratio, as in, "Make a 1:5 dilution of sodium hypochlorite in water." Colons are used in lieu of commas in the salutation line of a business document. Legal letters and personal correspondence use a comma after the salutation. In the documents familiar to a medical assistant, a colon is found in the reference notations, attention lines, subject lines, enclosure notations, copy notations, and postscripts.

Colons can be used to draw attention to a certain part of a sentence. For instance, a colon might be used after the word *therefore* in order to emphasize the insight that is to follow. Colons can also be effectively used in cases where the anticipatory phrase is not explicit, as in "Red foxes are beautiful creatures: long tails, keen eyes, and sleek pelts." Avoid using a colon when the anticipatory expression is at the beginning of an extremely long sentence.

Capitalization, Parentheses, and Quotation Marks

Capitalize the following words:

- First word in a sentence or list
- Independent questions within a sentence
- Proper nouns
- Adjectives derived from proper nouns
- Imaginative names and nicknames
- Each item in an outline
- The first word of a quoted sentence

Simple common nouns, like police officer or doctor, need not be capitalized.

Parentheses are used to set nonessential items apart, identify a citation, or to surround a brief explanation for example. Parentheses are often used for dates, references, authorities, or items on a list.

Quotation marks indicate the title of a piece of work. They may provide a special emphasis to certain words or phrases, or they may indicate that a person's exact words are being used. Any periods or commas at the end of a phrase inside quotation marks should be inside the quotation marks, though all semicolons and colons will go outside. Exclamation points and quotation marks should only go inside quotation marks when they are applied strictly to the quoted expression.

Greek Characters and Mathematical Symbols and Equations

To find Greek characters and mathematical symbols in Microsoft Word, choose *Insert* > *Symbol* > *More Symbols.* Scroll through the *Subsets.* To type the equation in Microsoft Word, choose *Insert* > *Equation* > and either *Built-In* or *Insert New Equation.*

Character	Pronunciation	Character	Pronunciation
α	alpha	ν	nu
β	beta	ξ	xi
γ	gamma	ο	omicron
δ	delta	π	pi
ε	epsilon	ρ	rho
ζ	zeta	σ	sigma
η	eta	τ	tau
θ	theta	υ	upsilon
ι	iota	φ	phi
κ	kappa	χ	chi
λ	lambda	ψ	psi
μ	mu	ω	omega

PROOFREADING ROUGH DRAFTS

To create accurate documents, a medical assistant must be adept at **proofreading**. The basic steps of proofreading a document are:

1. **Read backwards**: Three complete readings of a document are required. During the first reading, look for errors in punctuation and spelling, and word repetition with a software spellchecker. In the second reading, look for layout, grammar and style mistakes and add new words to the custom dictionary in the software's spellchecker. Here, it is helpful to read the document backwards, starting with the last sentence and working back up. This helps the author to see each sentence on its own. In the third reading, consider syntax. Ensure the document flows in logical sequence, and is easy to read and understand.
2. **Correct**: Check questionable words with the following references: Medical dictionary; English dictionary; drug compendium; spelling, grammar, and punctuation checking software; thesaurus; and directories (books or online) with the current addresses of relevant doctors, hospitals, and clinics.
3. **Revise**: Query the doctor in square or angle brackets or use Word's comment feature.
4. **Create an error analysis chart**: Keep a record of mistakes to save time in future.

TELEPHONE ETIQUETTE

Elements of appropriate telephone etiquette include the following:

- When starting work, ask the doctor which calls to put through immediately and which should be screened. Give messages to the doctor between appointments.
- Turn the lines over to a reliable answering service whenever out of the office. Record a detailed message (including where to go in an emergency and fax number for pharmacies) with music intervals whenever busy and check messages frequently.
- Get a landline number for the doctor when possible. Most hospitals forbid the use of cellular phones because they interfere with telemetry. They often permit pagers instead, but doctors cannot answer them in the OR.
- Write all telephone messages in a book with carbon copies, not on scrap paper. Include the caller's name, patient's name, phone number, a brief message, and the pharmacy or referring doctor's number.
- End personal calls immediately when a patient arrives. Acknowledge patients who arrive when on a medical call.

PRIORITIZING INCOMING TELEPHONE CALLS

The medical assistant answers the telephone within three rings. Identify oneself with, "Good morning/afternoon. Dr. Gentle's office, [your name] speaking." Record the caller's name, number, and detailed information in the day log. Do not put a call on hold until being certain that it is not an emergency.

Screen the call to determine if it is emergent, urgent, or routine. Do not interrupt the doctor, unless it is emergent or he or she instructs you to do so. If the doctor is occupied, instruct the emergent caller to go to the nearest emergency room. Phone 911 if the caller is unable to do so.

For routine and urgent calls, say, "The doctor is with a patient. May I give the doctor a message and ask him/her to return your call?" Most doctors allocate one hour per day to return phone calls and prepare prescriptions for the assistant to fax to pharmacies. The medical assistant must not give medical advice. Ask the routine or urgent caller to make an appointment. Do not release test results over the phone, unless instructed to do so by the doctor. Pass along urgent messages to the doctor before routine messages.

Managing Emergency Situations Via Telephone

Some states have very specific guidelines as to which healthcare professional are able to screen patients by telephone or to give directions, so the certified medical assistant must be aware of state guidelines. Medical assistants, who are not trained or licensed to diagnose or give medical advice, can generally screen telephone calls but must be knowledgeable about the types of questions to ask and should follow a screening manual when taking calls to ensure consistency. The screening manual should list the appropriate questions to ask depending on the patient's complaints/issues and indicate which responses require intervention of other healthcare providers, such as emergency medical personnel or an RN. When using a screening manual, the medical assistant should not deviate from the manual and should immediately consult a nurse or physician if the patient's complaints are not in the manual or the medical assistant has concerns (such as the inability to make an immediate appointment for a patient in distress).

Distribution of Test Results

Informing Patients of Test Results

Patients should be informed of diagnostic procedure results as soon as possible, as patients are often anxious when awaiting results. Once test results are received and the date entered into the diagnostic procedure tracking log, the test should be reviewed by the ordering healthcare provider before the patient is notified of the results. The healthcare provider should indicate who should notify the patient. When test results are negative, the medical assistant may be tasked with notifying the patient either by letter (standard format is generally utilized) or telephone. If test results are positive and/or follow-up is required, then the ordering healthcare provider or a nurse usually contacts the patient. In some cases, the medical assistant may need to make a follow-up appointment for the healthcare provider to discuss test results with the patient. For serious results, such as a positive finding of cancer, the physician should speak directly to the patient, in person if possible.

Handling Results Received from Outside Providers

Results from **outside providers** may include consultant reports and diagnostic test results. The physician should be immediately notified as per office protocol when a consultant report is received and a notation made in the patient's medical record. The diagnostic procedure tracking log is used to record all diagnostic procedures that are scheduled to ensure that no results are overlooked and that patients are informed of the results of all tests. Formats may vary somewhat. The diagnostic procedure tracking log should be filled out immediately when procedures are scheduled and again when results are received. The log should be checked every work day at the beginning of the day and again at the end so that calls to patients are made in a timely manner and recorded. The physician should be notified when diagnostic results are received and the results included in the patient's medical record.

Medical Transcription

Standard Set-Up for Medical Transcriptions

The standard set-up for any transcription includes the following:

- 8.5" x 11" white bond paper with black ink
- Margins at least 1" on all sides
- Portrait orientation
- Headings flush with the left margin, except for manuscripts, in which they are centered
- Double space between heading lines, paragraphs, and below the last line of the message
- Triple space before the memo, report, or chart message
- Most medical offices use full block style
- Double space drafts, with 5 spaces indented at the beginning of each paragraph
- Single space the body of the corrected message when it is ready to print and sign
- If the document is longer than one page, type the recipient's name, page number, date, and RE: Patient's Name at the top of each page.

Every document must contain:

- Date (and time if it is an Operating Room Report)
- Unique patient identifier (e.g., medical record number)
- Patient's name
- Dictator's name and credentials
- Typist's initials at the bottom left margin

Transcription Errors

The patient's health and life are at stake if a medical transcriptionist makes an **error**. One's reputation will be crippled if errors are discovered by accreditation surveyors or judges. Some of the most common errors found in medical records are incorrect usage, misspelling, added or omitted letters, grammatical errors, confusion of unfamiliar words, and confusion of similar-sounding words (homonyms). These errors can largely be avoided through careful proofreading and reference to the appropriate sources. Remember that the patient's health and life are also adversely impacted by transcription delays and slow turnaround time. Always find out which dictations are STAT before beginning the workday, and prioritize accordingly.

Difficulties for Novice Transcriptionists

Novice transcriptionists often have a hard time learning to understand medical dictation, especially if the doctor has a foreign accent or a strong local dialect. Medical recordings are frequently made in a loud setting with many distractions, so they are choppy, disjointed, and bursting with jargon and medical terminology. A transcriptionist's income and reputation depend on productivity and accuracy. New transcriptionists need to make use of medical dictionaries and other references in order to make sense of medical dictation. They should familiarize themselves with the dictionary or reference format for quick and effective use. In most medical dictionaries, the most commonly used noun is listed as the main entry and any related terms are subentries.

Reference Sources for Transcriptions

The ***Pharmaceutical Reference Guide*** and ***CPS*** are alphabetical indices of all the drugs that have been approved for prescription by the Food and Drug Administration. The entry for each drug will include the drug's method of administration, recommended dosage, classification, indications and contraindications of use, generic name, and brand names. These books are expensive and released annually, so it is more cost effective to pay for an up-to-date online subscription or check the FDA Orange Book, available for free on the FDA's website. Other useful reference books include the *Taber's Cyclopedic Medical Dictionary*, and the *Medical Word Book* and *Surgical Word Book*, both available from Saunders. Word books contain an alphabetical list of all the words that are commonly associated with medical and surgical procedures but do not contain definitions. Users should find the closest sounding entry that makes sense when they cannot understand a dictated word.

Transcribing Doctor's Dictation

Time permitting, a medical transcriptionist should listen to the entire dictation tape before he or she begins to transcribe a document. This helps the transcriptionist to get a general idea of the structure of the dictation and have an opportunity to notice any areas of difficulty or complexity. Resources should be used to identify difficult words; similar documents transcribed by predecessors can be used for comparison. Once the initial listening is complete, the transcriptionist can begin listening to small portions of the tape and transcribing them electronically. After the entire tape has been transcribed, he or she can begin the process of proofreading. Institutional regulations should be followed to erase and reuse a tape.

Operative Report and Postoperative Notes

Provided that surgery progressed well, the OR team transfers accountability for the patient to the recovery room team. The surgeon dictates a detailed **operative report**. The patient's physiological functioning generally returns to normal over 1-3 hours, depending on the type of surgery and anesthesia. The physician's assistant on the surgery usually dictates a brief **postoperative note**, which is not as detailed as a progress report, and can use abbreviations if the facility allows them. The following information should be included in the postoperative note:

- Date and time
- Unique patient identifier (e.g., medical record number)
- Patient's name
- Subjective symptoms (e.g., how the patient reports on the following: complaints of discomfort or anxiety, pain control, passing flatus, diet, comfort when ambulating)
- Objective signs (e.g., vital signs, edema, bowel sounds, chest sounds, incision status)
- Assessment (e.g., "The 42-year-old white female was alert and responsive after laparoscopic cholecystectomy…")
- Plan (e.g., remove Foley catheter, change from IV to oral pain control, advance to soft diet when flatus occurs, encourage ambulation)

Progress Reports

If the patient experienced complications during surgery or has difficulty recovering from anesthesia, he or she is transferred to the intensive care unit (ICU) for close monitoring. Vital signs (temperature, pulse, respirations, blood pressure, level of consciousness) are checked every 15-30 minutes. The interval increases as the patient's condition returns to baseline. The nurse may obtain central venous pressures and fluid balance (tracking all fluids that enter and exit the patient). The patient is stabilized before being moved to a step-down unit. The patient may move from step-down back to ICU or to an in-patient unit, according to his or her condition. The doctor, PA, or nurse practitioner dictates regular **progress reports** with more details than the Post Op Note. The progress report contains the following:

- Date and time
- Medical record number
- Patient's name
- Current level of functioning
- Amount of progress made
- Age appropriateness
- Assessments and plan
- The dictator's signature
- Avoid abbreviations and write in full sentences

Discharge Summary

The **discharge summary** is dictated at time of discharge. It contains the following:

- Admission and discharge dates
- Patient's name and medical record number
- Attending physician's name and contact information
- Chief complaint or reason(s) for admission
- History and physical examination
- Laboratory and x-ray findings
- Principal diagnosis
- Description of treatment
- Additional diagnoses
- Description of surgical procedure
- Disposition instructions given to the patient and/or caregivers (e.g., limit physical activity, medication timing, dietary restrictions, and follow-up appointment schedule)
- Prognosis for recovery
- Attending physician's signature and date

Documents required in the chart by law are the following:

- History and Physical Examination
- Operative Report
- Inpatient Progress Note
- Final Discharge Note

Discharge summaries are not required for routine births with a normal baby, including uncomplicated cesarean sections. If the patient's chart remains incomplete after 30 days, then the doctor's admitting privileges may be suspended.

FINAL DISCHARGE NOTE

The intermediate recovery period follows the immediate postoperative period and continues until the patient's hospitalization is complete. The patient has totally recovered from anesthesia and the emphasis shifts to healing, maintaining a nutritious diet, and regaining independence. The case manager arranges therapy with the rehabilitation team and home care with visiting nurses. The doctor dictates a **final discharge note** for any patient hospitalized longer than 24 hours. Do not use abbreviations in the final discharge note. It is not as detailed as the discharge summary. Include this information:

- Date and time
- Principal diagnosis that required hospital admission
- Complications that developed during hospitalization and extended length of stay
- Comorbidities present prior to admission that require follow-up and additional resources (e.g., diabetes)
- Principle procedure related to the diagnosis
- Discharge plan, including available resources for home care or community care
- Signature of attending physician

Business Practices

Office Equipment

The medical assistant operates the following standard office equipment:

- Calculator
- Photocopier
- Computer
- Fax
- Telephone
- Scanner

In larger facilities, engineering welds an identification tag to each piece of equipment. The facilities manager (CHFM) tracks its whereabouts. Security investigates theft and vandalism. Security controls traffic, access, identification of personnel, and creates an environment that is reassuring to persons with a legitimate reason for being at the facility. In a small office environment, the medical assistant records all serial numbers and photographs each piece of equipment for insurance purposes. The medical assistant creates a sign-out log to keep track of borrowed equipment, asks local police and fire officials to perform a review of office security and fire safety, and reports theft and vandalism to local police.

Managing Equipment with a Tickler File

File the manufacturer's recommendations for a preventative maintenance schedule when buying a new piece of equipment, and put the suggested date in the **tickler file** as a reminder. If there is no instruction guide provided when a second-hand machine was purchased, ask the vendor to provide one, or ask a biomedical engineer to write a manual as a resource for less skilled workers. Start a maintenance log for each new machine purchased, and keep it for the life of the machine or until its tax depreciation is finished, whichever comes later. Update the log with a description of each maintenance item performed, the name of the maintenance worker, the date and duration of maintenance, along with possible problems and feedback from the maintenance worker. Keep the log readily available with any relevant publications, such as service and operation manuals, and specialized tools for workers' use. Inspection and repair records, inspection schedules, and "as-built" drawings are also among the resources that should be available.

Processing of Work Orders When Equipment Fails or Must Be Moved

The medical assistant sends a **work order** to the maintenance department secretary by internal mail, fax, email, or phone. The maintenance secretary logs and time stamps the work order. The secretary alerts the supervisor if there are duplicate requests for the same work, and may phone the medical assistant to obtain clarification for the maintenance supervisor and to get the cost center number (if applicable). The supervisor reviews the work order to prioritize it. Work orders are not performed on a first-come-first-served basis. Work orders are prioritized as emergency (something that must be done at once), routine (something that should be done as quickly and efficiently as possible), and backlogged (something that must wait for parts, replacement, or cannot be done right away for some other reason). The supervisor may investigate who can do the work at the lowest cost. The supervisor signs the work order to authorize the work to begin as requested, and follows up to ensure it was completed.

MAINTENANCE AND REPAIRS OF MEDICAL AND OFFICE EQUIPMENT

In larger facilities, the facilities manager (CHFM) is responsible for equipment in all departments. In a small medical office, the medical assistant is responsible for ensuring the terms of a warranty or guarantee are fulfilled. The medical assistant deals with vendors and ensures that delivery dates and other specifications of purchase contracts are met. Careful record keeping lowers the risk of a warranty being voided based on poor maintenance. File all warranty records.

A large facility may have a **computerized maintenance management system (CMMS)** that contains illustrations and instructions for use of each piece of equipment. Scan the warranty into the facility's CMMS. In a small office, a manual **tickler file** is kept to prompt the medical assistant to schedule equipment maintenance on time. The tickler file helps reduce the costs associated with a piece of equipment by ensuring it is serviced according to the terms of its warranty. Include the expiration date of the warranty on the CMMS or tickler card.

MAIL

TYPES OF INCOMING MAIL

Types of incoming mail include the following:

Type of Mail	Example Carrier/Client
Routine letters and packages	United States Postal Service
Electronic money transfers	Western Union, chartered banks
Urgent letters and packages	Couriers such as DHL, FedEx, UPS; bike messengers
STAT specimens and drugs	Taxi-cab; armored vehicle (Brinks); Bus Express
Fax (facsimile)	Private offices, pharmacies, copy shops, postal outlets, hotels
Interoffice mail	Mailroom, porters, runners

HANDLING INCOMING MAIL

The modern medical assistant handles less paper today because email and voicemail have replaced most surface mail. The medical assistant can expedite processing so the doctor can deal with incoming mail efficiently by doing the following:

- Sign for insured or couriered mail and pay postage due from petty cash.
- Sort according to urgency the letters, bills, statements, interoffice, personal, newspapers and periodicals, ads and catalogs, and parcels.
- Open all mail except that marked "Personal and Confidential." If the addressee no longer works for the company, it goes to the successor if it is business-related. Forward personal mail to the last known home address.
- Inspect all business contents. If a date, signature, enclosure, or return address is missing, staple the envelope to the letter and annotate it. Tape torn letters. Discard most ads.
- Date and time stamp all mail for legal protection.
- Read and annotate each piece of mail, especially if it mentions an appointment date, a report being mailed separately, confirmation of a phone conversation, or requests a decision requiring more information.
- Present the doctor's mail to him or her covered in a folder to maintain confidentiality, with the most urgent on top.
- Distribute, route, or answer the remaining mail, as required.

Preventing Mail from Getting Delayed or Lost

The following are the five tools the medical assistant uses to prevent mail from getting delayed or lost on another employee's desk:

- **Expected mail record**: If the medical assistant reads in the incoming mail that a report or other item will arrive separately, he or she should make note of it. When the expected item arrives, retrieve the original correspondence and attach it behind the new mail.
- **Annotation**: If there is a discrepancy or problem with the letter, write a note to the addressee in the margin. Examples:
    - The amount on an enclosed check does not match the amount stated in the letter.
    - The writer asks for a specific appointment time that conflicts with an existing booking.
- **Routing slip**: If the manager wants everyone in the office to read an item, attach a slip listing all their names, the reading sequence, and the date by which they need the item returned. Instruct the readers to initial and date the routing slip when they read the item.
- **Action requested slip**: Give informal directions to the reader, such as, "Please handle this for Marie while she is on vacation."
- **Digest of incoming mail**: When the manager is away for more than two days, log mail by date, sender, content, and the action taken, such as forwarding a request for employment verification to Human Resources.

Processing Outgoing Mail

Cover outgoing mail at the desk with a folder or satchel to keep the addressee confidential. Delivery price is determined by size, weight, shape, urgency, destination, route (air or surface), insurance, signature verification, and contents. Price changes frequently, so check the USPS rate calculator on the USPS website. If insufficient postage is applied, then the item will be returned. If a return address is not included, then USPS will collect postage due from the recipient. Buy correct stamps and envelopes online at the USPS website.

Send items over 70 lb by freight carrier. The Department of Transportation (DOT) regulates shipping of diagnostic and biological specimens, infectious substances, and anything shipped on dry ice. Follow standards set by the International Air Transport Association (IATA), regardless of the distance the package is being shipped, or the transportation method (truck, rail, air, boat). The medical assistant needs the IATA Blue Pages to fill out the shipping manifest with the IATA shipping name, class, subsidiary risk, and UN codes. A Class 6.2 DOT sticker is also required, and if the biological is preserved with dry ice, a Class 9 DOT sticker.

Medical Inventory

The doctor and specialists inform the medical assistant which medical supply companies they purchase from routinely. Produce a list of required supplies, known as a **medical inventory**, including the following:

- Item name
- Size
- Color
- Number
- Units
- Cost
- Supplier's name
- Supplier's address
- Supplier's phone and fax numbers

This list tells the medical assistant how long an item lasts, when to reorder, and cost comparisons. Prescription pads and drug samples are available free from drug company sales reps.

Check the drug and supply cupboards against the supply list daily and weekly. Ensure the office always has adequate supplies available, but remember that reagents and drugs expire. Reorder before supplies are exhausted from the authorized suppliers only. Do not order large quantities without the doctor's authorization, as they may stale-date. Include the price quote on the purchase order (PO). Keep a copy of the PO in a pending file until the supplies arrive, for comparison to the packing slip.

Always lock the supply and drug cupboards. Drug addicts target painkillers, sleeping pills, tranquilizers, and syringes, so consult Pharmacy and Security about safe storage. Do not flush expired drugs down the toilet because they cause environmental harm. Call the hospital Pharmacy or drug rep to have the expired drugs incinerated.

Operating Systems and Software Used in Medical Offices

Most private medical offices use Windows **operating systems** on networked PCs. Most medical offices use Microsoft Office software, including Word, Outlook, Excel, Access, and PowerPoint. Common billing software packages are ABLEMed, EMR, Lytec, or Medisoft. The advantages of prepackaged software are that it is relatively cheap and many healthcare providers are already familiar with them. However, they are not customizable. The facility may hire programmers to write customized, proprietary software. Web-based scheduling and billing packages, such as Medical Office Online, are often much more expensive than prepackaged software.

If the clinic cannot afford prepackaged software, free alternatives to many of them are available, such as OpenOffice, an open-source software package that is largely compatible with Microsoft Office.

Safeguarding Patient Data

Medical office computers must comply with 1996 HIPAA Security Standards for the Protection of Electronic Protected Information. It is important for the medical assistant to recognize potential fraud and abuse. An unscrupulous user may sell a patient's information to a journalist or detective, or use it to stalk the patient, or alter the record to hide wrongdoing. **Safeguarding of patient data** includes the following:

- The medical assistant safeguards against computer viruses and hackers with regular antivirus and firewall updates.
- The supervisor ensures only authorized personnel access electronic health records (EHR) through an audit trail. The supervisor asks the IT Dept. to restrict access to a patient's EHR. The computer alerts the supervisor to a security breach (when someone attempts unauthorized access to the patient's EHR). The supervisor follows Standard ASTM E2147-01, which lists the specifications for audit trails in manual and EHR environments. Investigators will see who accessed a record, when, where, and previous versions.
- The IT programmer can restore the previous information through **versioning**, so that any tampering or falsification is not permanent.

Securing Electronic Applications Containing Patient Information

Measures to ensure the security of electronic applications containing patient information include:

- **Password**: Passwords should be strong but not so complex that users write them down because that increases risk of unauthorized access. Passwords should be changed on a regularly scheduled basis, such as monthly. Passwords should not be birthdates, anniversary dates, or names of children or pets.
- **Screen saver**: Medical screensavers should be set to automatically launch after a specified period of time to protect any information that may be left on the screen.
- **Encryption**: All information entered into the application or transmitted must be encrypted (protected by converting to code) so that it cannot be accessed without the proper password.
- **Firewall**: A computer application or hardware that blocks unauthorized access to computer programs and data and monitors incoming data to ensure its safety. Firewalls can also block internet users from accessing private networks (such as medical networks).

Protocols for Using Social Media

Some medical practices/organizations utilize **social media**, such as blogs, social networks, and websites, to communicate with patients and allow patients to set up appointments, obtain lab results, send messages, and receive messages. Strict protocols should be established for use of social media by healthcare professionals, including who has access, how access is obtained, the types of responses that are appropriate, and methods of dealing with inappropriate comments (such as from an angry patient). Personal social media, such as a personal Facebook account or Twitter account, should never be used to discuss any patient, patient care, or other healthcare-related issues associated with employment as this may violate HIPAA regulations regarding privacy and security and could place the practice/organization at risk for liability. Some healthcare organizations do not permit employees to even mention the place of employment on social media, so the medical assistant must review employment policies.

Principles of Ergonomics and Proper Body Mechanics

Ergonomics is the study of how to design work and products according to principles of body mechanics to avoid injury, especially in the workplace. **Proper body mechanics** include the following as it relates to lifting and carrying heavy objects:

- Avoid reaching for prolonged periods of time, overhead, or more than 20 inches
- Avoid pulling—push, roll, or slide instead
- Avoid lifting—pull, push, roll, or slide instead
- Lift with leg muscles, not back
- Hold weight close to body rather than at arm's length
- Flex at hips and knees, not waist
- Maintain a straight back and avoid twisting
- Assess weight and recognize limitations in lifting/carrying
- Get help when necessary and communicate every step with partner ("Lift on the count of three")
- Maintain firm base of support with feet apart (shoulder width) to stabilize stance
- Maintain line of gravity (imaginary line between center of gravity and ground) within the base of support
- Position oneself close to the object that is to be lifted or carried

Preventing Repetitive Strain Injuries Through Computer Work

Supporting the principles of ergonomics includes designing a work environment that promotes comfortable, safe, and injury-free work. Because some of a medical assistant's responsibilities require time behind the computer, the **set-up of the computer and desk** must be done so in a manner that encourages proper body mechanics, and therefore **prevents repetitive strain injuries**. Consider the following:

- The work area must allow for full range of motion, including sufficient knee and leg room.
- An ideal chair has five castors, an adjustable seat and back, a broad base, a foot bar and lumbar supports, armrests low enough that they are not used during keyboarding, and a shallow seat to permit leaning backwards.
- The medical assistant should sit with the thighs at or just above the knees, feet firmly planted on the floor, and head directly over the shoulders.
- Position the monitor with the top just below eye level and at a slightly backward incline.
- Position the keyboard at a height that allows for relaxed shoulders and forearms parallel to the floor.
- Protect oneself from eyestrain with an anti-glare screen and by looking away from the computer for 10 minutes every hour.
- Use more lighting for dark walls and paper handling than for light walls and working with computer monitors.
- Use a mouse pad with a gel wrist support.

Recordkeeping

Retention of Health Information

Health information is retained for predetermined periods of time, depending on the type of information:

Type of Information	AHIMA Recommended Retention Period
Adult medical record	10 years after the most recent encounter
Birth register	Permanently
Child (minor) medical record	Age of majority + statute of limitations
Death register	Permanently
Diagnostic images and x-rays	5 years
Disease index	10 years
Fetal heart monitor record	10 years after child reaches age of majority
Master patient index	Permanently
Operative index	10 years
Physician index	10 years
Surgical procedures register	Permanently

Consider federal and state statutes and regulations, the organization's policy, and the amount of storage space available before making a decision to purge. State and federal statutes of limitations determine the maximum of amount of time after an event that a lawsuit can be filed.

Permanently Retained Patient Information

Collaborate with the Medical Records manager on a retention and destruction schedule. Retain the following patient information permanently:

- Dates of admission, discharge, and encounters
- Physician names
- Diagnoses and procedures
- History and physical reports
- Operative and pathology reports
- Discharge summaries

Dispensation of Medical Records When a Facility Closes

In the event the medical facility closes, the medical assistant must carefully plan and articulate the **transfer of medical records**. If the facility is sold to another healthcare provider, then the records usually go to the new provider. If the employer is retiring and his or her practice will not be assumed by a successor, then arrange a storage contract with:

- Another healthcare provider
- The facility's attorney
- An appropriate storage facility

Scan the records so they remain accessible electronically. The State Department provides other options for dispensation of records. The medical assistant is responsible for ensuring that:

- The records are as complete as possible before transfer
- Living patients are kept informed if records are transferred

Identifying Theft Prevention

Elements of identity theft prevention include the following:

- **Answering machines/voicemail**: Never play messages aloud where they can be overheard. Use the receiver or earphones.
- **Fax**: Only dedicated lines should be used for faxes, and messages should be removed from the machine and properly filed immediately to prevent unauthorized access.
- **Email**: Never use emails to transmit information that should remain confidential.
- **Patient admission**: Greet patients in private if possible, but if the admission desk is in an open area, move the patient to a different area if personal questions must be asked, such as date of birth and Medicare number, or ask for the information needed in writing.
- **Computer**: All information should be password protected (with password changed frequently) and access limited to only those records the healthcare provider is authorized to use.
- **Telephone**: Conversations should be in private if possible. If not, care should be taken to avoid stating any identifying information that may be overheard.

Source-Oriented and Problem-Oriented Medical Records

Source-oriented medical records are as follows:

- They are paper-based.
- They are organized by practitioner.
- Source-oriented records keep information in reverse chronological order in each section, with the latest information at the beginning.
- If a record is kept in the same order during and after care, it has "universal" chart order.

Advantage: Particular aspects of patient care can be readily accessed, such as lab reports or patient response to medication

Disadvantage: Does not allow easy access to particular patient problems or the contributions of each department to a specific problem

Problem-oriented medical records are as follows:

- They are paper-based.
- Problem-oriented records contain four sections: A database of standard checklists, a problem list, an initial plan, and progress notes.
- The problems are numbered, and the plans and progress notes are numbered to match the problem.

Advantage: Provides holistic patient information by problem

Disadvantage: Difficult to maintain

Integrated vs. Electronic Health Records

Integrated health records are paper-based and primarily kept in reverse chronological order. Each episode of care is defined by date, with the latest information at the beginning.

- **Advantages**: Integrated medical records provide easy access to current information, and the chronology of patient care is quickly apparent.
- **Disadvantage**: Integrated medical records do not allow easy access to particular aspects of patient care, by problem or by practitioner.
- **Note**: Some integrated medical records do divide lab reports from Progress Notes, making them more user-friendly.

Electronic health records are computer-based. Any chart order format can be the default in an electronic health record, with other formats available through data manipulation.

- **Advantages**: Electronic health records up less storage space, and can be parsed (arranged and rearranged) for specific kinds of access.
- **Disadvantages**: Software and hardware may become obsolete, so a paper back-up is legally required, expensive equipment and training are required, and stringent security is required to protect from hackers.

Electronic Health Records

The healthcare industry developed a foundational technology infrastructure with plans for expansion with added technological developments. Its primary component is the electronic health record (EHR), developed to share medical information easily among patients, providers, payers/insurers, and government agencies. The EHR includes:

- **Electronic medical records (EMRs)** generated by healthcare providers for individual patients
- **Point-of-care clinical information systems**, which allow caregivers to collect and input data at the bedside or service area on monitors and electronically transmit it by modem
- A **Decision Support System (DSS)**, a computerized system that gathers information from various sources and uses analytical models to assist providers in clinical decision-making

HIPAA requires standardized data formats for easy, secure information transfer.

Data Types and Data Interface Standards

The following represent the basic types of data included in an electronic health record (EHR) and the sort of information that might typically be expressed by these types:

- **Text**: Reports, such as discharge summary, history and physical, and operative
- **Numbers**: ICD-10-CM codes, CFI codes, and blood pressure values
- **Voice**: Stored dictation accessed by phone or personal computer, voice recognition, or radiology images
- **Images**: Radiology film and document images
- **Video**: Echocardiograms
- **Drawings**: Rule of 9s charts showing burn distribution on the patient's skin surface
- **Signal**: EEG or EKG tracings

Data-interface standards, such as those developed by X12 and HL7 standard development organizations, are standardized data formats that allow data to be transferred between units or facilities. HIPAA legislation imposes standards on data exchange of billing data to reduce administrative costs associated with the billing process. Certain coding systems and an X12 schema for data transfer are required.

Privacy, Confidentiality, and Security

Privacy refers to the rights of individuals to control disclosure of their personal information. It is the principle behind HIPAA, mandated confidentiality requirements, and responding data security measures. **Confidentiality** is endorsed by health professionals as a legal and ethical obligation to meet the expectation of privacy from patients. **Data security** refers to the technical and procedural methods that manage and control confidential information.

Medical assistants oversee confidentiality matters and update organizational policies and procedures. It is important to review policies and procedures in light of the health record system, particularly if procedures have been developed around a paper-based environment, but the facility is moving to an electronic environment. Remember that the protection of confidentiality and patient privacy is not only a systems issue, but also a personnel issue in that training and oversight of facility personnel provide a distinguishing measure of security above and beyond system security.

Thinning Paper Records and Coding Health Records

In a paper-based environment, hard copy health records must be thinned during a patient's long-term stay when the file has become too cumbersome to handle on a regular basis. **The thinned portions** are not destroyed but are returned to the main file room and should still be accessible.

Health records must be **coded**, which is the process of applying facility and professional coding, usually for billing purposes. In an electronic health record (EHR) environment, coding is done in the EHR on an ongoing basis and should be available when needed. In a paper or partial-paper environment, hospital information management (HIM) departments must be diligent about getting codes applied to paper records; paper records arrive in HIM for coding a period of time after the patient is discharged. HIM professionals also need to develop procedures for a combined environment, using electronic and hand coding.

Authentication of Patient Records

The Joint Commission requires the following health records to be **authenticated with a date and signature**: History and physical (H&P), operative reports, consultations, and discharge summaries. Individual facilities may require authentication of additional records. All records requiring authentication must be signed by the original author, not a delegate. Some require countersignatures (e.g., the department head or admitting cashier). Consult federal, state, and facility regulations for authentication policies. The following considerations must be made:

- Basic authentication requires only an initial and a last name. Eliminate error by using full first names for staff with similar or duplicate last names.
- Keep a historical legend accessible in the facility to match initials and signatures with names, because staff rotate, quit, or retire.
- Signature stamps are unsafe. Keep a disclaimer on file, stating the doctor/owner takes legal responsibility for the stamp's use and storage.
- Electronic signatures may include an email signature; a digitized image of the signature; a unique PIN number; a biometric identifier, such as a fingerprint; and/or an encryption.

Look Back

A look back refers to record checking, often on microfilm or microfiche, to find old contacts and disease vectors. For example, when a patient tests positive for HIV, the doctor is responsible for notifying public health authorities, which then check blood transfusion records to find out if the patient was a blood donor. If the patient did donate blood, those authorities attempt to find the recipients. Many years can elapse between donation and HIV diagnosis. The medical assistant may be required to "look back" through the patient's chart for clues to assist in this process.

To make the chart useful for a look back, document the following:

- A copy of all lab requisitions and test results, including the date and time
- Any no-shows
- Name and contact information of translators used to explain tests, if any
- Signed and witnessed consent forms
- Copies of any patient preparation or aftercare instructions
- Adverse reactions
- Patient refusal of tests and person in authority that was notified
- When and to whom the results were reported

Procedures for Disaster Recovery of Medical Documents and Supplies

Disaster recovery refers to the salvaging of medical records, equipment, and insurance papers. Most disasters affecting medical records are water-based, like leaks and floods. Before using machinery to test or treat patients, ensure that a qualified Biomedical Engineer checks it for safety. Most supplies (blankets, gloves, bandages, medications, and needles) are unsalvageable. Arrange for their safe disposal.

Prevent disaster-induced record damage by training staff where sprinkler shut-off valves are located and how to close them. Take these post-damage steps:

1. For small amounts of paper, simply separate and dry out in a confidential area.
2. For larger amounts, contact a disaster recovery specialist through the Association of Specialists in Cleaning and Restoration (ASCR). Outside service providers need to know what kinds of paper are involved, such as printer paper or coated paper for electrocardiograms.
3. Reduce the chance of mildew by keeping the temperature down and the air as dry as possible.
4. Develop a reasonable estimate for the amount of time needed for recovery, and plan accordingly.

Professionalism

Traits Important to Display in Professional Situations

The following traits are important to display in professional situations:

- **Tact**: Speaking in such a manner to avoid giving offense. Being tactful can mean addressing issues in private rather than public, choosing the best time to address an issue, and softening criticisms by choosing words carefully.
- **Diplomacy**: Having skills in handling people and negotiating. Diplomacy usually includes keeping an end-goal in mind. For example, a medical assistant may need to use diplomacy if advocating for different work benefits for staff members.
- **Courtesy**: Being thoughtful and polite. Courteous behavior includes always remembering to say *please*, *thank you*, and *excuse me*, and treating others with respect and consideration.
- **Integrity**: Being honest and having high moral standards. This includes admitting errors, reporting errors, and acknowledging the need for more education/knowledge.

Responding Professionally to Criticism

Responding professionally to criticism includes:

- **Avoiding an emotional response**: Whether criticism is good or bad, responding with anger or enthusiasm should be avoided. If the criticism seems unfair, the best thing may be to take a deep breath and avoid responding right away, to allow time to calm down.
- **Accepting benefits of feedback**: Consider how the criticism can help to improve skills or relationships with others.
- **Understanding the message**: The medical assistant should listen attentively and ask clarifying questions that show that they are interested in what the person is saying. Ask for specific examples of any problems discussed and ask for suggestions as to how the situations might have been handled differently.
- **Asking about follow-up**: Be sure to understand what is expected, when, and how. If there is a timeframe or deadline, it should be clearly outlined.
- **Expressing appreciation**: Thank the person for providing feedback (even if you don't agree with the feedback). Always react with tact and courtesy.

Job Searching

The methods of job searching include the following:

- Personal contacts
- School career planning and placement offices
- Cold-calling employers
- Classified advertisements
- Internet job sites and message boards
- Professional associations
- Labor unions
- State employment service offices
- US Office of Personnel Management (OPM)
- Community agencies
- Private employment agencies and career consultants
- Internships

The essentials of a good resume and cover letter include the following:

- An objective tailored to the target job
- Correct spelling and grammar
- Relevant skills, experience, education, and training
- Highlights of accomplishments and qualifications
- Truthfulness
- Chronological work history

The essentials of a good interview include the following:

- Research and rehearse
- Dress appropriately
- Stay calm
- Address the interviewer's concerns effectively
- If it is a behavioral interview, answer in a STAR pattern, stating the **s**ituation, **t**ask, **a**ction, and **r**esults achieved.

Performance Appraisal

The supervisor conducts a performance appraisal (PA) with a staff member to:

- Confirm hiring
- Promote
- Schedule training or remediation
- Reward
- Refer to the Employee Assistance program
- Discipline

A human resources representative or the union shop steward may be present, particularly if discipline may result. The employee's first PA occurs at the end of the probationary period (3 months or 6 months) and annually thereafter. The written appraisal may include a rating scale, checklist, productivity studies, and narrative.

The supervisor must be acquainted with the employee and observe him or her at work. The PA is based on objective data from performance improvement measures. The employee must comply with published standards. The job description should include expectations and goals related to performance. The written PA should indicate compliance with performance expectations. The supervisor discusses the PA results with the employee and allows him or her to respond with new goals, based on findings from performance improvement measures and related to the organization's strategic plans.

Chapter Quiz

Ready to see how well you retained what you just read? Scan the QR code to go directly to the chapter quiz interface for this study guide. If you're using a computer, simply visit the bonus page at **mometrix.com/bonus948/certmedasst** and click the Chapter Quizzes link.

CMA Practice Test #1

Want to take this practice test in an online interactive format?
Check out the bonus page, which includes interactive practice questions and much more: **mometrix.com/bonus948/certmedasst**

1. Title I of the Americans with Disabilities Act (ADA) mandates that individuals with disabilities are:

a. To be provided access to public services
b. To be given opportunities for public housing
c. Not to be discriminated against in obtaining employment
d. To be provided means of telecommunication

2. Which of the following health care issues is NOT covered under the Health Insurance Portability and Accountability Act (HIPAA)?

a. Increasing the portability of health insurance
b. Addressing health care fraud and abuse
c. Standardizing the electronic transmission of health data
d. Outlining payment of Medicare and Medicaid

3. Which of the following constitutes a breach of contract by a health care provider?

a. Discontinuing treatment because the patient did not pay in a timely manner
b. Discontinuing treatment because it is no longer needed
c. Being formally discharged by the patient
d. Withdrawing from the case due to patient noncompliance or an inability to serve the patient

4. Under the doctrine of *respondeat superior*, which of the following CANNOT potentially be held legally responsible for an act of negligence by a medical assistant?

a. The medical assistant
b. The medical assistant's supervisor
c. The medical assistant's education provider
d. The medical assistant's employer

5. Touching a patient in a manner to which they have not consented is considered a tort of:

a. Invasion of privacy
b. Battery
c. Libel
d. Slander

6. All of the following minors (under age 18) are considered emancipated EXCEPT a minor who is:

a. A member of the armed forces
b. Financially responsible and no longer under parental care
c. Married
d. Being treated for a sexually transmitted disease

7. Unless public safety is involved, what is required in all cases to release patient medical records after a subpoena is issued?

a. The patient's written consent
b. A court order
c. A deposition
d. An interrogatory

8. According to typical statutes of limitations involving negligence or malpractice, which of the following time points is NOT used as a starting point?

a. When the negligent act occurred
b. When the negligent act was revealed
c. When the litigant filed a claim
d. When treatment was terminated

9. What normal patient right is suspended upon discovery of child abuse?

a. Privacy
b. Confidentiality
c. Documentation
d. Standard of care

10. A POLST form is a type of:

a. Document declaring durable power of attorney for health care
b. Document releasing a provider from liability under Good Samaritan laws
c. Living will or advance directive
d. PSDA

11. Generally, medical assistants are permitted to do certain clinical procedures only under the supervision of an employer/provider because they are NOT

a. Certified
b. Registered
c. Licensed
d. Certified, registered, or licensed

12. Which of the following best describes ethics?

a. Individual choices relating to conduct
b. Personal values governing an individual's perceptions of right and wrong
c. Laws defining acceptable behavior
d. Creeds to live by

13. Bioethics is defined as:

a. Any ethical matter that pertains to life and/or health care
b. Issues regarding abortion and the use of fetal tissue
c. Dealings with individuals who have committed sexual abuse or exploitation
d. Dealings with individuals who have committed physical or emotional abuse

14. Which of the following is NOT set forth by the American Association of Medical Assistants (AAMA) Code of Ethics?

a. Respect for the confidentiality of patient information
b. Performance of service while respecting all patients
c. Continuous professional improvement
d. Specific ways of dealing with certain situations

15. At present, what is the main difference between reporting child abuse and reporting elder or intimate partner abuse?

a. Child abuse must be reported to authorities in all 50 states, while other types of abuse do not always need to be reported.
b. Sexual abuse is the main offense related to child abuse, but not to elder or intimate partner abuse.
c. Physical abuse is more predominant in elder and intimate partner abuse than in child abuse.
d. Child abuse is more likely to involve another reportable criminal act.

16. A provider is dealing with a patient with HIV or AIDS. Which of the following statements regarding the provider's legal or ethical requirements is NOT true?

a. The provider cannot withhold treatment to the HIV-positive patient.
b. The provider should protect the patient's confidentiality.
c. The provider can ethically deny treatment.
d. The patient's intimate partner should be notified by the patient, the provider, or authorities.

17. What is the time frame during which an abortion can be legally performed in all states?

a. There is no universal time frame for all states.
b. Abortion can be performed during the first trimester.
c. Abortion can be performed during the first trimester only in cases of rape.
d. Abortion can be performed during the first and second trimesters.

18. Therapeutic communication injects what element into communication?

a. Empathy
b. Advice
c. Recommendations
d. Knowledge of the process of communication

19. Which of the following adequately describes the qualities necessary for active listening?

a. Being alert and interested in what the other person is saying
b. Maintaining eye contact with the other person
c. Being attuned to what is said and what is communicated nonverbally
d. Being able to respond quickly with a corrective action

20. In order for verbal communication between two people to be effective, the sender's message must be:

a. Complete
b. Clear and concise
c. Cohesive
d. All of the above

21. In the United States, what do most people consider a comfortable personal space for dealing on a personal (not intimate) level with another individual?

a. Between 0 and 1.5 feet
b. Between 1.5 and 4 feet
c. Between 4 and 12 feet
d. Between 12 and 15 feet

22. The use of a defense mechanism in which a person unconsciously ascribes their own undesirable acts or impulses to someone else is known as:

a. Sublimation
b. Repression
c. Projection
d. Compensation

23. According to Maslow's hierarchy of needs, what is the first level of need that people must satisfy before all others?

a. Physiological and survival needs
b. Necessities for safety and security
c. Needs related to loving and belonging
d. Conditions promoting prestige and esteem

24. A cultural broker is someone who:

a. Acts as a medical interpreter for a family member
b. Is responsible for a non-English-speaking relative
c. Acts as an intermediary or advocate for another person or cultural group within the health care community
d. Interviews non-English-speaking patients and later conveys the information to a medical professional

25. When interviewing a patient, which of the following types of question prompts only a yes or no response?

a. Indirect statement
b. Closed question
c. Open-ended question
d. Active question

26. Which of the following does NOT initially occur when a person is exposed to an acute stressor?

a. Triggering of the parasympathetic nervous system
b. Activation of the fight-or-flight response
c. Releasing of adrenaline and other hormones into the bloodstream
d. Increased respiration rate

27. The four stages of job burnout, in order, are:

a. Value, ambiguity, overload, conflict
b. Value, reality, dissatisfaction, detachment
c. Dissatisfaction, reality, crisis, devaluation
d. Honeymoon, reality, dissatisfaction, crisis

28. Which of the following activities does NOT relieve stress?

a. Goal setting
b. Meditation
c. Gladly accepting all assigned work
d. Taking time off for lunch or a break

29. The symptoms lethargy and weight loss can be associated with which of the following conditions?

a. AIDS
b. Cancer
c. End-stage renal disease
d. All of the above

30. According to Dr. Kubler-Ross, what are the most likely stages of grief experienced by a patient with a life-threatening illness, in order?

a. Denial, bargaining, anger, depression, acceptance
b. Denial, anger, bargaining, depression, acceptance
c. Acceptance of reality, experience of pain, adjustment, development of a new reality
d. Denial, followed by any number of stages, leading to acceptance in the end

31. Which of the following management styles offers rewards to subordinates in terms of teamwork, recognition by other workers, and self-actualization?

a. Authoritarian management
b. Micromanagement
c. Participatory management
d. Management by walking around

32. If an office manager is using a teamwork approach, what is the first step in getting the team started?

a. Brainstorming with the team
b. Developing a work statement with the team
c. Looking at benchmarks from other institutions
d. Developing a time frame and standards for goal achievement

33. As an office manager, when is the best time to carry out a salary review for employees?

a. At the same time as their performance evaluation
b. When the employee asks for a salary review
c. At the beginning of each year
d. When the office experiences changes in funding

34. A medical assistant who functions as a human resources manager is responsible for developing and updating which of the following documents?

a. Office policy manual
b. Office procedure manual
c. HIPAA manual
d. Safety data sheets

35. Which of the following actions during an initial employment interview is discouraged?

a. Providing a time frame for decisions on hiring or additional interviews
b. Using predetermined questions during the interview
c. Providing a quiet and private environment for the interview
d. Offering the applicant the job on the spot

36. The standard rate of overtime pay for administrative or clinical medical assistants is generally:

a. Twice the regular hourly rate for each hour over 40 in a week
b. At least 1.5 times the regular hourly rate for each hour over 40 in a week
c. Not applicable because most medical assistants are considered exempt employees
d. Only applicable in terms of increasing benefits outside pay

37. Medical assistants and other individuals who handle finances in the medical office should:

a. Be bonded
b. Maintain liability insurance
c. Be registered
d. Be licensed

38. When must federal and state taxes related to employee wages be paid?

a. Monthly
b. Quarterly
c. At the end of the year
d. Upon filing of W-2 form

39. What types of nutrients can be converted into energy?

a. Carbohydrates
b. Fats
c. Proteins
d. All of the above

40. Unhealthy trans unsaturated fatty acids are found in:

a. Olive and canola oils
b. Linoleic acid
c. Stick margarine
d. Unhydrogenated oils

41. Which of the following statements is NOT true regarding a person's basal metabolic rate (BMR)?

a. It is the level of energy needed when the body is resting.
b. It is higher in people who have a large percentage of body fat.
c. It is elevated in children during growth spurts.
d. It is increased when a woman is pregnant.

42. Which of the following summarizes the US Department of Agriculture's diagram of dietary recommendations?

a. Recommendations are divided by category, with recommended intake of each category in the form of a food pyramid.
b. Recommendations are represented by a plate diagram, which is divided to show the proportion of each food group that should make up every meal.
c. Statements of recommended intake for each food group, based on age, weight, and comorbidities, are presented in the form of a color-coded chart.
d. Statements of recommended intake are divided into four sections of a box diagram based on age and gender.

43. What are the main inorganic nutrients that act as antioxidants?

a. Vitamin K and folic acid
b. Vitamin D and the minerals calcium and phosphorus
c. Vitamins A, C, and E, and the mineral selenium
d. Several B-complex vitamins and the minerals phosphorus, magnesium, and sulfur

44. What type of diabetes mellitus requires the individual to take insulin regularly throughout life?

a. Type I only
b. Type II only
c. Types I and II
d. Gestational

45. What is the cardiovascular disease in which arteries narrow due to inner deposition of cholesterol and fat?

a. Hypertension
b. Atherosclerosis
c. Arteriosclerosis
d. Myocardial infarction

46. Cancerous cells that are derived from epithelial cells are known as:

a. Carcinomas
b. Sarcomas
c. Lymphomas
d. Germ cell tumors

47. Which of the following characteristics does NOT distinguish a virus from all other types of microorganisms?

a. A virus can only reproduce within another type of living cell
b. Viruses are pathogenic
c. Viruses produce spores
d. Viruses cannot be observed directly under a light microscope

48. An organism that serves as a carrier of a disease to another organism, such as a human, is known as a(n):

a. Fomite
b. Vector
c. Bloodborne carrier
d. Exudate

49. Which of the following currently available vaccines are contraindicated in pregnant women, immunocompromised patients, and those with active AIDS?

a. Measles, mumps, rubella (MMR)
b. MMR and influenza
c. MMR, varicella, and zoster
d. Hepatitis A and B

50. Pathogenic microorganisms, cancer cells, and transplanted tissues are initially recognized as foreign by:

a. Macrophages and helper T cells
b. B cells
c. Memory and killer T cells
d. Immunoglobulins

51. The biggest concern regarding the infectious diseases of methicillin-resistant *Staphylococcus aureus* (MRSA) infection and tuberculosis is that:

a. Identification of the infectious agent is difficult.
b. They are highly drug-resistant, limiting antibiotic treatment options.
c. They are viral and cannot be cured.
d. Symptoms are hard to identify.

52. Which of the following is NOT a characteristic of hepatitis A infection?

a. It is spread via the oral-fecal route.
b. It can be prevented by an available vaccine.
c. Patients usually develop jaundice, dark urine, and flu-like symptoms.
d. It becomes a chronic infection.

53. Which of the following is a progressive neurologic disorder in which brain cells degenerate due to an absence of dopamine in the brain, causing rigid muscles and akinesia?

a. Multiple sclerosis
b. Meningitis
c. Parkinson's disease
d. Sciatica

54. Which of the following is the neurotransmitter released at the neuromuscular junction between axons of motor neurons and the motor end plate?

a. Acetylcholine
b. GABA
c. Serotonin
d. Dopamine

55. A streptococcal infection might be linked to all of the following circulatory disorders EXCEPT:

a. Rheumatic fever
b. Mitral valve stenosis
c. Congestive heart failure
d. Varicose veins

56. Which of the following types of anemia can be controlled by injecting the patient with vitamin B12?

a. Iron deficiency anemia
b. Pernicious anemia
c. Sickle cell anemia
d. Hodgkin's disease

57. What layer of the skin contains blood vessels, nerve endings, and glands?

a. Epidermis
b. Dermis
c. Hypodermis
d. Integumentary

58. Which of the following is a contagious skin disorder characterized by pustules and caused by staphylococci and/or streptococci?

a. Dermatitis
b. Dermatophytosis
c. Impetigo
d. Psoriasis

59. Which of the following statements is NOT true regarding herpes zoster infection?

a. It is caused by the same virus associated with varicella or chicken pox in children.
b. It usually presents as a linear area of a skin rash.
c. A later symptom can be postherpetic neuralgia.
d. Since it is caused by a virus, there is no available vaccine.

60. The purpose of immunotherapy for allergies is to use extracts of allergens to:

a. Induce production of blocking IgG-class antibodies toward the allergens.
b. Induce production of IgE-class antibodies toward the allergens.
c. Generally build up the immune system.
d. Use immunomodulation to suppress the immune system.

61. Which of the following urinary tract disorders should be suspected if a patient has chills, fever, abrupt back pain, and tenderness in the suprapubic region?

a. Cystitis
b. Glomerulonephritis
c. Pyelonephritis
d. Renal calculi

62. Which of the following functions is NOT performed by the kidneys?

a. Regulation of water and acid-base balance
b. Filtration of the blood to remove waste
c. Regulation of blood pressure
d. Collection and storage prior to urinary excretion

63. Gastroesophageal reflux disease (GERD) is caused by:

a. Lesions in the mucous membranes in the stomach or duodenum
b. Return of stomach acid due to leakage of the valve leading to the stomach
c. Inflammation of diverticula
d. Inflammation of the ileum

64. Which of the following statements about the pancreas is NOT true?

a. It functions as both an endocrine and an exocrine gland.
b. It is involved in the secretion of insulin.
c. It can develop stones, causing pain.
d. It can become inflamed, which can be life-threatening.

65. Which of the following correctly lists the parts of the large intestine, in order?

a. Cecum, colon, and rectum
b. Duodenum, jejunum, and ileum
c. Ascending, transverse, descending, and sigmoid colons
d. Liver, gall bladder, and pancreas

66. What is the chief cause of blindness in the United States?

a. Retinal detachment
b. Glaucoma
c. Diabetic retinopathy
d. Presbyopia

67. The gel occupying space between the lens and retina of the eye is called the:

a. Fovea centralis
b. Vitreous body
c. Sclera
d. Aqueous humor

68. In patients with myopia, light rays entering the eye focus:

a. On several areas of the retina
b. In front of the retina
c. Beyond the retina
d. On the retina

69. When a person moves their head, their equilibrium is usually maintained by:

a. The vestibular system in the inner ear
b. The tympanic cavity in the middle ear
c. The auricle
d. The cochlea

70. Hearing loss due to hardening of the stapes of the middle ear is known as:

a. Tinnitus
b. Otitis media
c. Otosclerosis
d. Meniere's disease

71. Which of the following is NOT a possible cause of epistaxis?

a. Allergic rhinitis
b. Blunt force
c. Hypertension
d. Childbirth

72. In the respiratory system, gas exchange between oxygen breathed in and carbon dioxide to be removed takes place in the:

a. Pharynx
b. Trachea
c. Bronchi
d. Alveoli

73. The main characteristic that distinguishes asthma from forms of chronic obstructive pulmonary disease (COPD) is that asthma:

a. Does not cause dyspnea
b. Is characterized by a permanent narrowing of the airways
c. Can usually be reversed either spontaneously or through use of agents such as bronchodilators
d. Is caused by a loss of elasticity of the alveoli

74. Which of the following can cause pneumonia?

a. Bacteria
b. Fungi
c. Viruses
d. All of the above

75. Which of the following is a spinal defect in which there is a sideways curvature of the spine?

a. Lordosis
b. Kyphosis
c. Paget's disease of bone
d. Scoliosis

76. A fracture in which the bone is broken into a number of fragments is described as:

a. Greenstick
b. Comminuted
c. Oblique
d. Transverse

77. The main type of arthritis (joint inflammation) that is considered a systemic autoimmune disease is:

a. Osteoarthritis
b. Rheumatoid arthritis
c. Gout
d. Psoriatic arthritis

78. Which of the following is NOT true of endochondral ossification?

a. It is responsible for the growth in length of long bones.
b. The cell types involved are bone cells, their progenitors, and cartilage.
c. It begins during embryonic development and continues until the late teens and early twenties.
d. It is direct deposition of bone into the mesenchyme.

79. Of the two bones connecting the kneecap to the foot, the larger one is the:

a. Patella
b. Femur
c. Tibia
d. Fibula

80. The human vertebral column normally consists of:

a. 24 articulating vertebrae and the spinal cord
b. 24 articulating vertebrae and 9 fused vertebrae
c. The vertebral body and the vertebral arch
d. Clearly separated regions

81. The cervical region of the spinal cord controls certain movement in the:

a. Neck, diaphragm, shoulder, arm, wrist, and hand
b. Trunk and abdomen
c. Abdomen, thigh, leg, and toes
d. Leg, foot, and toes

82. Viral infections have been associated with which of the following neurologic disorders?

a. Cerebral palsy
b. Trigeminal neuralgia
c. Reye's syndrome
d. Huntington's disease

83. Which of the following is NOT characteristic of cerebrovascular accident (CVA)?

a. A loss of blood to the brain, depriving it of oxygen
b. Direct impairment of cranial nerves
c. Symptoms like loss of consciousness and paralysis
d. Being caused by hemorrhage or blockage of a blood vessel

84. Which of the following portions of the brain is primarily responsible for maintaining homeostasis?

a. Cerebellum
b. Cerebral cortex
c. Hypothalamus
d. Hippocampus

85. Which of the following injuries and conditions is NOT known to cause paralysis?

a. Spinal cord injury
b. Stroke
c. Poliomyelitis
d. De Quervain's syndrome

86. When a patient is covered by more than one insurance policy, the total amount paid is limited by policy language regarding:

a. Preauthorization
b. Assignment of benefits
c. Coordination of benefits
d. The deductible

87. What is capitation?

a. A payment system in which the health care provider is paid a fixed fee per patient
b. A payment system in which the health care provider is paid a specific fee for a particular service
c. Payment for the full fee for health care services by the patient
d. Payment for health care services by the government through Medicare

88. The managed care organization model, in which a network of providers and hospitals sign agreements to provide patient services at a discount to the insurance company nonexclusively, describes a(n):

a. Point-of-service (POS) plan
b. Preferred provider organization (PPO)
c. Exclusive provider organization (EPO)
d. Integrated delivery system (IDS)

89. What health care services are covered under Medicare Part B?

a. Hospital stays, home health care, and hospice care
b. Outpatient expenses
c. Prescription drug coverage
d. All of the above

90. The resource-based relative value scale (RBRVS) is used to:

a. Coordinate with Medigap policies.
b. Determine whether a Medicare payment is PAR or non-PAR.
c. Calculate Medicare payments.
d. Determine practice overhead.

91. Which of the following groups is NOT a mandatory eligibility group to receive medical care under the Medicaid program?

a. Low-income families
b. Individuals with tuberculosis
c. Individuals receiving supplemental security income
d. Disabled adult children

92. Which of the following is the medical insurance program that covers active-duty military service members?

a. CHAMPVA
b. TRICARE Prime
c. TRICARE Extra
d. TRICARE Standard

93. Workers' compensation insurance covers which of the following expenses for a person injured on the job?

a. All medical expenses
b. All medical expenses plus lost wages
c. All medical expenses plus lost wages, and an automatic settlement for pain, suffering, and other punitive damages
d. Some medical expenses and lost wages, as determined by state laws

94. If a usual, customary, and reasonable (UCR) fee structure is used for billing, an insurance carrier that pays fees that are considered customary will pay the provider:

a. The top fee in the customary range for that region
b. The full fee as long as it falls within the customary fee range
c. The RBRVS-calculated fee
d. An adjustment

95. When is patient health information that is transmitted via telephone call or fax subject to the security rule under the Health Insurance Portability and Accountability Act (HIPAA) regarding electronic transmission?

a. Always
b. Never
c. When that information was derived from electronically stored information
d. When the patient has signed a privacy agreement

96. The relative value units (RVUs) issued for a particular service fee under Medicare are computed using which of the following factors?

a. Rates determined by a senate subcommittee
b. The provider's rate for the service, practice expenses, malpractice expenses, and adjustors like the geographic practice cost index and the Budget Neutrality Adjuster
c. Standard national codes
d. Sliding fees within an acceptable range

97. According to the CPT system, what is the procedure to change a code for billing a medical procedure to reflect that the service lasted longer than described?

a. Enter the code twice.
b. Add a plus sign (+) before the code.
c. Use an unlisted code and add a report.
d. Use a Category III code.

98. Under the CPT system of coding, what type of modifier should be added to a code to indicate a slight difference in the description (for example, using a surgical team instead of one surgeon)?

a. Indicate both the described code and 09999.
b. Put a -99 after the described code.
c. Use a code beginning with 099 and ending with the two-digit modifier.
d. Add the modifier 09966.

99. Which medical insurance coding system should be used when billing Medicare or Medicaid?

a. ICD-10-CM
b. CPT
c. HCPCS
d. V codes

100. Which of the following is the general format for describing a diagnosis due to disease under the ICD-10-CM system?

a. Three-character coding for the diagnosis, starting with a letter; may be followed by a decimal point with a one- or two-digit modifier
b. Three-digit coding for the diagnosis, followed by a decimal point, and then a one- or two-digit modifier
c. A five-digit numeric code plus two-digit modifiers if required
d. A seven-digit alphanumeric code

101. Which of the following is the standard claim form to be completed for situations such as inpatient admissions, emergency department services, and walk-in facilities?

a. CMS-1500 (08-05)
b. Uniform Bill 04 (UB-04)
c. Authorization for Release of Medical Information
d. Encounter form

102. When can Medicare patients be held responsible for paying out-of-pocket expenses in addition to what is paid by the government?

a. Never
b. If they sign a written waiver
c. If they sign an Advance Beneficiary Notice (ABN)
d. In any situation that is beyond the scope of Medicare

103. Which of the following is the most commonly used manual system of managing a patient's account?

a. Patient ledger
b. Encounter form
c. Posting system
d. Pegboard system

104. In a patient's account or ledger, what should be posted as a credit?

a. The services provided and the charges for each
b. Payments by the insurance company or patient
c. Payments by the insurance company or patient and adjustments
d. The difference between charges and payments

105. The primary reason to keep day sheets and month-end sheets is to maintain accurate records of:

a. Accounts receivable for the practice
b. Accounts payable for the practice
c. Individual patient accounts
d. Receipts

106. Which of the following is NOT generally included in monthly billing statements generated in computerized account systems?

a. Contact information for both the practice and the patient
b. History of all past services performed
c. Aging of past-due balances
d. Itemized charges, payments, and a running balance

107. Which of the following types of check endorsement will prevent cashing by anyone else?

a. Rubber endorsement stamp
b. Daily depositing
c. Blank endorsement
d. Restrictive endorsement

108. In order to comply with the Truth in Lending Act, what must be done by a provider who allows a patient to pay using installment payments?

a. Always have the patient sign a written agreement outlining cost of services rendered and outstanding terms of the agreement, including interest.
b. Have the patient sign a written agreement outlining cost of services rendered and outstanding terms of the agreement, including interest, only if there are at least five installments.
c. Explain to the patient when payments are due and whether there will be interest charged if they do not comply.
d. Explain to the patient at the time of service that they must pay any insurance-required co-pay at that time, and that further payments will be assessed after the insurance company pays their portion of the bill.

109. Which of the following tools is used to measure how rapidly patient accounts are being paid?

a. Collection ratio
b. Accounts receivable (AR) ratio
c. Account aging
d. Number of accounts with balances over two months old

110. Which of the following is generally the last resort for collection of an overdue bill?

a. Telephone collections
b. Collection letters
c. Outside collection firm
d. Filing in small claims court

111. When a patient has declared bankruptcy under Chapter 7, what should the medical office do regarding their unpaid account?

a. Write off the outstanding charges.
b. Send a proof-of-claim and a copy of the patient's debt to bankruptcy court.
c. File a claim to the individual's attorney as an outstanding unsecured debt.
d. File a claim in probate court.

112. An accounting software package that computerizes every aspect of running a medical facility is known as a:

a. Single-entry system
b. Double-entry system
c. Computer service bureau
d. TPMS

113. Which of the following is an accounting system designed to generate information for governmental or other external organizations?

a. Managerial accounting
b. Cost accounting
c. Cost analysis
d. Financial accounting

114. If a practice uses an accrual basis for income reporting, when is the income recorded?

a. The date the money was collected
b. The date the charges were accrued
c. The completion date for treatment
d. A convenient date every month

115. Which of the following is a fidelity bond purchased to guard against embezzlement or other financial loss caused by any employee of a practice?

a. Position-schedule bond
b. Personal bond
c. Blanket-position bond
d. Total-practice bond

116. When closing the facility, an administrative medical assistant should lock up:

a. Cabinets used for record storage
b. Cabinets used for storage of drugs named under the Controlled Substances Act
c. Petty cash and the day's receipts
d. All of the above

117. Which of the following is a good estimate of the number of chairs needed in a waiting room?

a. As many as will fit
b. One and a half seats per examination room
c. Two seats per provider per their hourly turnover
d. Two seats per appointment scheduled per hour

118. Which of the following is the type of internal computer memory that is used for temporary storage of data and programs until saved?

a. Read-only memory (ROM)
b. Random-access memory (RAM)
c. Data storage memory
d. Redundant array of independent disks (RAID) storage

119. Which of the following is a sign that an Internet site is secure?

a. Site address includes "www"
b. Site address is located on a ".org" domain
c. Site address is located on a ".gov" domain
d. Site address begins with "https://"

120. The combination of various sources into a comprehensive electronic database for patient information is known as a(n):

a. Electronic medical record (EMR)
b. Electronic health record (EHR)
c. Medical office simulation software (MOSS)
d. Total practice management system (TPMS)

121. Where is a good place to position a computer monitor relative to incoming light from windows or artificial lighting?

a. Such that the light is directed at a downward angle toward the top of the monitor
b. Such that the light is directed at a downward angle toward the individual's face
c. Such that the light is to the individual's side, parallel to the sight line to the monitor
d. At the same height but at an angle to the incoming light

122. Which of the following types of calls CANNOT be handled by the medical assistant and should be referred to the provider?

a. Obtaining information such as date of birth and insurance carrier from a new patient
b. Scheduling an appointment
c. Scheduling patient tests
d. Authorizing a prescription refill

123. When needed for administrative or medical purposes, a medical assistant can always discuss information about a patient with the patient's:

a. Parent or legal guardian
b. Employer
c. Insurance carriers
d. Attorney

124. Which of the following is NOT true of encrypted email?

a. It is a good way to send medical data via email.
b. It utilizes a virtual private network (VPN) for security.
c. It requires a digital ID consisting of public and private keys and a digital signature.
d. It is more secure than unencrypted email.

125. The patient scheduling style in which several patients are scheduled in the first half hour of each hour and then seen on a first-come, first-served basis is:

a. Double booking
b. Clustering
c. Wave scheduling
d. Stream scheduling

126. What should a medical assistant do when a patient cancels an appointment or is a no-show?

a. Cross out no-shows with a red X and cancellations with a red line on a paper appointment sheet.
b. Keep a permanent record and count these up so the provider is aware.
c. Input this information using computer scheduling software to remove the name and document the missed appointment.
d. Do any of the above, depending on the system used.

127. If an error in an electronic medical record is discovered shortly after entry, how should it be corrected?

a. Draw a single red line through the error, add the correction, indicate "Corr." or "Correction" above the error, and initial and date the area.
b. Erase or white-out the error and put in the correct information.
c. Set the computer software to track the error slot, line out the error with the dash key, make the correction to the right of the lined-out error, key in "Corr." or "Correction," and initial and date the error.
d. Create a new citation identifying and correcting the error, sign and date it, and insert it into the original record.

128. What is an accession record?

a. A cross-reference method used in a numeric filing system
b. A record in a numeric filing system in which a journal or computer listing with predetermined numbers assigns patient or other records
c. The order of filing used in alphabetic filing
d. The rationale for the filing system used in subject filing

129. Which of the following is the letter style in which all of the lines commence at the left margin except the date, complimentary closure, and keyed signature, which start near the center?

a. Simplified
b. Full block
c. Standard modified block
d. Indented modified block

130. Which of the following statements regarding mail sent under the postal class of bulk mail is NOT true?

a. Use of bulk mail requires the organization to pay an annual fee.
b. Bulk mail can be sent by first-class mail, standard mail, parcel post mail, or as bound printed matter.
c. Bulk mail can be picked up by the postal service at the medical facility.
d. There are rules regarding the format of bulk mail.

131. The turnaround time for transcription and return to the provider of a STAT report should be no more than:

a. 12 hours
b. 24 hours
c. 48 hours
d. 72 hours

132. The OSHA Bloodborne Pathogens Standard applies to contact with:

a. Blood and all body fluids
b. Blood and all body fluids, secretions, and excretions
c. The items in response B plus non-intact skin and mucous membranes
d. The items in response C plus unfixed human tissue and tissue culture, cells, or fluid known to be positive for HIV, HBV, or HCV

133. The CDC guidelines for isolation of patients with highly transmissible diseases are to use:

a. Standard Precautions
b. Personal protective equipment (PPE)
c. Transmission-Based Precautions
d. Standard Precautions and the applicable type of Transmission-Based Precautions

134. The preferred method for disposal of sharps is to:

a. Use the scoop technique.
b. Put them into a puncture-proof sharps container marked "biohazard."
c. Put them in a metal pan for later sterilization.
d. Recap the sharp and then put it in a sharps container.

135. According to the OSHA Bloodborne Pathogens Standard, what is required if an employee is accidentally exposed to blood or other potentially infectious materials?

a. The employer must conduct an immediate medical evaluation of the employee.
b. The incident must be reported to a superior and documented within 48 hours.
c. The employer must offer to test the employee for HBV, HCV, and HIV.
d. The employer must submit an ISO 9001 form.

136. Which of the following is NOT an acceptable method of hand-washing as part of infection control?

a. Medical asepsis hand wash using an antimicrobial soap
b. Medical asepsis hand wash using a non-antimicrobial soap
c. Antibacterial wipes
d. Alcohol-based hand rub

137. Which of the following best describes the use of chemical germicidal agents on surfaces to kill most microorganisms?

a. Sanitization
b. Disinfection
c. Sterilization
d. Antisepsis

138. What is the sequence for removing potentially contaminated personal protective equipment when exiting an isolation room?

a. Remove gown and gloves, remove goggles, remove mask, wash hands
b. Remove gown, remove goggles, remove mask, remove gloves, wash hands
c. Remove mask, remove goggles, remove gloves, remove gown
d. Remove gloves, wash hands, remove gown, remove mask

139. When applying sterile gloves or assisting in a sterile procedure, where should the hands and/or sterile objects be held?

a. In front, at a distance from the body
b. In front, at a distance from the body and above waist level
c. Above waist level
d. Toward the sterile field

140. Which statement regarding the differences between surgical hand cleansing and medical hand cleansing is NOT true?

a. Surgical hand washing takes longer.
b. During rinsing, hands should be down for medical hand cleansing and up for surgical hand cleansing.
c. Lotion can be applied after medical hand cleansing, but not after surgical hand cleansing.
d. Medical hand cleansing includes the forearm to the elbow, while surgical hand cleansing focuses only on the hands.

141. Which of the following sterilization processes is most appropriate for a heat-sensitive item such as a fiber-optic endoscope?

a. Gas sterilization
b. Dry heat sterilization
c. Chemical sterilization
d. Steam sterilization

142. When sterilizing instruments using an autoclave, what parameters should be achieved for wrapped instrument packages or trays?

a. 212 °F, 15 psi, 30 min exposure
b. 270 °F, 15 psi, 30 min exposure
c. 270 °F, 15 psi, 15 min exposure
d. 270 °F, 20 psi, 20 min exposure

143. Which of the following types of quality control is recommended by the CDC for checking the effectiveness of steam sterilization by an autoclave?

a. Autoclave tape
b. Sterilization strips placed in the wrapped package
c. Biological indicators with strips or ampules containing bacteria, which are later cultured
d. Biological indicators with strips or ampules containing heat-resistant bacterial spores, which are later cultured

144. Which of the following chemicals is usually used to destroy tissues using cryosurgery?

a. Silver nitrate
b. Sodium hydroxide
c. Liquid nitrogen
d. Nitrous oxide

145. Which of the following designates the smallest suture material available?

a. Swaged
b. Gauge 6-0
c. Gauge 0
d. Gauge 4

146. Which of the following features on an instrument locks it closed and is situated between the handle rings?

a. Serration
b. Tooth
c. Ratchet
d. Serrated loop

147. How do Mayo dissecting scissors differ from all other types of surgical scissors?

a. Their tips have beveled, not blunt or sharp, edges.
b. They are actually knives used to cut skin.
c. One of the tips has a notched blade.
d. Their blades are very delicate.

148. All hemostatic forceps have which of the following features?

a. Straight tips and serrations
b. Ratchets and serrations
c. Ring handles and bent shape
d. Ratchets and teeth

149. Which of the following is NOT true of scopes?

a. They are lighted.
b. They are used to visualize inside body orifices.
c. They have parts that are disposable or must be disinfected.
d. They are long and rigid.

150. Which of the following should NOT be done when using an ultrasonic cleaner to sanitize surgical instruments after use?

a. Put the instruments in an open position.
b. Completely submerge the instruments.
c. Mix stainless steel instruments with those composed of other metals.
d. Process the instruments for at least five minutes.

151. Which of the following is a sterile cream designed for topical application on burns and other abrasion wounds?

a. Povidone-iodine
b. Silver sulfadiazine
c. Chlorhexidine
d. Hydrogen peroxide

152. Which of the following bandage-wrapping techniques should be utilized at a joint where movement is necessary?

a. Spiral turns
b. Reverse spiral turns
c. Figure-eight turns
d. Circular turns

153. Epinephrine is often added to injectable anesthetics because it is a:

a. Vasoconstrictor
b. Vasodilator
c. Mild anesthetic
d. Monitor of anesthesia effectiveness

154. Which of the following is a type of open wound in which skin structures are torn off or away?

a. Laceration
b. Avulsion
c. Puncture
d. Incision

155. What is the appropriate usage of gloves when changing a surgical dressing?

a. Non-sterile gloves throughout the process
b. Sterile gloves throughout the process
c. Sterile gloves for removal of the dressing, non-sterile gloves for cleaning of the wound, and then sterile gloves for the application of sterile cream and dressing
d. Non-sterile gloves for removal, ungloved hand washing, and then sterile gloves for cleaning of the wound and application of sterile cream and dressing

156. In which of the following types of fever does the person's body temperature swing between being elevated and being at or below baseline?

a. Continuous
b. Intermittent
c. Remittent
d. Febrile

157. When using a temporal artery (TA) thermometer to measure a patient's temperature, how is the probe generally used?

a. Used behind the earlobe
b. Inserted into the ear
c. Attached to an electronic thermometer and inserted orally or rectally
d. Pressed against the forehead and then slid across the forehead to the temple area while scanning

158. How is a temperature in degrees Celsius converted into degrees Fahrenheit?

a. Multiply by 9/5
b. Multiply by 9/5 and then add 32
c. Multiply by 5/9
d. Subtract 32 and then multiply by 5/9

159. Which of the following pulse sites is normally used to take a pulse rate in emergencies?

a. Radial pulse
b. Brachial pulse
c. Carotid pulse
d. Apical pulse

160. An adult with a pulse rate of 70 beats per minute has:

a. A normal pulse rate
b. Bradycardia
c. Tachycardia
d. Arrhythmia

161. All of the following abnormalities of respiration are associated with a period of complete absence of breathing EXCEPT:

a. Voluntarily holding one's breath
b. Orthopnea
c. Sleep apnea
d. Cheyne-Stokes respiration

162. Which of the following breath sounds occurs with many lung diseases, sounds like rattling, and should be documented when taking a respiration rate?

a. Stridor
b. Stertorous respiration
c. Rales
d. Wheezing

163. Blood pressure is a function of all of the following EXCEPT:

a. How strong the heart muscle is
b. The elasticity of the arteries
c. The size of the lumen of the arteries
d. The ejection fraction

164. The major difference between electronic and other types of sphygmomanometers used to measure blood pressure is that electronic types:

a. Do not use a pressure cuff
b. Do not require simultaneous use of a stethoscope
c. Tend to lose calibration and accuracy
d. Can only read systole or diastole measurements in one take

165. When using a mercury or aneroid sphygmomanometer for blood pressure reading on an adult, the systolic pressure reading is recorded:

a. During the first phase of deflation when a sharp tapping sound is heard
b. During the auscultatory gap
c. As tapping and muffled sounds begin to fade
d. When all sounds cease

166. How should a blood pressure measurement be recorded on an adult patient's chart?

a. Systolic pressure/diastolic pressure
b. Systolic pressure/diastolic pressure, arm used, patient position
c. Diastolic pressure/systolic pressure
d. Diastolic pressure/systolic pressure, arm used, patient position

167. An adult whose blood pressure is 125/85 is considered to have:

a. Normal blood pressure
b. Prehypertension
c. Hypertension
d. Secondary hypertension

168. A traditional beam balance scale includes a lower measuring bar, with stops set at 50-pound increments, and an upper measuring bar that slides freely between 0 and 50 pounds. To weigh a patient, the medical assistant begins by setting the lower bar to the closest 50-pound increment below the patient's weight, and then moves upper bar until the beam is centered. What additional steps are needed to find the patient's weight in kilograms?

a. Add the measurements on the upper and lower measuring bars.
b. Subtract the measurement on the upper bar from the one on the lower bar.
c. Add the measurements on the upper and lower bars, then multiply by 2.2.
d. Add the measurements on the upper and lower bars, then divide by 2.2.

169. In which of the following physical examination methods is a stethoscope used to listen for lung and heart sounds?

a. Palpation
b. Percussion
c. Auscultation
d. Mensuration

170. A patient with a probable cardiovascular or respiratory problem should be positioned on the examination table in what position?

a. Dorsal recumbent or lithotomy
b. Semi- or high Fowler's
c. Trendelenburg
d. Sims'

171. During a physical examination, the provider may use a tongue depressor and light source to check for any of the following EXCEPT

a. Dental hygiene along the teeth and gums
b. Swelling of the tonsils and uvula
c. Functioning of cranial nerve XI
d. Functioning of cranial nerves IX and X

172. During examination of the abdomen, which of the following observations is NOT a cause for concern?

a. Palpable liver or spleen
b. Presence of bowel sounds
c. Presence of masses
d. Abdominal distension

173. During the prenatal visit, a woman's obstetrical history should be recorded as:

a. One number for gravidity, then one number for parity
b. One number for gravidity, then four numbers separated by dashes under the FPAL system for parity
c. Either A or B
d. One number for gravidity, then one number for total previous live births

174. Which of the following laboratory tests commonly done at the initial prenatal visit is NOT part of a urinalysis?

a. Venereal disease research laboratory (VDRL)
b. Human chorionic gonadotropin (hCG)
c. Glucose
d. White and red blood cell counts

175. The pregnancy disorder in which the placenta is positioned over the cervical opening, potentially causing bleeding during labor and fetal anoxia and death, is:

a. Eclampsia
b. Placenta previa
c. Placenta abruptio
d. Incompatibility

176. The provider is inserting an intrauterine device (IUD) for pregnancy prevention. While assisting, the medical assistant might do all of the following EXCEPT:

a. Assist the patient into the lithotomy position and drape her.
b. Hand the speculum to the provider.
c. Swab the cervix with an antiseptic and inject a local anesthetic if needed.
d. Document the procedure in the patient's chart.

177. Which of the following is NOT true of a breast self-examination (BSE)?

a. The examination should be done standing up.
b. The three middle fingers should probe for lumps or abnormalities in the opposite breast.
c. Each breast should be checked using an up-and-down pattern.
d. The individual should also check for abnormalities or redness in the mirror.

178. According to the Bethesda system of classifying Pap tests, how should potential malignancy, defined as squamous cell carcinoma, be classified?

a. CIN 3
b. Category 2, subgroup 1a
c. Category 2, subgroup 1c
d. Category 3

179. Wet preps/mounts and potassium hydroxide preps are performed in order to:

a. Screen for chlamydia and gonorrhea.
b. Ascertain the cause of vaginitis in women or urethritis in men.
c. Diagnose conditions such as endometriosis or fibroids.
d. Biopsy for malignancies.

180. What is always administered to children who experience an allergic reaction to a vaccine?

a. Oral pseudoephedrine once, at a dose of 0.05 mg/kg body weight
b. Subcutaneous epinephrine once, at 1:1,000 dilution and a dose of 0.01 mg/kg body weight up to three times, in 10–20-minute intervals
c. Oral or intramuscular diphenhydramine, 1 mg/kg body weight for up to 30 mg
d. Cardiopulmonary resuscitation (CPR)

181. The preferred intramuscular vaccine injection site for toddlers, older children, adolescents, and adults is the:

a. Anterolateral aspect of the thigh
b. Gluteal muscle
c. Deltoid muscle
d. Triceps muscle

182. Growth charts for newborns, infants, and toddlers are differentiated according to percentiles for:

a. Length and weight versus age in months
b. Length and weight versus age in months, separated according to sex
c. Length, weight, and chest circumference versus age in months
d. Length, weight, and chest circumference versus age in months, separated according to sex

183. When taking the pulse rate for children up to 5 years old, which of the following is the preferred pulse site?

a. Radial pulse
b. Brachial pulse
c. Apical pulse
d. Dorsalis pedis pulse

184. When checking a patient for prostate cancer, which of the following tests is NOT typically performed?

a. Prostatic MRI
b. Prostatic ultrasound
c. Biopsy
d. Prostate-specific antigen (PSA)

185. When performing a urinary catheterization on a female patient, which of the following should NOT be done?

a. Use sterile gloves to maintain sterility of both hands throughout.
b. Wipe each portion of the labia with antiseptic-soaked cotton balls in a front-to-back motion.
c. Have the patient in a dorsal lithotomy position during the procedure.
d. Use sterile lubricant on the catheter tip prior to insertion.

186. When developing a fecal occult blood test, a positive result is indicated by:

a. Immediate appearance of a blue color around the periphery of the stool smear
b. Appearance of a blue color around the periphery of the stool smear as well as the positive control within 30-60 seconds
c. Immediate appearance of a red color around the periphery of the stool smear and all controls
d. Patches of red in the stool sample

187. Which of the following pulmonary function tests is a good indication of the extent of someone's asthma or other respiratory disorder?

a. Forced vital capacity (FVC)
b. Forced expiratory volume at one second (FEV1)
c. Mean expiratory flow rate (MEFR)
d. Peak expiratory flow rate (PEFR)

188. Which of the following is NOT true of an erythrocyte sedimentation rate (ESR)?

a. A value of 25 mm/hour is always considered abnormal.
b. An ethylenediaminetetraacetic acid (EDTA) or sodium citrate venous blood sample is used.
c. The test must be read at precisely 60 minutes.
d. The test should be performed within two hours of the blood draw.

189. A patient who cannot walk or lift himself is to be transferred. He should be lifted:

a. By the arms
b. Under the armpits
c. By gripping his gait belt from underneath and lifting
d. By his waist

190. A patient can bear only partial weight on one leg. Which of the following types of gait should this patient use with a crutch?

a. Two-point gait
b. Three-point gait
c. Four-point gait
d. Swing-to gait

191. Which of the following is a range of motion (ROM) exercise that involves a motion directed away from the body's midline?

a. Flexion
b. Rotation
c. Abduction
d. Adduction

192. Which of the following best describes the current American Heart Association guidelines for emergency cardiopulmonary resuscitation (CPR) on an adult?

a. Perform rescue breathing using one breath every 10 seconds.
b. For circulation, use a ratio of 30 fast compressions to two breaths.
c. Shock with an automated external defibrillator (AED) prior to CPR.
d. Initiate CPR starting with rescue breaths followed by compressions.

193. Under the Controlled Substances Act, a special Drug Enforcement Agency (DEA) form must be utilized to order which of the following types of drugs in a medical setting?

a. Schedule I
b. Schedule II
c. Schedule III
d. Schedule IV

194. Of the cardiac-related drugs that should be kept on hand in an ambulatory setting, which one is used for angina pectoris?

a. Nitroglycerin
b. Atropine
c. Digoxin
d. Isoproterenol

195. A provider must administer a certain number of units of a drug. The drug is available at a particular concentration in units/mL. How should the provider calculate the number of mL to administer?

a. Multiply the units/mL concentration of the available dose by 16.
b. Divide the number of units ordered by the concentration (units/mL) of the available drug.
c. Divide the concentration (units/mL) of the available drug by the number of units ordered.
d. Convert mL to mg, then divide the number of units ordered by the concentration (units/mg) of the available drug.

196. When taking a standard electrocardiogram (ECG), where should the bipolar leads be placed?

a. Between the left and right arms, the left leg and right arm, and the left leg and left arm
b. Between the middle of the left arm to left leg and the right arm, the middle of the right arm to left leg and the left arm, and the middle of the right arm to left arm and the left leg
c. Between six different points on the chest and a point on the right arm to left leg lead
d. Between six different points on the chest and the intersection of the left arm/right arm/left leg leads

197. An irregular electrocardiogram (ECG) characterized by closely spaced premature ventricular contractions (PVCs), a lack of P waves, and distorted QRS complexes, indicates:

a. Atrial fibrillation
b. Paroxysmal atrial tachycardia
c. Ventricular tachycardia
d. Ventricular fibrillation

198. A "3" in the blue diamond on a chemical label indicates that the chemical is:

a. A flammable liquid
b. Reactive with water
c. A corrosive or toxic health hazard
d. Potentially explosive near a spark or if heated

199. The basic metabolic panel that is approved by the Centers for Medicare & Medicaid Services (CMS) consists of laboratory tests for:

a. Carbon dioxide, potassium, chloride, and sodium
b. Carbon dioxide, potassium, chloride, sodium, blood urea nitrogen (BUN), total calcium, creatinine, and glucose
c. Carbon dioxide, potassium, chloride, sodium, blood urea nitrogen (BUN), total calcium, creatinine, glucose, albumin, total bilirubin, total protein, SGOT, and SGPT
d. Albumin, alkaline phosphatase, direct bilirubin, total bilirubin, total protein, SGOT, and SGPT

200. If the laboratory tests to be performed require a serum sample, a venipuncture specimen should be collected in a tube with what color top?

a. Red top or red-gray mottled top
b. Lavender top or blue top
c. Dark green top
d. Light gray top

Answer Key and Explanations for Test #1

1. C: There are five titles outlined in the ADA. Title I covers prohibition of discrimination in employment for those individuals with physical or mental disabilities. The other answers describe the content of Titles II, III, and IV. Title V covers insurance and definitions of exclusions, among other things.

2. D: HIPAA covers all of the issues discussed in choices A through C as well as a number of others, such as tax breaks for medical savings accounts, in its five titles. However, the only reference in HIPAA to Medicare type plans is that they must coordinate with other plans to prevent duplication of coverage.

3. A: Discontinuation of treatment by a health care provider merely because the patient has not paid in a timely manner would be considered a breach of contract. The other choices describe the three instances in which the provider can legally discontinue treatment. Choices C and D require the professional to send a notice to the patient (by certified mail with return receipt) describing the situation.

4. C: Under the doctrine of *respondeat superior*, both the medical assistant's employer and supervisor (usually a doctor, nurse, or some other licensed professional) are responsible for the employee's actions to a degree and can be sued in instances of negligence by the medical assistant. However, the medical assistant can also be sued, because they are considered responsible for providing a reasonable standard of care.

5. B: All of the given choices are types of torts, which are wrongful actions that culminate in injury to the other person (in this case, the patient). Battery is the touching of a patient in a manner to which they have not consented. Invasion of privacy includes a number of situations in which a patient's privacy is invaded, such as releasing information about them without permission or failing to shield them properly during examination. Libel and slander are two types of defamation of character: false and malicious writing or speaking about someone, respectively.

6. D: The minors described in A, B, and C, as well as minors who are parents, are considered to be emancipated and are capable of signing their own consent. In most states, minors being treated for sexually transmitted diseases, as well as those who are pregnant or have a drug or alcohol addiction, can also sign their own consent, but in this case, they are considered mature (not emancipated) minors.

7. A: A subpoena is a court-issued request for access to part or all of a patient's medical record. Unless public safety is involved, the basic requirement for record release to anyone is the patient's written consent. A court order is sometimes also required when sensitive issues are involved, such as AIDS, other sexually transmitted diseases, or mental illness. Choices C and D refer to later processes during the discovery phase of litigation, dealing with oral and written testimony, respectively.

8. C: The time point most often used as the starting point for the statute of limitations on negligence is generally choice A, when the act occurred, but choices B and D are sometimes utilized. However, choice C, the date the litigant filed the claim, is not a valid starting point for the statute of limitations to apply.

9. B: When a health care provider or other professional observes an instance of suspected child abuse, they are legally required to report this to the police, a social services agency, and parents; this suspends the normal patient right to confidentiality. The right to privacy is slightly different. The provider must still properly document the case and provide the expected standard of care.

10. C: The POLST (Physician Orders for Life-Sustaining Treatment) form, which is available in some configuration in the majority of states, is a type of living will or advance directive for level of care when a patient is near death. This may also be referred to as a MOLST (Medical Orders for Life-Sustaining Treatment). A durable power of attorney designates another individual for decisions regarding the patient's health care. PSDA refers to the federal Patient Self-Determination Act, which is related in that it discusses Medicare/Medicaid payments and availability of advance directives in institutions. POLST forms are unrelated to the Good Samaritan laws.

11. C: Medical assistants are only allowed to do certain clinical procedures because they are not a licensed profession, as opposed to doctors and nurses, who must fulfill specified educational requirements and pass a state-administered examination. Many medical assistants choose to voluntarily become certified.

12. B: Ethics refers to the set of personal values that shape an individual's perceptions of right and wrong, which is different from morals. Ethics are not laws defining acceptable behavior or creeds to live by, although the latter generally are derived from ethics.

13. A: Bioethics is an overall term relating to all ethical matters pertaining to life and/or health care. The other responses describe particular situations in which bioethics might be invoked.

14. D: The AAMA Code of Ethics for medical assistants does not outline specific ways of dealing with certain situations, but it does expound five things that should be strived for. These include choices A, B, and C, as well as upholding the principles and disciplines of the profession, and taking part in further service activities related to the betterment of the community.

15. A: Not all states have legislation related to reporting of elder (60 years of age or older) or intimate partner abuse. All three types of abuse could potentially be sexual, physical, or emotional. Other types include neglect in cases of child or elder abuse, financial in cases of elder abuse, and sexual exploitation and incest in cases of child abuse. All types could also potentially involve a reportable criminal act, such as rape.

16. C: The provider cannot withhold treatment to an HIV-positive patient, so C is the correct answer. In addition, patient confidentiality should be maintained, and any intimate partners notified.

17. A: The majority of states allow elective abortion during the first trimester. It is important to know the law in the state in which you work. Regardless of the circumstances under which state law permits abortions, a health care provider is not required to perform or participate in an abortion procedure if he or she is ethically opposed.

18. A: Therapeutic communication is distinguished from normal social communication in that it injects empathy toward the other person, not advice or recommendations. A person effective at therapeutic communication is often knowledgeable about the process of communication, but that is not required.

19. C: Active listening requires the receiver to be attuned not only to what the other person is saying, but also to what they may be hinting at through body language or nonverbal communication. Being alert and interested is helpful but does not in itself constitute active listening. Maintaining eye contact can be helpful at times but is neither essential nor sufficient. Making a quick response defining a corrective action is generally thought to be detrimental to communication.

20. D: According to references such as *Legal Nurse Consulting Principles and Practices*, effective verbal communication occurs when the message is complete, clear, concise, cohesive, and also courteously delivered.

21. B: There are cultural differences in what is considered a comfortable personal space, but generally in the United States, between 1.5 and 4 feet is considered comfortable space for personal interaction with another individual. The other responses represent the personal spaces generally considered necessary for intimate communication, social communication, and in public spaces.

22. C: All of the listed responses are types of defense mechanisms, but choice C is the described mechanism. Sublimation is diverting a socially unacceptable behavior into one that is socially acceptable. Repression is subconsciously forgetting an event. Compensation is disguising a real or imagined undesirable trait by overemphasizing one that is considered healthy or acceptable. Other types of defense mechanisms include regression, denial, displacement, rationalization, and undoing.

23. A: The most basic needs on the base of Maslow's hierarchy are those related to physiology and survival, such as food, water, and air. Maslow describes five levels of needs. Choices B, C, and D represent levels two, three, and four, respectively. The fifth and final level is self-actualization, the achievement of one's potential.

24. C: A cultural broker is an intermediary or advocate for another person or cultural group. A cultural broker can act as a medical interpreter; generally, a family member is not the best choice for a medical interpreter because they may not comprehend the medical terminology. When acting as a medical interpreter, the cultural broker should never interview the patient independently, but rather act as a direct interpreter.

25. B: A question that is designed to prompt only a yes or no response is a closed question. An open-ended question is one designed to prompt more information and therefore facilitate therapeutic communication. An indirect statement, which can also encourage therapeutic communication, is posed in a form such as "Tell me about..." Active listening is a good way of observing what a patient is communicating nonverbally.

26. A: When a person is exposed to an acute stressor, the sympathetic nervous system (not the parasympathetic) is initially triggered in the fight-or-flight response, which includes things like release of hormones, increase of respiration rate, and short-term memory loss. After the body is exhausted by these reactions, the parasympathetic nervous system is triggered to allow the body to resume normal functions.

27. D: Response D describes, in order, the four stages a person goes through on the way to job burnout. The four characteristics in response A, when preceded by the word "role," are features associated with job burnout.

28. C: If a worker accepts a workload that is too heavy, beyond their skill level, or not clearly differentiated from work others are doing, the worker can experience frustration, stress, and potentially burnout. The activities in options A, B, and D are all good ways to relieve stress.

29. D: AIDS, cancer, and end-stage renal disease are all potentially life-threatening illnesses that can result in lethargy and weight loss in addition to other symptoms.

30. B: Response B illustrates the most likely scenario, according to Dr. Kubler-Ross, although she emphasized that everyone's experience is unique; not everyone experiences all five stages, and not always in the same order. Response C, known by the acronym TEAR (to accept the reality, experience the pain, adjust to the new environment, and reinvest in the new reality), is another way of looking at the stages of grief.

31. C: The type of management technique that offers subordinates these types of rewards is participatory management. Authoritarian management is essentially the same as micromanagement; managers practicing this style plan everything on their own and offer subordinates only monetary rewards. Management by walking around (MBWA) is a style in which the manager visits employees to collect data about how smoothly the organization is running.

32. B: The first step as a manager in getting a team started is development of a work statement with the team, which should include mutually established (not pre-established) time frames and standards. Brainstorming should be done after development of the work statement, and it often includes looking at benchmarks from other institutions to determine feasibility. The later steps are planning, implementation, and recognition.

33. C: The best time to carry out a salary review for all employees is the beginning of each year because that ensures equality and continuity for each employee. This is fairer than waiting for the individual to ask for a salary review, which can result in much longer time periods between reviews. It is best to keep salary reviews separate from performance evaluations. Practice funding is important, but it is more cost-effective to retain good employees than to hire new ones.

34. A: The only responsibility listed that applies strictly to a medical assistant who functions as a human resources manager is developing and updating the office policy manual. The other responsibilities apply to medical assistants acting as office managers.

35. D: The only response that is discouraged is D, offering the potential employee the job at the time of the initial interview, because the interviewer should review all candidates before making any decisions. The other responses are all suggested behaviors during the initial interview of a potential employee.

36. B: Although overtime may be paid at twice the regular hourly rate, the general standard rate is at least 1.5 times the regular hourly rate for each hour over 40 in a week. Some medical assistants may be exempt employees, but those are usually functioning in higher grade levels, such as managers.

37. A: The act that guarantees that a provider will get back any monies an employee embezzles is to buy a bond that covers losses in that employee's name. Professional liability insurance should be purchased by practicing medical assistants, but in that case things like malpractice are covered. Registration, while desirable, is not required for handling finances, and medical assistants are not licensed.

38. B: A medical assistant functioning as an office manager must pay federal and state taxes related to employee wages quarterly.

39. D: All these nutrients can be converted into energy, although carbohydrates are the primary source. Proteins are mainly used to generate amino acids, which can be utilized as building blocks of structural proteins, enzymes, and hormones.

40. C: Trans unsaturated fatty acids are solid at room temperature and found in things like stick margarine. These fats elevate the bad type of cholesterol, low-density lipoprotein (LDL), and lower the good type of cholesterol, high-density lipoprotein (HDL). Olive and canola oils both have healthier types of unsaturated and saturated fats. Linoleic acid is the one essential fatty acid needed in the human diet.

41. B: All of the statements are true except for B. BMR is actually higher in people with lean body mass or relatively more muscle because it takes more energy to fuel muscles than to store fat.

42. B: The USDA uses MyPlate as a diagram to present dietary recommendations. This graphic has replaced the formerly used food pyramid. In this diagram, fruits and vegetables take up half the plate, with grains and protein taking up the other half. Dairy is shown in a circular shape outside the plate (like a cup). Rather than listing explicit amounts, MyPlate demonstrates the proportion that each food group should make up for each meal.

43. C: Antioxidants attack free radicals in the body that can harm DNA and blood vessel cells. The main antioxidants are vitamins A, C, and E, and the mineral selenium. Vitamin K and folic acid contribute to blood clotting and formation of red blood cells and DNA. Vitamin D and the minerals calcium and phosphorus contribute to bone growth. Several B-complex vitamins and the minerals phosphorus, magnesium, and sulfur contribute to energy metabolism.

44. A: People with type I diabetes mellitus are insulin-dependent because they do not produce insulin, a hormone needed to signal to cells that glucose is available for conversion to energy. If they do not receive insulin, carbohydrates will not be metabolized. People with type II diabetes are not insulin-dependent and can usually control their disease through diet because they produce insulin, but in insufficient quantities. Gestational diabetes is a temporary situation in which a woman develops glucose intolerance while pregnant.

45. B: Atherosclerosis is the correct answer, but all of these cardiovascular conditions can be interrelated. Hypertension is high blood pressure, which can be due to things like high bodily water levels due to high sodium intake, but can also occur with atherosclerosis. Arteriosclerosis is the hardening of the arteries due to reduced elasticity of the vessel, often as a result of atherosclerosis. A myocardial infarction (heart attack) is an interruption of the blood supply to a coronary artery due to eruption of an atherosclerotic plaque.

46. A: Cancer is the general term for unregulated cell growth. Cancers derived from epithelial cells are the most common type and are known as carcinomas. Cancers derived from connective tissues such as bone are called sarcomas. Cancers derived from blood-forming hematopoietic cells are called lymphomas and leukemias. Cancers derived from pluripotent stem cells are called germ cell tumors.

47. C: Viruses do not produce spores, but a number of other types of microorganisms do, including certain bacteria, fungi, and protozoa. Viruses can only reproduce within another type of living cell. They are pathogenic, like most microorganisms (but not all bacteria are). They cannot be observed directly under a light microscope, although their effects may be.

48. B: Vectors are disease carriers, such as ticks or mosquitoes, that carry a microorganism to ultimately infect a human or other organism; most are associated with transmission of rickettsiae, which are small, nonmotile bacteria that are intracellular parasites. The other answers are other modes of transmission for microorganisms. A fomite is an inanimate object, such as a piece of equipment, on which a microorganism lives until it is transmitted. Bloodborne transmission is a common mode in which infection occurs through exposure to blood. An exudate is wound drainage, which often transmits a microorganism through direct contact. Other transmission modes include airborne transmission and ingestion.

49. C: MMR, varicella, and zoster vaccines are all contraindicated in the described patient categories, because all of these vaccines contain live attenuated viruses and the patients have low immune responses. The other vaccines are safer because they contain either inactivated virus or only viral proteins.

50. A: Foreign invaders are initially recognized by macrophages and helper T cells. After they are recognized, the two types of immunity directed against specific antigens, cellular and humoral, are activated. Cellular immunity involves activation of helper T cells to develop memory and killer T cells; along with macrophages, the killer T cells surround and kill the foreign organism or cell. Humoral immunity involves activated B cells, which divide into memory B cells and plasma cells. These produce specific immunoglobulins called antibodies, which bind to the antigens.

51. B: MRSA infection, caused by methicillin-resistant *Staphylococcus aureus*, and tuberculosis, caused by *Mycobacterium tuberculosis*, are both highly drug-resistant bacterial infections, thus limiting antibiotic treatment options. There are a number of ways to diagnose each, and they are not viral.

52. D: All of the statements are true except for D. The other two major hepatitis virus infections, hepatitis B and C, usually become chronic, but hepatitis A is generally resolved within two months of contraction and patients do not become carriers of the virus.

53. C: This is a description of Parkinson's disease. Multiple sclerosis is demyelination of nerve fibers, resulting in symptoms such as visual disruptions and muscle weakness. Meningitis is inflammation in the brain or spinal cord, caused by a viral or bacterial infection and resulting in symptoms like headache, fever, and stiff neck. Sciatica is sharp leg pain along the sciatic nerve due to its compression by a severed intervertebral disk or osteoarthritis.

54. A: These are all neurotransmitters of some type, but acetylcholine is the one released at the neuromuscular junction. Gamma-aminobutyric acid (GABA) is an inhibitory transmitter in the brain. Serotonin is found primarily in the intestinal tract and central nervous system, and contributes to feelings of well-being. Dopamine activates a number of receptors in the brain. There are a number of other neurotransmitters as well.

55. D: The major circulatory disorder associated with a streptococcal infection is rheumatic fever. This can, in turn, cause narrowing or stenosis of the mitral value, thwarting blood flow between the atrium and ventricle of the heart. It can also cause carditis, or inflammation of the heart muscle, which could manifest as congestive heart failure or other heart conditions. The correct answer, varicose veins, is completely different; these enlarged veins are caused by impaired venous return.

56. B: The term *anemia* refers to any disorder characterized by low circulating red blood cells and hemoglobin, resulting in symptoms like pallor, weakness, and malaise. There are three variations: iron deficiency anemia due to decreased levels of iron; pernicious anemia, due to lack of intrinsic factor which results in an inability to absorb vitamin B12; and sickle cell anemia, a hereditary disorder in which the red blood cells are shaped like sickles and often lyse and clump in blood vessels. Hodgkin's disease is a type of cancer of the lymphatic system.

57. B: The skin consists of three layers: the epidermis (outer layer), made up of squamous epithelium, keratin, and melanin; the dermis (middle layer), which contains the blood vessels, nerve endings, glands, and some connective tissue; and the hypodermis (deepest layer), with subcutaneous connective and adipose tissue. Integumentary is the inclusive name for the system of the skin and its connected structures, like hair, nails, nerve endings, and oil and sweat glands.

58. C: The contagious skin disorder described is impetigo. Dermatitis is erythema (redness) due to an irritant. Dermatophytosis is a contagious fungal infection causing skin to flake, scale, and itch, most often in the foot area (also called athlete's foot or tinea pedis). Psoriasis is a chronic autoimmune type of dermatitis, the most common presentation of which is red and white scaly patches.

59. D: All these statements regarding herpes zoster infection (shingles) are true except for option D. There is an available vaccine recommended for adults over 50.

60. A: There are various types of immunotherapy, including immunomodulation for instances such as cancer. However, when the term is applied to allergic diseases, it refers to the injection of increasing amounts of allergens (to which the patient is allergic) to induce production of blocking IgG-class antibodies—not IgE-class antibodies, which are the type causing the allergy in the first place. The goal is not general buildup of the immune system.

61. C: Pyelonephritis presents with these types of symptoms after a pyogenic bacterial infection. It is usually located in the bladder and kidneys. Pyelonephritis can occur due to pregnancy or renal calculi (kidney stones). The main symptom of kidney stones is excruciating pain when they are lodged in and move within the ureter. Cystitis is inflammation of the bladder due to a urinary tract infection. It is characterized by signs like urinary frequency and burning. People with glomerulonephritis have chills, fever, and hypertension due to inflammation of the glomeruli, or small blood vessels in the kidneys; streptococcal infection is one cause.

62. D: As the final part of the urinary system, the bladder collects and stores urine prior to excretion. The kidneys perform all of the functions listed in A, B, and C, as well as others, such as releasing certain hormones.

63. B: GERD occurs when there is valve leakage in the area between the esophagus and stomach, which brings up stomach acid and causes heartburn. Response A describes gastric (stomach) and duodenal ulcers, which can be caused by things like *Helicobacter pylori*, salicylates, alcohol, and too much secretion of hydrochloric acid. Response C refers to diverticulitis in diverticula of the colon. Response D refers to Crohn's disease in the ileum, the final section of the small intestine.

64. C: Pain due to stones is generally associated with the gallbladder. The other statements all pertain to the pancreas. Inflammation of the pancreas is pancreatitis, which can be life-threatening because pancreatic enzymes can cause the organ to necrose and hemorrhage.

65. A: Response A lists the parts of the large intestine in order. Response B is the order of structures within the small intestine. Response C lists the parts of the colon. The structures described in response D are organs that are associated with the digestive system.

66. C: Diabetic retinopathy, the chief cause of blindness in the United States, is injury to the retina in individuals with diabetes due to vascular changes. Retinal detachment, separation of the retina from the choroid layer, can also cause blindness. Untreated glaucoma, high intraocular pressure due to accumulation of aqueous humor, can impair vision significantly. Presbyopia is the loss of elasticity in the lens, which occurs as people age, impairing close vision.

67. B: This gel between the lens and the retina on the inner surface of the eye is the vitreous body or vitreous humor. This differs from the aqueous humor, which is a watery substance occupying the space between the lens and the cornea on the front of the eye. The fovea centralis is the spot in the middle of the central macula region of the retina, which is responsible for sharp central vision. The sclera is the outer white layer of the eye.

68. B: Myopia, also known as nearsightedness, occurs because the eyeball is elongated, causing light rays to focus in front of the retina. Astigmatism is due to non-uniform lens curvature or cornea shape. Farsightedness is due to shortening of the eyeball, causing light rays to focus beyond the retina. Response D describes normal vision.

69. A: Equilibrium is maintained by the vestibular system in the inner ear. The cochlea is also in the inner ear, but it is associated with hearing. The middle ear is made up of three bones (the malleus, incus, and stapes) carrying waves from the outer ear, as well as the hollow space called the tympanic cavity. The auricle is the external ear.

70. C: This is a description of hearing loss called otosclerosis. Tinnitus is hearing sound within the ear in the absence of external sound, which could be due to something like impacted cerumen (ear wax). Otitis media is a middle-ear infection resulting in symptoms like pain, discharge, and hearing loss. Meniere's disease is a composite of the symptoms of hearing loss, vertigo, tinnitus, and nausea, probably due to swelling of the labyrinth in the inner ear.

71. D: *Epistaxis* is another word for nosebleed. This could be caused by a variety of factors, including those listed in options A, B, and C, as well as low humidity in the environment, nasal infections, and many others. Childbirth has nothing to do with this condition, but an episiotomy (which sounds similar) is sometimes done during childbirth. Hormones in pregnancy cause dilation of the blood vessels in the nose, increasing blood supply and pressure on the vessels, and at times causing epistaxis.

72. D: Gas exchange takes place in the alveoli, which are the tiniest air sacs in the lungs. When air is taken in during the inspiration phase of respiration, the order of intake is nose or mouth, pharynx, trachea, bronchi, bronchioles, and then the alveoli.

73. C: Asthma is usually reversible because it involves inflammation but not actual airway narrowing, whereas in the two types of COPD, emphysema and chronic bronchitis, there is permanent narrowing of the airways. Dyspnea, shortness of breath, is a common symptom of both asthma and COPD. Loss of elasticity of the alveoli (most commonly due to smoking) is the hallmark of emphysema.

74. D: Pneumonia is inflammation of the lungs resulting in symptoms like chills, fever, cough, and yellow sputum. It can be caused by various bacteria, fungi, viruses, and sometimes chemical irritants.

75. D: Three of the options are abnormal curvatures of the spine, with scoliosis being a sideways curvature to the right or left. Lordosis is an inward curve to the lower spine, resulting in swayback. Kyphosis is an outward curve to the upper portion, resulting in hunchback. Paget's disease of bone is characterized by localized, irregularly shaped, weakened bones, resulting from relatively excessive bone destruction followed by their irregular repair.

76. B: Comminuted fractures involve bone splintering into a number of fragments; if those fragments are forced into another bone, they are said to be impacted. A greenstick fracture is a fracture in which the bone bends and partially breaks, usually found in soft, young bones. An oblique fracture is a fracture in which the break is diagonal to the bone's long axis. A transverse fracture is a fracture at a right angle to the bone's long axis.

77. B: There are many types of arthritis. A number of these are either proven or suspected to be autoimmune diseases, the most prevalent being rheumatoid arthritis. Osteoarthritis is a chronic joint inflammation due to degeneration and overgrowth of bone and cartilage. Gout is joint inflammation due to deposition of uric acid crystals through a defect in purine metabolism. Psoriatic arthritis is joint inflammation in individuals with the skin condition psoriasis.

78. D: Direct deposition of bone cells into the primitive connective tissue mesenchyme is the other type of bone formation, intramembranous ossification. The other characteristics listed are associated with endochondral ossification.

79. C: There are two bones connecting the knee cap (the patella) to the foot; the larger is the tibia and the narrower one is the fibula. The femur is the thigh bone.

80. B: The vertebral column consists of 24 articulating vertebrae and 9 fused vertebrae in the sacrum and coccyx. It does house and protect the spinal cord, but that is not part of it. Individual vertebrae are made up of the anterior vertebral body and the posterior vertebral arch. The vertebral column is continuous, not clearly separated into regions, although there is normally a characteristic curvature to the spine, and the fused areas look different from the articulating ones.

81. A: The cervical region is the top portion of the spinal cord; it consists of seven levels (C1 to C7) and controls movements in the areas listed in response A. There is some overlap with the functions in other regions. However, response B describes movements controlled by the next section, the thoracic (T1 to T12); response C describes those controlled by the next lower section, the lumbar (L1 to L5); and response D describes movements controlled by the sacral region (S1 to S5).

82. C: Viral infections have been associated with neurological disorders such as Reye's syndrome, meningitis, encephalitis, and shingles. Cerebral palsy is a developmental disorder. Trigeminal neuralgia is a pain disorder, believed to be caused by excess pressure on the trigeminal nerve. Huntington's disease is a genetic disorder.

83. B: All of the choices except response B, direct impairment of cranial nerves, are characteristic of CVA, or stroke. Regarding response D, there are two types of CVA: hemorrhagic, caused by hemorrhage of a blood vessel in the brain, and ischemic, whose potential causes include obstruction by a blood clot (thrombosis) or embolus from somewhere else (embolism), systemic hypoperfusion, and venous thrombosis.

84. C: The hypothalamus is the brain portion primarily responsible for maintaining homeostasis, equilibrium of the internal environment. Located within the temporal lobe, the hippocampus is involved in memory and learning processes. The cerebellum modulates things like motor function and cognition, and the cerebral cortex or gray matter controls functions such as memory and language.

85. D: Paralysis can be caused by spinal cord injury, stroke, and poliomyelitis, as well as a number of other means of interfering with nerve function, such as the drug curare, and conditions like multiple sclerosis, spina bifida, meningitis, and Guillain-Barré syndrome. De Quervain's syndrome is a musculoskeletal disorder that does not cause paralysis.

86. C: Coordination of benefits (COB) refers to policy language that describes how multiple applicable policies will be coordinated to limit the amount paid to no more than 100% of the fee.

This is different than assignment of benefits, which means the signing over of benefits to someone else. Preauthorization is the carrier's consent prior to care, which, depending on the policy, may or may not be required. The deductible is the amount of out-of-pocket medical expenses a person must pay before the policy starts to pay, generally on a yearly basis.

87. A: Capitation is a payment system in which the health care provider is paid a fixed fee per patient, a common method used by managed care organizations, as opposed to a specific fee for a particular service, which is more common with traditional insurance.

88. B: This is a description of the PPO model of a managed care organization. Health maintenance organizations (HMOs) are similar but usually require use of only physicians in the system and selection of a primary care provider for payment as well. A POS plan allows the patient to use HMO provider services or non-HMO providers at higher rates. An EPO consists of providers and facilities under exclusive contract. An IDS uses associated service providers that work together to reduce cost.

89. B: Medicare Part B covers outpatient expenses, such as provider charges, laboratory tests, and durable medical equipment. Hospital stays and home health and hospice care are covered to an extent under Medicare Part A, and prescription drug coverage is the essence of Medicare Part D, if purchased. Medicare Part C (Medicare Advantage) plans are private plans approved by Medicare that usually cover the same things as Parts A, B, and sometimes D.

90. C: RBRVS, which is a comprehensive regional scale of fees for Medicare services, is used to calculate Medicare payments. Response B is a related answer in that *PAR* and *non-PAR* signify whether the provider is a regular Medicare provider or not, which influences how Medicare payments are determined. Medigap policies, which are supplemental insurance policies addressing non-covered fees, are not taken into account.

91. B: Mandatory eligibility groups are those identified by the federal law as qualifying for Medicaid. Examples include low-income families, individuals receiving supplemental security income (SSI), and disabled adult children. Each state has the option to expand coverage to categorically needy groups, such as individuals with tuberculosis.

92. B: The TRICARE program offers three levels of medical insurance for active-duty service members, National Guard members, reserves, military retirees, their families, and survivors. TRICARE Prime is the level for active-duty service members and is administered mostly in military hospital facilities. TRICARE Extra uses civilian preferred providers, and TRICARE Standard uses fee-for-service providers. CHAMPVA stands for Civilian Health and Medical Program of the Department of Veterans Affairs, which provides insurance to spouses and dependents of veterans who were disabled or killed in the line of duty.

93. B: Workers' compensation insurance always covers all medical expenses and lost wages as defined by state minimum standards. The company may pay a settlement at a later date as well, but that is not part of workers' compensation per se.

94. B: When using a customary fee system, the insurance carrier will pay the full fee the provider charges, providing it falls within the customary fee range charged in that geographical region. Anything above that range will have to be written off by the provider as an adjustment. The top fee is not automatically paid. The RBRVS-calculated fee, as determined relative to Medicare, may be the actual fee paid, but not necessarily.

95. C: HIPAA laws govern patient health information that is generated, transmitted, received, or stored electronically. Therefore, when information in an electronic record is transmitted via phone or fax, it becomes subject to the HIPAA security rule.

96. B: RVUs are computed using a complex equation involving all of these factors, which is then multiplied by a conversion factor to convert the RVU into dollars.

97. B: The addition of a plus sign before the code indicates the service lasted longer than described in the original code. The provider should not enter the code twice, use an unlisted code with an attached report (which is used for services for which a code cannot be clearly identified), or use a Category III code (which is temporary and designed for emerging technologies).

98. C: While the correct modifier for use of a surgical team would be 09966, the question asks for the general method of determining the modifier. This is described in response C: using a code beginning with 099 and ending with the appropriate two-digit modifier. The other responses describe coding options if multiple modifiers are required.

99. C: When billing for Medicare or Medicaid patients, HCPCS codes should be used. ICD-10-CM codes are widely used but they are not specific to Medicare/Medicaid; V codes are part of this system. The CPT coding system is also widely used.

100. A: Response A is the general format for an ICD-10-CM description of the disease diagnosis. The format in response B was the format used under ICD-9-CM. Response C describes the general format used for coding under the Current Procedural Terminology (CPT) or Healthcare Common Procedure Coding System (HCPCS) systems. Seven-digit alphanumeric codes are used for the International Classification of Diseases, 10th Revision, Procedure Coding System (ICD-10-PCS).

101. B: The correct answer in this case is the UB-04 form. The claim form generally used for office visits is A, the CMS-1500 (08-05), which derives information from the initially completed encounter form. The Authorization for Release of Medical Information form is usually signed by a patient to allow for transmission of medical information.

102. C: Medicare patients can be held responsible for some out-of-pocket expenses if they have signed an ABN.

103. D: Although the majority of facilities now use computerized financial systems, the most commonly used manual system is the pegboard system, also called the write-it-once method. This system incorporates the patient ledger, the encounter form, and other things like charge and deposit slips, day sheets, and checks. Posting is the term for the recording of financial transactions into the bookkeeping system.

104. C: All payments by the insurance company or patient, as well as adjustments (which include discounts and write-offs), should be posted as credits. The ledger should also include all debits and a running balance.

105. A: In a manual pegboard-type system, day sheets and month-end sheets are used to reconcile practice balances with patient ledgers. Accounts payable are promises to pay suppliers for expenses incurred and are not part of day or month-end sheets. Receipts are given to patients to record their payments.

106. B: Typically, computerized account systems will generate bills that include contact information for both the practice and the patient, itemized charges for recent services, payments, a running balance, aging of past-due balances, account number, date of billing, and possibly other information. A history of all past services performed is not generally included.

107. D: The only way to prevent cashing of a check by anyone else is restrictive endorsement, which means that in addition to a signature, the words "for deposit only" or "pay to the order of..." are added. Further information, such as the account number for deposit, should also be included. A blank endorsement is the signature alone, which does not ensure safety. Daily depositing of a practice's checks is a good idea, but not sufficient.

108. B: All of these practices are good ways of guaranteeing payment, but response B describes what is required under the Truth in Lending Act for making installment payments.

109. B: Rapidity of patient account payment is calculated by an accounts-receivable (AR) ratio. AR ratios have several forms depending on the scale that is being observed, whether it is looking at the daily, weekly, monthly, or yearly level. For instance, at the monthly level, it is common for an AR ratio of about two or less to be considered good. This ratio means that, on average, practice account balances are past due by two months or less. Aging is similar, but it refers to a specific patient account. The collection ratio is an indication of the effectiveness of billing procedures.

110. C: Generally, the order of attempting to settle overdue bills is telephone collections, followed by one or more collection letters, and then use of an outside collection firm. Occasionally, a tactic might be filing in small claims court, but only small claims can be brought and the process is time-consuming.

111. B: There are two types of bankruptcy that can be declared. Under Chapter 7, the debtor is cleared of all debts, so the office may need to write-off the charges; however, the required procedures are outlined in response B. Answer C describes what should be done if the patient has declared Chapter 13 bankruptcy, in which they come up with a plan to pay off some of their debt; unfortunately, a medical provider is low on the list of payees because their services are unsecured debt. Probate court is the court that deals with debt related to an estate.

112. D: An accounting software package that computerizes every aspect of running a medical facility, including patient data, electronic records, and accounting procedures, is known as a total practice management system (TPMS). A computer service bureau utilizes an outside company to coordinate data, billing services, etc. The other two options are manual methods of bookkeeping. In the single-entry system, a daily log and various records are kept and then posted to a ledger. In the double-entry system, assets are balanced against the sum of liabilities and owner's equity.

113. D: This type of accounting is financial accounting. Managerial accounting is designed to provide data that improves internal management, and cost accounting is a subset that focuses on what particular services cost. Cost analysis is the method of determining the costs of services, which are a composite of fixed and variable costs.

114. B: When using an accrual basis for income reporting, the income is recorded at the time the charges were produced. Response A describes the cash basis for income reporting, which is more commonly used.

115. C: There are three categories of fidelity bonds that can be purchased. The type that covers any employee is a blanket-position bond. A position-schedule bond pertains to a specific position but not a named employee. A personal bond covers one named employee.

116. D: When closing the facility, an administrative medical assistant should routinely do all of the things listed, and put rooms in order for the next day. An alternative to locking up the day's receipts is to take them and a bank deposit to the bank that day.

117. C: A good way of estimating the number of chairs needed in the waiting room is to add up the hourly turnover of all providers and multiply by two. Another good estimate is two and a half seats per examination room. The medical assistant or receptionist must be able to see all of the people in the waiting room. Seats should not be based on the number of appointments scheduled, because that value can change significantly over time. Having as many chairs as will fit may be excessive or dangerous in terms of egress in the case of an emergency.

118. B: RAM is the type of internal memory used for temporary storage of data and programs; it can be both written to and read from. ROM is data that cannot be altered—for example, data permanently stored in the computer motherboard on chips, or on a CD-ROM. Data storage refers to long-term storage, as with data on internal or external hard drives. RAID storage is a type of storage system.

119. D: A site address that begins with "https://" indicates a secure site. Note that a site being secure is not the same as a site being trustworthy.

120. B: An EMR is an electronic medical record from a single source, such as a medical practice, but when EMRs from various sources are combined to generate a comprehensive electronic patient database, they constitute an EHR. MOSS is a type of TPMS.

121. C: Glare from incoming light is prevented with the relative positioning described in response C. The other positions can result in some type of glare, either directly into the eyes or indirectly from reflection off the monitor. The monitor should be placed just below eye level.

122. D: A medical assistant can take a call regarding a prescription refill. However, they cannot authorize the refill themselves, so the information must be given to the provider for authorization. The other listed calls can be handled by the medical assistant.

123. A: Under the right to confidentiality, the only type of individual listed that a provider is allowed to discuss information about a patient with in all circumstances is their parent or legal guardian. A medical assistant should never discuss a patient with the patient's employer, and discussions with insurance carriers or attorneys are allowed only if a signed release is obtained from the patient.

124. B: All of these statements are true of encrypted email except choice B. A virtual private network (VPN) is a special protocol for establishing a protected connection to website or server.

125. C: This style is wave scheduling, a variation of which is modified wave scheduling, in which several patients are scheduled at the top of the hour plus single appointments at approximately 15-minute intervals thereafter. Double booking involves scheduling two or more patients simultaneously but performing different functions on each, such as seeing the doctor versus laboratory tests. Clustering is a style in which patients with similar types of issues are booked one after another. Stream scheduling is continuous booking of patients within discrete time frames. Other scheduling styles include open hours, in which patients are seen without appointments on a first-come, first-served basis, and customized practice-based scheduling.

126. D: Depending on whether scheduling is done on a daily appointment sheet or via computer, any combination of these things should be done. The important thing for legal and other purposes is to document cancellations and no-shows in some type of permanent record.

127. C: When using an electronic medical record, this is the way of correcting errors discovered promptly. Response D describes how to make these corrections later, after the software locks out the method in response C. Responses A and B describe right and wrong ways, respectively, to make corrections on paper medical records.

128. B: An accession record is a journal or computer listing with predetermined numbers, used in a numeric filing system to assign a number (rather than a name) to a file in order to protect patient confidentiality. The alphabetic card file is used as a cross-reference and contains patient name and other information. There are two other types of filing systems, alphabetic and subject, which are useful in research settings.

129. C: Modified block letter styles put some components, including those listed, in approximately the center. The standard modified block style is described. The indented modified block differs in that paragraphs are indented five spaces. In a full block letter, every component begins flush with the left margin. A simplified letter is similar, except that the salutation and complimentary closure are left out.

130. C: All these statements are true except choice C. Bulk mail must be delivered to the bulk mail entry unit at the post office and cannot be picked up.

131. A: Facilities have varying requirements, but generally a STAT report is something containing needed information (such as a laboratory report) that should be transcribed and returned in less than 12 hours. The 24-hour turnaround time is generally for current reports, an example of which is a history and physical examination (H&P) report. The 72-hour turnaround is generally for old or aged reports, such as discharge summaries.

132. D: Response C applies to CDC recommendations for use of Standard Precautions, but the OSHA Bloodborne Pathogens Standard goes further to include the items in response D.

133. D: If a patient has or may have a highly transmissible disease, both Standard Precautions and the applicable type of Transmission-Based Precautions should be used. Transmission-Based Precautions depend on whether the infectious disease is spread via the airborne route, physical contact, or respiratory droplets. The hallmark of Standard Precautions is use of personal protective equipment, which includes gloves, gowns, and mouth, nose, and eye protection, but they also include proper hand hygiene, as well as care with other potentially infectious materials, such as laundry.

134. B: The preferred disposal method is to put the sharp directly into a sharps container after use. Sharps and other biohazard containers have an orange or red-orange biohazard sticker. The scoop technique is a way to recap the needle for transport only if the sharps container is not nearby. Sharps and other forms of infectious waste are later burned or sterilized before disposal, usually by a company specializing in this disposal.

135. C: If an employee is accidentally exposed to blood or other potentially infectious materials, they should be tested for HBV, HCV, and HIV (assuming they consent to the test) and offered prophylaxis if a test is positive. The employer must offer the employee a confidential medical evaluation, but the employee has the right to refuse this as well. The incident must be immediately reported to a superior and documented. Additional requirements include testing of the source blood if the patient consents, counseling of the employee, and submission of an OSHA 301 form.

136. C: The preferred method of hand-washing is the procedure in responses A or B. The procedure in response D is acceptable, but the use of antibacterial wipes is not.

137. B: The use of chemical germicidal agents on surfaces by wiping or soaking is known as disinfection; it destroys most pathogens, but not spores. Sanitization is the use of techniques such as enzymatic detergents and ultrasonic cleaners to reduce microbial load on instruments and equipment. Sterilization is the use of techniques such as steam sterilization to kill all microbes, including spores. Antisepsis is the use of topical chemicals on the skin to kill or inhibit microbes.

138. A: The sequence recommended by the CDC for PPE removal is gown and gloves (together), then goggles, then mask, and finally washing the hands. This process is optimal for ensuring the prevention of exposure to pathogens. If taking off gown and gloves separately, gloves should be removed before the gown. After each type of PPE is removed, it should be disposed of in a biohazard container.

139. B: In order to maintain sterility, both hands should be held in front of the body, at a distance from the body, and above waist level.

140. D: Surgical hand cleansing extends to the elbows, while medical hand cleansing is focused on the hands. Surgical hand washing takes longer and hands are held up during rinsing. Hands are held down during medical hand cleansing, and lotion can be applied after. Additional differences include that alcohol-based products can be substituted for medical washing but are only used after other steps in surgical washing, and that gloves are always applied after surgical hand cleansing.

141. C: Heat-sensitive items, such as fiber-optic endoscopes, as well as certain items that will not fit in an autoclave for steam sterilization, should be sterilized using chemical or so-called "cold" sterilization. In this process, the object is immersed in a chemical solution that can kill certain microorganisms, and then it is rinsed with sterile water. The other methods are either impractical or use too high a temperature.

142. B: Response B describes the parameters that must be achieved for steam sterilization of wrapped instrument packages or trays. Response C applies if sterilizing unwrapped items (20 minutes for unwrapped objects covered with cloth). After the autoclave cycle is done, the door can be opened slightly when the temperature goes down to 212 °F, but the pressure at that point should be zero.

143. D: Use of biological indicators that are later cultured is recommended for quality control for autoclaves. These indicators contain heat-resistant bacterial spores, such as those from the thermophile *Geobacillus stearothermophilus*, not a generic type of bacteria. Sterilization tapes, which contain a thermolabile dye that gets darker upon sterilization, do indicate that the proper parameters have been achieved but not whether spores have been killed. Autoclave tape should be placed on packages to be autoclaved; they develop stripes, which indicate that a high temperature has been achieved.

144. C: Cryosurgery destroys tissues, namely things like superficial lesions, by freezing them. Usually, liquid nitrogen is used because it gets very cold, making it quite destructive. Nitrous oxide can also be utilized for most applications, except things like removal of cancerous lesions that require complete destruction. Silver nitrate is commonly used for cautery of broken blood vessels in nosebleeds, and sodium hydroxide is commonly used for destruction of toenail growth plates after removal of toenails.

145. B: The smallest suture material available is gauge 6-0, and it is commonly used in ambulatory settings. Gauge 0 is larger, and gauge 4 is the largest. *Swaged* is a term referring to suture materials that come pre-attached to a needle.

146. C: The feature described is a ratchet. Serrations are generally at the other end of the instrument and are a series of narrow slits that secure gripping without tearing the tissue; they are found on instruments like hemostats or loops. By contrast, teeth are sharp and puncture the tissue.

147. A: Mayo dissecting scissors have beveled edges instead of some combination of blunt and/or sharp edges, characteristic of standard operating scissors. The other types of cutting instruments described are scalpels, suture or stitch removal scissors, and iris scissors.

148. B: All hemostatic forceps (or hemostats), which are utilized to grasp and clamp blood vessels, have ratchets and serrations. Most, but not all, are straight, and some have teeth in addition to serrations. Response C describes several types of forceps, used for ear and nose procedures, and response D characterizes the Allis tissue forceps.

149. D: Scopes may be long or short, and they are flexible devices that allow visual access to both superficial and deep aspects of the human body. They are equipped with a light and a camera or lens to allow visualization using minimally invasive measures. Due to the scope's entrance into the body, they must be capable of being disinfected. If that is not a capability for the scope or the facility, then there are disposable scopes available for use. Examples of scopes are otoscopes (used in the ear), proctoscopes, anoscopes, and sigmoidoscopes (used to look at the rectum, anus, and sigmoid part of the large intestine).

150. C: Of the choices, the only thing that should not be done is to mix instruments composed of different types of metals. The processing time varies depending on the instrument, but is usually at least five minutes.

151. B: The topical antibacterial cream used for burns and other abrasion wounds is silver sulfadiazine. Povidone-iodine (which can be used as a surgical scrub), chlorhexidine, and hydrogen peroxide are skin antiseptics.

152. C: Figure-eight turns, which alternate crossing on either side of the joint, should be used. Spiral turns are circular turns that overlap when going up a body part. Reverse spiral turns are turns that reverse or twist each turn on a limb that gets increasingly large. Circular turns are turns that wrap around the body part several times. All bandages are non-sterile. They may be used over a sterile dressing to anchor it, or as support.

153. A: The property of epinephrine that makes it a frequent addition to injectable anesthetics is that it is a vasoconstrictor. When restricted blood flow to the area of surgery is desired, epinephrine is a good additive.

154. B: Response B describes the type of open wound known as an avulsion. A laceration is the tearing of body tissue by a sharp object. A puncture is a small hole or wound caused by a pointed object. An incision is an intentional cut made during surgery with a scalpel.

155. D: This is the correct use of gloves for changing a surgical dressing, as well as for removal and wound irrigation prior to putting on a new dressing.

156. B: Fevers in which there are significant fluctuations in body temperature are either intermittent, as described here, or remittent, in which the temperature never returns to baseline. A continuous fever is one in which the body temperature stays above baseline pretty consistently. Febrile is the general term for any presence of fever, a body temperature elevated above the normal range, which for an adult is an average of 98.6 degrees Fahrenheit.

157. D: Response D is the primary way in which a TA thermometer probe is used, although the probe can be used behind the earlobe if there is a great deal of perspiration on the forehead. Probe insertion into the ear is used with tympanic thermometers, which measure the aural temperature. Probe attachment to an electronic thermometer and insertion orally or rectally is commonly used today but employs a different type of thermometer.

158. B: This is the correct method for changing a temperature from Celsius to Fahrenheit. The correct formula for converting Fahrenheit to Celsius is expressed in response D.

159. C: During emergency situations, the pulse site used is normally the carotid pulse, which is located on either side of the front of the neck, between the larynx and sternocleidomastoid muscle. In other situations, the radial pulse above the base of the thumb on the wrist, and the brachial pulse in the antecubital space on the inner side of the elbow, are commonly used sites. The apical pulse is located at the apex of the heart, can only be found using a stethoscope, and is typically used only in cardiac patients or infants. Other pulse sites include the temporal, femoral, popliteal, and dorsalis pedis artery sites.

160. A: A pulse rate of 70 beats per minute is considered a normal pulse rate for an adult (range 60-80 beats per minute). However, in infants and children this would be considered too low, because average normal pulse rates steadily decline from birth through infancy and childhood. The other choices are abnormalities. Bradycardia is a pulse rate of less than 60 beats per minute. Tachycardia is a pulse rate of more than 100 beats per minute. Arrhythmia is any abnormal electrical activity in the heart, resulting in alteration of the interval between pulsations.

161. B: Orthopnea, or labored breathing, is difficulty breathing unless standing or sitting erect; it occurs in conditions like angina pectoris, heart failure, and various pulmonary conditions. The other situations do involve a period of complete absence of breathing known as apnea. Sleep apnea is characterized by periods of more than 10 seconds in which breathing stops during sleep, depleting the brain of oxygen and potentially causing a variety of cardiac and neurologic defects. Cheyne-Stokes respiration is a respiration cycle in which there is approximately 10-60 seconds of apnea, then deep and rapid breathing, and then a decreased rate.

162. C: This is a description of rales, which is indicative of secretions in the lung passageways. Stridor and wheezing are similar in that they are high-pitched sounds caused by some type of airway obstruction; stridor sounds more like crowing, while wheezing sounds more like whistling. Stertorous respiration is labored breathing, similar to snoring, usually due to some upper respiratory obstruction.

163. D: Blood pressure is a function of how strong the heart muscle is and the elasticity of the arteries, as well as blood volume and blood viscosity. The size of the lumen of the arteries is directly related to their peripheral resistance, which also impacts blood pressure. Ejection fraction represents the volume of blood that is released from the heart with every contraction, but does not directly affect blood pressure.

164. B: The only one of these characteristics that distinguishes an electronic sphygmomanometer is that it does not necessitate simultaneous use of a stethoscope because there is a digital readout.

There are three types of manometers, all of which use a pressure cuff: electronic, aneroid, and the traditional mercury type, which is being phased out. Response C is true of the aneroid type, which uses a dial attached to the rubber bladder pressure cuff.

165. A: There are five phases generally observed during deflation of the pressure cuff when taking blood pressure readings. The systolic pressure is the highest pressure, representing the force exerted on arterial walls during cardiac contraction, and it is heard as the first Korotkoff sound. In subsequent phases, more blood passes through the blood vessels. Generally, the sounds heard include swishing, then rhythmic tapping, and lastly muffled tapping sounds. Sometimes there is an auscultatory gap sometime after phase I, in which no sounds are heard; but they later reappear. The diastolic pressure, which represents the force during cardiac relaxation, is taken when all sounds cease in phase V. In children, diastolic pressure may be recorded in phase IV, as some tapping may be heard down to pressure zero.

166. B: A blood pressure measurement in itself is written as "systolic pressure/diastolic pressure" (for example: 110/75), but it is preferable to also note the arm used and the patient position (for example: right arm, supine).

167. B: An adult with this blood pressure (BP) reading is considered to have prehypertension, which can lead to hypertension if not controlled. Normal blood pressure for an adult is a systolic pressure less than 120 and a diastolic pressure less than 80. Any BP above 140/90 is considered hypertension. Secondary hypertension is high blood pressure due to some underlying cause, such as atherosclerosis. If atherosclerosis is treated, the BP can return to normal or close to normal.

168. D: Once the scale has been balanced, the medical assistant needs to add the number from the upper bar to that of the lower bar. This gives the patient's weight in pounds. If you need the patient's weight in kilograms, divide the number of pounds by 2.2 to convert pounds to kilograms.

169. C: This examination is auscultation. Palpation is the use of touch to feel for things like body parts, masses, and skin texture. Percussion is tapping with the fingers or a percussion hammer to listen for characteristic dull or hollow sounds. Mensuration is taking measurements such as height, weight, and circumference of a body part. Other examination methods include observation of things like symmetry and posture, and manipulation to check for range of motion.

170. B: Patients with cardiovascular or respiratory problems should be positioned in either the semi-Fowler's or high Fowler's position, which are at 45- and 90-degree angles sitting up, respectively, to help them breathe. The dorsal recumbent or lithotomy position has patients lie on their back with their knees flexed and their feet either on the table or in attached stirrups. This position is used for genital and pelvic examinations, urinary catheterization, and other examinations. The Trendelenburg position has patients lie supine on their back with their feet elevated. This position is used to increase blood flow to the brain in emergencies and during abdominal or pelvic surgery. The Sims' position has patients lie laterally on their left side. This position is used for situations like vaginal and rectal exams, sigmoidoscopy, etc.

171. C: The provider can check for dental hygiene, swollen tonsils and uvula, and gag reflex using a tongue depressor and light source during the mouth and throat examination. Dental hygiene issues of note include caries and pus discharge at the gums, indicating infection. Swollen tonsils and uvula may also indicate infection. The gag reflex, a reflection of cranial nerves IX and X, should occur when the soft palate is touched; absence of the gag reflex could indicate neurologic issues. Cranial nerve XI is tested by asking the patient to shrug their shoulders.

172. B: All of these are a cause for concern, except the presence of bowel sounds if they are within expected levels.

173. C: Depending on the system used, either response A or B could be applied. Gravidity refers to the total number of pregnancies, regardless of outcome. Parity is the number of pregnancies carried to the point of viability, generally considered to be 24 weeks after conception or the attainment of one pound of body weight. Parity is not dependent on whether or not there was a live birth, or on the number of children born. The FPAL system for parity reflects the number of full-term deliveries (F), pre-term or premature deliveries (P), abortions prior to 20 weeks (A), and current number of living children (L).

174. A: A urinalysis tests for all of the listed things except VDRL, which is a blood test for syphilis. Urinalysis is done to screen for diabetes, hypertension, infection, renal disease, and pregnancy. A number of other blood tests, smears, or cultures for infectious diseases, immunity, etc., are done as part of a prenatal visit. Glucose in the blood is measured as well, to check for gestational diabetes.

175. B: This is a description of placenta previa. Eclampsia is hypertension, edema, and proteinuria induced by pregnancy, which can endanger the fetus. Placenta abruptio is sudden premature pulling away of the placenta from the uterus, which can cause fetal hypoxia and possibly death, as well as maternal shock and possibly death. Incompatibility is a situation in which the mother is Rh-negative and the fetus Rh-positive and the mother develops anti-Rh antibodies to the fetus's red blood cells, which can then be depleted and cause fetal death.

176. C: The only thing listed that must be done by the provider, not the medical assistant, is swabbing of the cervix with an antiseptic and injection of a local anesthetic. The medical assistant should be prepared to assist the patient into the lithotomy position and drape her, to hand the speculum to the provider, and to document the procedure in the patient's chart.

177. A: The only false statement is that the actual breast examination should be done standing up, because it should be performed while supine in order to spread out the breast tissue. Other portions of the examination can be done standing up, such as checking in the mirror and feeling the underarm area for swollen lymph nodes.

178. C: The Bethesda system of classifying Pap tests has three categories. Category 1 is a Pap test negative for intraepithelial, precancerous, or cancerous cells or other abnormalities. Category 2 is presence of epithelial cell abnormalities; it is subdivided into four groups, of which the ones represented here are subgroup 1a (atypical squamous cells of uncertain significance) and subgroup 1c (squamous cell carcinoma). Category 3 is the presence of other malignancies, such as melanoma. CIN 3 would be correct under the other classification system, which grades the amount of cervical intraepithelial neoplasia into three types of increasing dysplasia (CIN 1, CIN 2, and CIN 3).

179. B: These procedures are used to ascertain the cause of female vaginitis or male urethritis. The medical assistant often assists by mixing the discharge sample in saline and putting it on the microscope slide (wet prep/wet mount), and later adding potassium hydroxide (KOH) and preparing another slide. These are used by the provider to identify yeast, bacteria, and trichomonas, and later for fungi with KOH addition. Amplified DNA probe tests are used to screen for chlamydia and gonorrhea, laparoscopy or ultrasound help diagnose endometriosis and fibroids, and cervical punch or cervical cone biopsies are used to diagnose malignancies.

180. B: Subcutaneous epinephrine is always administered as described until the emergency medical services (EMS) arrive or symptoms subside. Diphenhydramine may also be necessary if the child is experiencing anaphylaxis, and CPR may be needed in such a case to maintain the airways.

181. C: The deltoid muscle is the preferred intramuscular site for all ages, except infants younger than 12 months, who should be vaccinated in the anterolateral aspect of the thigh or, if necessary, the gluteal muscle. The triceps muscle, which is lower along the arm, is the preferred site for subcutaneous injections. Intramuscular injections are done at a 90-degree angle to the skin, while subcutaneous ones are done at a 45-degree angle.

182. B: Growth charts up to age 36 months generally are separated according to sex and have a series of curves for both length and weight versus age in months. Typically, these measurements are recorded in one corner along with the date, age, and head (not chest) circumference. The head-circumference-for-age curves are usually on a chart that also shows percentiles for weight-for-length.

183. C: The preferred site to take a pulse rate in pediatric patients 5 years or younger is the apical pulse.

184. A: Prostatic ultrasound, biopsy, and prostate-specific antigen (PSA) are all used in conjunction to provide a diagnosis of prostate cancer.

185. A: All of these apply to doing a urinary catheterization on a female patient except for choice A. While the provider should use sterile gloves, only the dominant hand retains sterility throughout, because once the provider starts wiping the genitalia, the other hand becomes contaminated.

186. B: The developer in a fecal occult blood test contains guaiac, which, when combined with blood, will turn a blue color seen at the periphery within 30-60 seconds. The positive control, but not the negative control, should also show this blue halo to constitute a valid test.

187. D: All of the choices are pulmonary function tests (also known as spirometry) used to assess respiration, but the PEFR is particularly useful for determining the extent of asthma or another disorder because it is depressed during an attack.

188. A: The only statement that is not universally applicable to an ESR is response A. This statement is true for all male patients and women under 50, but the normal range for women over 50 is 0-30 mm/hour. The ESR is a relatively simple test in which blood is put in a tube in an upright rack and allowed to settle, separating the plasma on top from the settled blood and red blood cells (RBCs) on the bottom; many disease states cause RBC and fibrinogen alterations that result in greater settling. There are two methods, the Wintrobe and Westergren.

189. C: The only correct way to lift a patient who cannot walk or lift themselves is by gripping their gait belt from underneath and then lifting. Injuries to the provider or the patient can result from using any of the other listed methods.

190. B: In all of these types of gaits, except the three-point gait, there is some point at which the patient is bearing weight on both legs.

191. C: This type of ROM exercise is abduction. The opposite, in which motion is toward the midline, is called adduction. Flexion is the bending of a body part, and rotation is the turning of a body part around its central axis. Other types of ROM include extension, pronation, and eversion. Every joint has a certain amount of ROM, or amount of movement possible, and is measured in degrees using a device called a goniometer.

192. B: CPR, or cardiopulmonary resuscitation, is indicated when an individual is found unresponsive and pulseless (or with a dangerously low pulse). Per AHA guidelines, CPR should be initiated as quickly as possible for maximum effect, starting with chest compressions. For circulation, 30 chest compressions should be administered rapidly, at a depth of 2" to 2.5", followed by 2 rescue breaths, with this cycle repeating until help has arrived and/or the defibrillator has been applied, charged, and is prepared to deliver a shock.

193. B: There are five schedules of drugs under the Controlled Substances Act. Schedule I applies to drugs of abuse that are not available medicinally, such as heroin. Schedule II drugs have abuse potential, but they have accepted medical uses, such as cocaine. These drugs might be used medically, but they require the DEA form along with a non-renewable prescription. Schedules III through V drugs have decreasing potential for abuse and can be ordered via prescription.

194. A: Nitroglycerin, a vasodilator, is used to treat an attack of angina pectoris or chest pain due to chronic heart disease. Atropine is used to increase heart rate. Digoxin is used in congestive heart failure or arrhythmias. Isoproterenol is used to treat heart blocks. Other types of drugs should also be available, such as albuterol (bronchodilator), epinephrine (vasoconstrictor for anaphylactic shock), and prochlorperazine (an antiemetic).

195. B: The correct method is response B; response C has the calculation reversed. Do not convert to mg because this type of drug is a liquid and units will probably not be related to mg, a measurement of mass or weight. Multiplying by 16 is an approximate way to convert mL to another unit called minims (there are about 16 minims in a mL), but that is not necessary here.

196. A: Of the choices for ECG leads given, response A describes the bipolar or standard limb leads, response B describes the augmented leads, and response D describes the chest or precordial leads.

197. C: All of the listed irregularities are types of arrhythmias. This pattern is seen in ventricular tachycardia, which is a very fast heart rate originating in the ventricles. Both ventricular tachycardia and ventricular fibrillation, which looks like an irregular up-and-down pattern on an ECG, can indicate myocardial infarction and life-threatening situations. Atrial fibrillation can be associated with conditions like mitral valve prolapse, and is indicated on an ECG by irregularly spaced patterns without distinguishable P waves. Paroxysmal atrial tachycardia is a sudden pattern of more rapid beating that lasts briefly; it can be seen in cardiac patients but often occurs in healthy people.

198. C: All chemical labels have composite National Fire Protection Association ratings on them in the form of four diamonds of different colors, with numbers from 0-4 on three of these diamonds indicating an increasing seriousness of the hazard. The blue diamond rates the health hazard, and a "3" in that diamond means the chemical is a corrosive or toxic health hazard. Flammability is rated in the red diamond; a "3" would mean that it is a flammable liquid. Reactivity or instability is rated in the yellow diamond; a "3" would mean that it is potentially explosive near a spark or if heated. The fourth diamond is white; any symbol there would give information on a special hazard (such as "W" for water reactive) or appropriate protective equipment.

199. B: Response B is the approved basic metabolic panel of laboratory tests, while C is the approved comprehensive metabolic panel. Response A is the electrolyte panel, while response D is the hepatic function panel. There is often overlap between panels.

200. A: In order to collect a serum sample, the provider must use a tube that promotes clot formation, such as a red top, which contains no additives, or a red-gray mottled top, which contains a clot activator and serum separating tube. All of the other listed choices contain additives that prevent clot formation at some step in the cascade to give either plasma or whole blood.

CMA Practice Tests #2, #3 and #4

To take these additional CMA practice tests, visit our bonus page: **mometrix.com/bonus948/certmedasst**

How to Overcome Test Anxiety

Just the thought of taking a test is enough to make most people a little nervous. A test is an important event that can have a long-term impact on your future, so it's important to take it seriously and it's natural to feel anxious about performing well. But just because anxiety is normal, that doesn't mean that it's helpful in test taking, or that you should simply accept it as part of your life. Anxiety can have a variety of effects. These effects can be mild, like making you feel slightly nervous, or severe, like blocking your ability to focus or remember even a simple detail.

If you experience test anxiety—whether severe or mild—it's important to know how to beat it. To discover this, first you need to understand what causes test anxiety.

Causes of Test Anxiety

While we often think of anxiety as an uncontrollable emotional state, it can actually be caused by simple, practical things. One of the most common causes of test anxiety is that a person does not feel adequately prepared for their test. This feeling can be the result of many different issues such as poor study habits or lack of organization, but the most common culprit is time management. Starting to study too late, failing to organize your study time to cover all of the material, or being distracted while you study will mean that you're not well prepared for the test. This may lead to cramming the night before, which will cause you to be physically and mentally exhausted for the test. Poor time management also contributes to feelings of stress, fear, and hopelessness as you realize you are not well prepared but don't know what to do about it.

Other times, test anxiety is not related to your preparation for the test but comes from unresolved fear. This may be a past failure on a test, or poor performance on tests in general. It may come from comparing yourself to others who seem to be performing better or from the stress of living up to expectations. Anxiety may be driven by fears of the future—how failure on this test would affect your educational and career goals. These fears are often completely irrational, but they can still negatively impact your test performance.

Review Video: 3 Reasons You Have Test Anxiety
Visit mometrix.com/academy and enter code: 428468

Elements of Test Anxiety

As mentioned earlier, test anxiety is considered to be an emotional state, but it has physical and mental components as well. Sometimes you may not even realize that you are suffering from test anxiety until you notice the physical symptoms. These can include trembling hands, rapid heartbeat, sweating, nausea, and tense muscles. Extreme anxiety may lead to fainting or vomiting. Obviously, any of these symptoms can have a negative impact on testing. It is important to recognize them as soon as they begin to occur so that you can address the problem before it damages your performance.

Review Video: 3 Ways to Tell You Have Test Anxiety
Visit mometrix.com/academy and enter code: 927847

The mental components of test anxiety include trouble focusing and inability to remember learned information. During a test, your mind is on high alert, which can help you recall information and stay focused for an extended period of time. However, anxiety interferes with your mind's natural processes, causing you to blank out, even on the questions you know well. The strain of testing during anxiety makes it difficult to stay focused, especially on a test that may take several hours. Extreme anxiety can take a huge mental toll, making it difficult not only to recall test information but even to understand the test questions or pull your thoughts together.

Review Video: How Test Anxiety Affects Memory
Visit mometrix.com/academy and enter code: 609003

Effects of Test Anxiety

Test anxiety is like a disease—if left untreated, it will get progressively worse. Anxiety leads to poor performance, and this reinforces the feelings of fear and failure, which in turn lead to poor performances on subsequent tests. It can grow from a mild nervousness to a crippling condition. If allowed to progress, test anxiety can have a big impact on your schooling, and consequently on your future.

Test anxiety can spread to other parts of your life. Anxiety on tests can become anxiety in any stressful situation, and blanking on a test can turn into panicking in a job situation. But fortunately, you don't have to let anxiety rule your testing and determine your grades. There are a number of relatively simple steps you can take to move past anxiety and function normally on a test and in the rest of life.

Review Video: How Test Anxiety Impacts Your Grades
Visit mometrix.com/academy and enter code: 939819

Physical Steps for Beating Test Anxiety

While test anxiety is a serious problem, the good news is that it can be overcome. It doesn't have to control your ability to think and remember information. While it may take time, you can begin taking steps today to beat anxiety.

Just as your first hint that you may be struggling with anxiety comes from the physical symptoms, the first step to treating it is also physical. Rest is crucial for having a clear, strong mind. If you are tired, it is much easier to give in to anxiety. But if you establish good sleep habits, your body and mind will be ready to perform optimally, without the strain of exhaustion. Additionally, sleeping well helps you to retain information better, so you're more likely to recall the answers when you see the test questions.

Getting good sleep means more than going to bed on time. It's important to allow your brain time to relax. Take study breaks from time to time so it doesn't get overworked, and don't study right before bed. Take time to rest your mind before trying to rest your body, or you may find it difficult to fall asleep.

Review Video: <u>The Importance of Sleep for Your Brain</u>
Visit mometrix.com/academy and enter code: 319338

Along with sleep, other aspects of physical health are important in preparing for a test. Good nutrition is vital for good brain function. Sugary foods and drinks may give a burst of energy but this burst is followed by a crash, both physically and emotionally. Instead, fuel your body with protein and vitamin-rich foods.

Also, drink plenty of water. Dehydration can lead to headaches and exhaustion, especially if your brain is already under stress from the rigors of the test. Particularly if your test is a long one, drink water during the breaks. And if possible, take an energy-boosting snack to eat between sections.

Review Video: <u>How Diet Can Affect your Mood</u>
Visit mometrix.com/academy and enter code: 624317

Along with sleep and diet, a third important part of physical health is exercise. Maintaining a steady workout schedule is helpful, but even taking 5-minute study breaks to walk can help get your blood pumping faster and clear your head. Exercise also releases endorphins, which contribute to a positive feeling and can help combat test anxiety.

When you nurture your physical health, you are also contributing to your mental health. If your body is healthy, your mind is much more likely to be healthy as well. So take time to rest, nourish your body with healthy food and water, and get moving as much as possible. Taking these physical steps will make you stronger and more able to take the mental steps necessary to overcome test anxiety.

Mental Steps for Beating Test Anxiety

Working on the mental side of test anxiety can be more challenging, but as with the physical side, there are clear steps you can take to overcome it. As mentioned earlier, test anxiety often stems from lack of preparation, so the obvious solution is to prepare for the test. Effective studying may be the most important weapon you have for beating test anxiety, but you can and should employ several other mental tools to combat fear.

First, boost your confidence by reminding yourself of past success—tests or projects that you aced. If you're putting as much effort into preparing for this test as you did for those, there's no reason you should expect to fail here. Work hard to prepare; then trust your preparation.

Second, surround yourself with encouraging people. It can be helpful to find a study group, but be sure that the people you're around will encourage a positive attitude. If you spend time with others who are anxious or cynical, this will only contribute to your own anxiety. Look for others who are motivated to study hard from a desire to succeed, not from a fear of failure.

Third, reward yourself. A test is physically and mentally tiring, even without anxiety, and it can be helpful to have something to look forward to. Plan an activity following the test, regardless of the outcome, such as going to a movie or getting ice cream.

When you are taking the test, if you find yourself beginning to feel anxious, remind yourself that you know the material. Visualize successfully completing the test. Then take a few deep, relaxing breaths and return to it. Work through the questions carefully but with confidence, knowing that you are capable of succeeding.

Developing a healthy mental approach to test taking will also aid in other areas of life. Test anxiety affects more than just the actual test—it can be damaging to your mental health and even contribute to depression. It's important to beat test anxiety before it becomes a problem for more than testing.

Review Video: Test Anxiety and Depression
Visit mometrix.com/academy and enter code: 904704

Study Strategy

Being prepared for the test is necessary to combat anxiety, but what does being prepared look like? You may study for hours on end and still not feel prepared. What you need is a strategy for test prep. The next few pages outline our recommended steps to help you plan out and conquer the challenge of preparation.

Step 1: Scope Out the Test

Learn everything you can about the format (multiple choice, essay, etc.) and what will be on the test. Gather any study materials, course outlines, or sample exams that may be available. Not only will this help you to prepare, but knowing what to expect can help to alleviate test anxiety.

Step 2: Map Out the Material

Look through the textbook or study guide and make note of how many chapters or sections it has. Then divide these over the time you have. For example, if a book has 15 chapters and you have five days to study, you need to cover three chapters each day. Even better, if you have the time, leave an extra day at the end for overall review after you have gone through the material in depth.

If time is limited, you may need to prioritize the material. Look through it and make note of which sections you think you already have a good grasp on, and which need review. While you are studying, skim quickly through the familiar sections and take more time on the challenging parts. Write out your plan so you don't get lost as you go. Having a written plan also helps you feel more in control of the study, so anxiety is less likely to arise from feeling overwhelmed at the amount to cover.

Step 3: Gather Your Tools

Decide what study method works best for you. Do you prefer to highlight in the book as you study and then go back over the highlighted portions? Or do you type out notes of the important information? Or is it helpful to make flashcards that you can carry with you? Assemble the pens, index cards, highlighters, post-it notes, and any other materials you may need so you won't be distracted by getting up to find things while you study.

If you're having a hard time retaining the information or organizing your notes, experiment with different methods. For example, try color-coding by subject with colored pens, highlighters, or post-it notes. If you learn better by hearing, try recording yourself reading your notes so you can listen while in the car, working out, or simply sitting at your desk. Ask a friend to quiz you from your flashcards, or try teaching someone the material to solidify it in your mind.

Step 4: Create Your Environment

It's important to avoid distractions while you study. This includes both the obvious distractions like visitors and the subtle distractions like an uncomfortable chair (or a too-comfortable couch that makes you want to fall asleep). Set up the best study environment possible: good lighting and a comfortable work area. If background music helps you focus, you may want to turn it on, but otherwise keep the room quiet. If you are using a computer to take notes, be sure you don't have any other windows open, especially applications like social media, games, or anything else that could distract you. Silence your phone and turn off notifications. Be sure to keep water close by so you stay hydrated while you study (but avoid unhealthy drinks and snacks).

Also, take into account the best time of day to study. Are you freshest first thing in the morning? Try to set aside some time then to work through the material. Is your mind clearer in the afternoon or evening? Schedule your study session then. Another method is to study at the same time of day that you will take the test, so that your brain gets used to working on the material at that time and will be ready to focus at test time.

Step 5: Study!

Once you have done all the study preparation, it's time to settle into the actual studying. Sit down, take a few moments to settle your mind so you can focus, and begin to follow your study plan. Don't give in to distractions or let yourself procrastinate. This is your time to prepare so you'll be ready to fearlessly approach the test. Make the most of the time and stay focused.

Of course, you don't want to burn out. If you study too long you may find that you're not retaining the information very well. Take regular study breaks. For example, taking five minutes out of every hour to walk briskly, breathing deeply and swinging your arms, can help your mind stay fresh.

As you get to the end of each chapter or section, it's a good idea to do a quick review. Remind yourself of what you learned and work on any difficult parts. When you feel that you've mastered the material, move on to the next part. At the end of your study session, briefly skim through your notes again.

But while review is helpful, cramming last minute is NOT. If at all possible, work ahead so that you won't need to fit all your study into the last day. Cramming overloads your brain with more information than it can process and retain, and your tired mind may struggle to recall even previously learned information when it is overwhelmed with last-minute study. Also, the urgent nature of cramming and the stress placed on your brain contribute to anxiety. You'll be more likely to go to the test feeling unprepared and having trouble thinking clearly.

So don't cram, and don't stay up late before the test, even just to review your notes at a leisurely pace. Your brain needs rest more than it needs to go over the information again. In fact, plan to finish your studies by noon or early afternoon the day before the test. Give your brain the rest of the day to relax or focus on other things, and get a good night's sleep. Then you will be fresh for the test and better able to recall what you've studied.

Step 6: Take a practice test

Many courses offer sample tests, either online or in the study materials. This is an excellent resource to check whether you have mastered the material, as well as to prepare for the test format and environment.

Check the test format ahead of time: the number of questions, the type (multiple choice, free response, etc.), and the time limit. Then create a plan for working through them. For example, if you have 30 minutes to take a 60-question test, your limit is 30 seconds per question. Spend less time on the questions you know well so that you can take more time on the difficult ones.

If you have time to take several practice tests, take the first one open book, with no time limit. Work through the questions at your own pace and make sure you fully understand them. Gradually work up to taking a test under test conditions: sit at a desk with all study materials put away and set a timer. Pace yourself to make sure you finish the test with time to spare and go back to check your answers if you have time.

After each test, check your answers. On the questions you missed, be sure you understand why you missed them. Did you misread the question (tests can use tricky wording)? Did you forget the information? Or was it something you hadn't learned? Go back and study any shaky areas that the practice tests reveal.

Taking these tests not only helps with your grade, but also aids in combating test anxiety. If you're already used to the test conditions, you're less likely to worry about it, and working through tests until you're scoring well gives you a confidence boost. Go through the practice tests until you feel comfortable, and then you can go into the test knowing that you're ready for it.

Test Tips

On test day, you should be confident, knowing that you've prepared well and are ready to answer the questions. But aside from preparation, there are several test day strategies you can employ to maximize your performance.

First, as stated before, get a good night's sleep the night before the test (and for several nights before that, if possible). Go into the test with a fresh, alert mind rather than staying up late to study.

Try not to change too much about your normal routine on the day of the test. It's important to eat a nutritious breakfast, but if you normally don't eat breakfast at all, consider eating just a protein bar. If you're a coffee drinker, go ahead and have your normal coffee. Just make sure you time it so that the caffeine doesn't wear off right in the middle of your test. Avoid sugary beverages, and drink enough water to stay hydrated but not so much that you need a restroom break 10 minutes into the test. If your test isn't first thing in the morning, consider going for a walk or doing a light workout before the test to get your blood flowing.

Allow yourself enough time to get ready, and leave for the test with plenty of time to spare so you won't have the anxiety of scrambling to arrive in time. Another reason to be early is to select a good seat. It's helpful to sit away from doors and windows, which can be distracting. Find a good seat, get out your supplies, and settle your mind before the test begins.

When the test begins, start by going over the instructions carefully, even if you already know what to expect. Make sure you avoid any careless mistakes by following the directions.

Then begin working through the questions, pacing yourself as you've practiced. If you're not sure on an answer, don't spend too much time on it, and don't let it shake your confidence. Either skip it and come back later, or eliminate as many wrong answers as possible and guess among the remaining ones. Don't dwell on these questions as you continue—put them out of your mind and focus on what lies ahead.

Be sure to read all of the answer choices, even if you're sure the first one is the right answer. Sometimes you'll find a better one if you keep reading. But don't second-guess yourself if you do immediately know the answer. Your gut instinct is usually right. Don't let test anxiety rob you of the information you know.

If you have time at the end of the test (and if the test format allows), go back and review your answers. Be cautious about changing any, since your first instinct tends to be correct, but make sure you didn't misread any of the questions or accidentally mark the wrong answer choice. Look over any you skipped and make an educated guess.

At the end, leave the test feeling confident. You've done your best, so don't waste time worrying about your performance or wishing you could change anything. Instead, celebrate the successful completion of this test. And finally, use this test to learn how to deal with anxiety even better next time.

Review Video: 5 Tips to Beat Test Anxiety
Visit mometrix.com/academy and enter code: 570656

Important Qualification

Not all anxiety is created equal. If your test anxiety is causing major issues in your life beyond the classroom or testing center, or if you are experiencing troubling physical symptoms related to your anxiety, it may be a sign of a serious physiological or psychological condition. If this sounds like your situation, we strongly encourage you to seek professional help.

Tell Us Your Story

We at Mometrix would like to extend our heartfelt thanks to you for letting us be a part of your journey. It is an honor to serve people from all walks of life, people like you, who are committed to building the best future they can for themselves.

We know that each person's situation is unique. But we also know that, whether you are a young student or a mother of four, you care about working to make your own life and the lives of those around you better.

That's why we want to hear your story.

We want to know why you're taking this test. We want to know about the trials you've gone through to get here. And we want to know about the successes you've experienced after taking and passing your test.

In addition to your story, which can be an inspiration both to us and to others, we value your feedback. We want to know both what you loved about our book and what you think we can improve on.

The team at Mometrix would be absolutely thrilled to hear from you! So please, send us an email at tellusyourstory@mometrix.com or visit us at mometrix.com/tellusyourstory.php and let's stay in touch.

Additional Bonus Material

Due to our efforts to try to keep this book to a manageable length, we've created a link that will give you access to all of your additional bonus material:

mometrix.com/bonus948/certmedasst

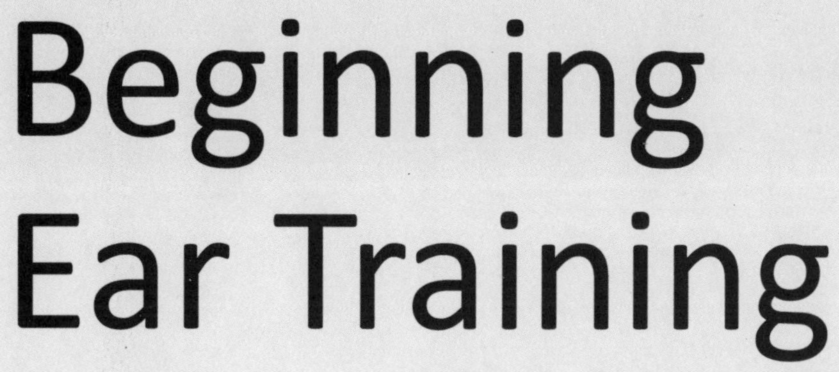

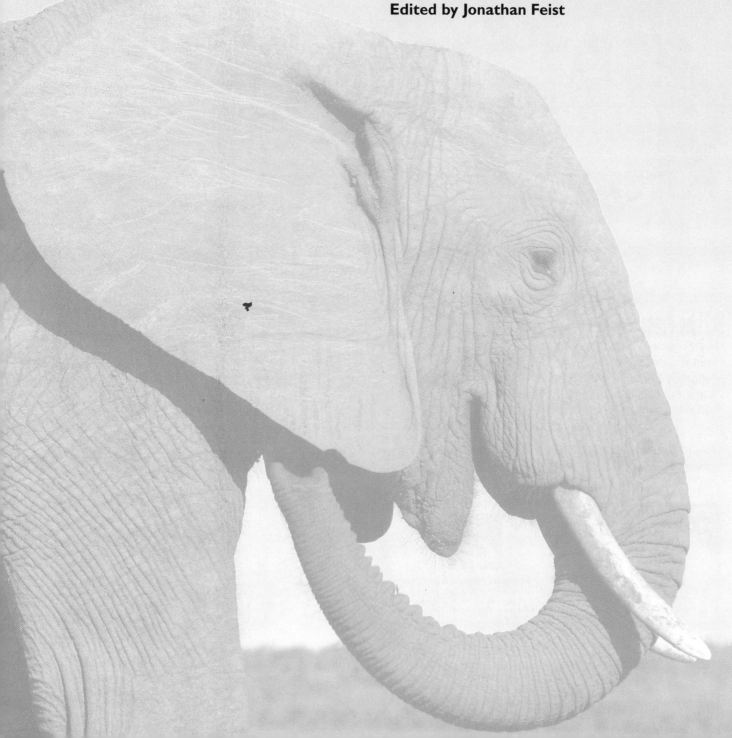

Beginning Ear Training

by Gilson Schachnik

Edited by Jonathan Feist

Berklee Press
Vice President: David Kusek
Dean of Continuing Education: Debbie Cavalier
Managing Editor: Jonathan Feist
Director of Business Affairs: Robert F. Green
Senior Designer: Robert Heath
Editorial Assistants: Rajasri Mallikarjuna, Anna Rochinsky, Jonathan Whalen

ISBN-13: 978-0-87639-081-8
ISBN-10: 0-87639-081-5

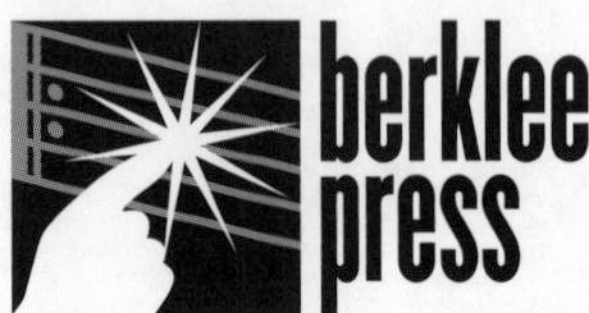

1140 Boylston Street
Boston, MA 02215-3693 USA
(617) 747-2146

Visit Berklee Press Online at
www.berkleepress.com

DISTRIBUTED BY

HAL•LEONARD®
CORPORATION
7777 W. BLUEMOUND RD. P.O. BOX 13819
MILWAUKEE, WISCONSIN 53213

Visit Hal Leonard Online at
www.halleonard.com

CONTENTS

PREFACE

Great musicians seem to have very little in common. Some start very early, some not that early. Some start with classical music, some with popular, jazz, or gospel. The disparity in their technique is even greater. Consider the techniques of Keith Jarrett, Chick Corea, and Herbie Hancock—three completely different approaches to piano playing. But one commonality between them is that *they all learned to play by ear*! Particularly for popular music styles, such as jazz, Brazilian, Latin, and funk, the ability to play by ear is critical.

Though it seems an obvious path, the reality of playing by ear is not that easy. Often, beginning musicians get overwhelmed when they try to learn a solo or a tune by ear. They give up, opting to the easier and faster route of using a fake book or written transcription. Though they might learn the notes, they never learn the nuances and soul of the music's language.

This book's purpose is to introduce the process of learning music by ear, serving as a bridge between hearing music and being able to notate it.

It is my sincere hope that after mastering this material, you will feel motivated and empowered to start learning music by ear.

—Gilson Schachnik

ACKNOWLEDGMENTS

Many thanks to Roberta Radley, Steve Prosser, Scott McCormick, and Charlie Banacos. I can't even count how many hours you spent helping me learn how to teach.

To Jonathan Feist for the invaluable help in putting all these ideas in a coherent package.

To Scott DeOgburn for "digitizing" all the dictation examples.

Finally to my father Israel, my wife Luciana, and my daughters Marina and Julia for the constant love and support.

INTRODUCTION

This book covers the Ear Training 1 curriculum at Berklee College of Music.

Berklee uses "movable Do" solfege. In this system, the tonal center is always considered Do and the other notes of the scale follow. Here are the solfege syllables set on a C major scale, in the key of C.

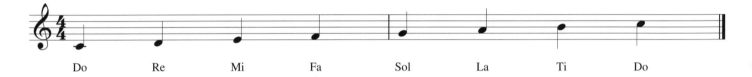

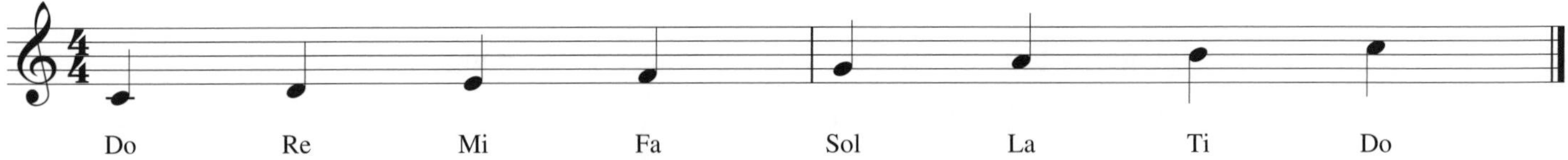

Here are the solfege syllables for a D major scale in the key of D major.

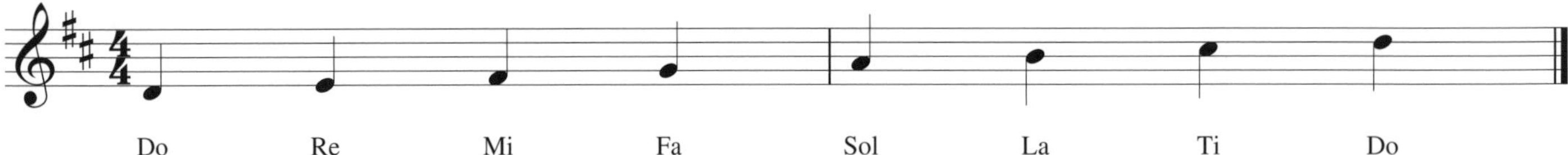

Although the notes are different, the solfege syllables are the same. D is now the tonal center, and therefore Do. The relationships between Do and the other notes are always the same, in all keys.

The warm-up exercises in this book will help you internalize these relationships and prepare you for the dictation examples. Each chapter focuses on an expanding set of rhythms, pitches, keys, and other musical elements.

HOW TO USE THIS BOOK

Each chapter has three types of exercises: melody and rhythm warm-ups, leading to a dictation example.

Melody Warm-Ups

Melody warm-ups—what we call "Sol Fa" exercises at Berklee—will help you to become familiar with note relationships and to develop relative pitch. Detailed instructions on how to practice are given in each warm-up section, but in essence, each melody is a series of solfege syllables followed by a breath mark (/), like this:

Do Re Mi / Mi Re Do / Re Mi Re / Mi Re Mi Do Re Mi /

Choose any key, and sing the solfege syllable for each note. Periodically, check your pitch against a keyboard by playing Do, while you sing the other solfege syllables. This will help you to keep in tune and reinforce the relationship of the notes to Do.

Refrain from playing the notes before or while you are singing! In the beginning, it's okay to check occasionally whether you sang the correct pitch. As you advance, you will not need to check as often. Remember to breathe between phrases!

Rhythm Warm-Ups

This book focuses on basic rhythms. Use a metronome when you practice the rhythm exercises. Conducting while you sing will help you to keep your place in the measure. Practice each of these patterns with a metronome before you begin the rhythm exercises.

Here are the conducting patterns for 2/4, 3/4, and 4/4 (S = Strong, W = Weak, LS = Less Strong).

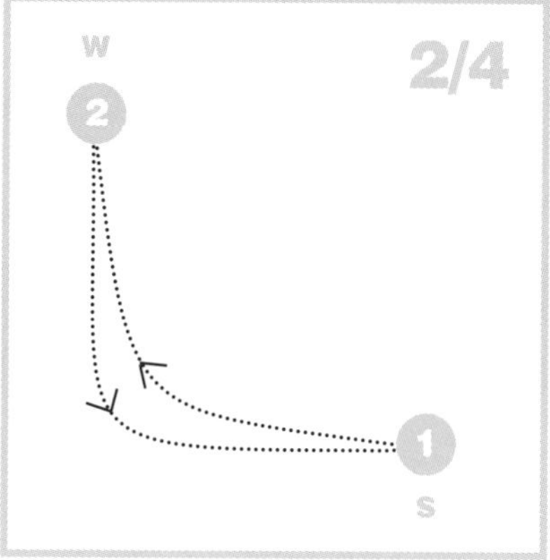

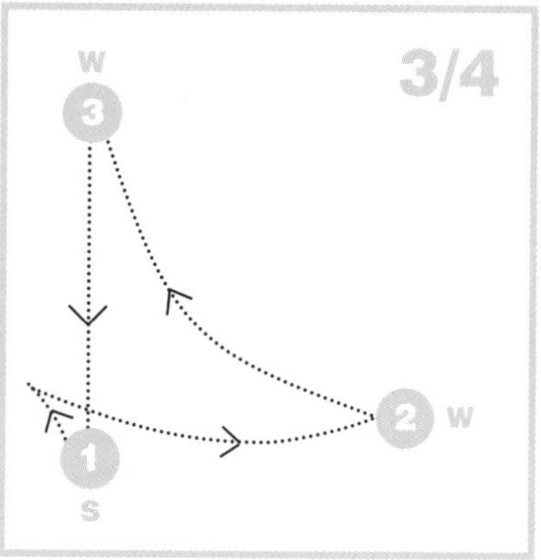

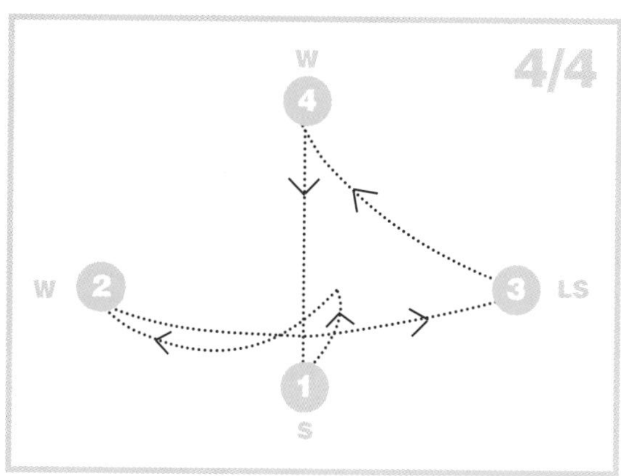

Other ways to help keep track of where you are in the meter include clapping or tapping the beats. Whatever method you choose, always be aware of what beat you are on. A good tip is to write the beats and subdivisions above the staff. While you count the beats, clap the notated rhythm.

Dictation

Follow this strategy for the dictation exercises. As an example, the following melody is in E-flat major, treble clef, 4/4.

1. Listen to the whole track as many times as you need to in order to memorize it. This step is very important towards developing your music memory. The more you do it, the faster you will be at memorizing music.
2. On a staff, write down the rhythm.

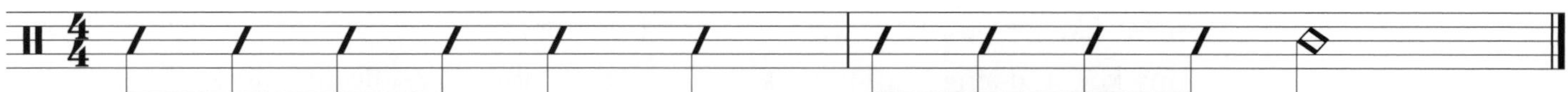

3. Write the solfege syllable under each note. At this point you are basically done with the ear training aspect of dictation. You now have the example notated in its "pure form." All you have to do is transform it into actual notated music.

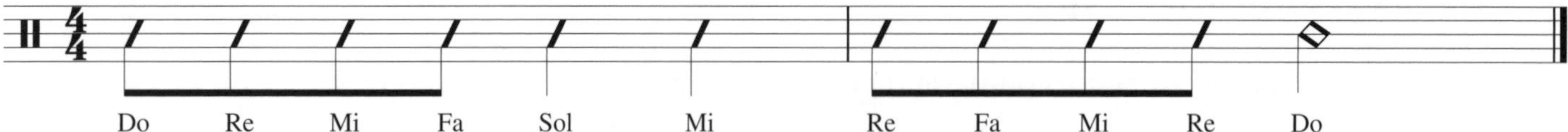

4. Note the given key (E♭), then determine the octave. (Finding the correct octave gets easier with practice.) If necessary, look at the E♭ major scale in the treble clef, and find the corresponding pitches. Then write out the final notation in your chosen key.

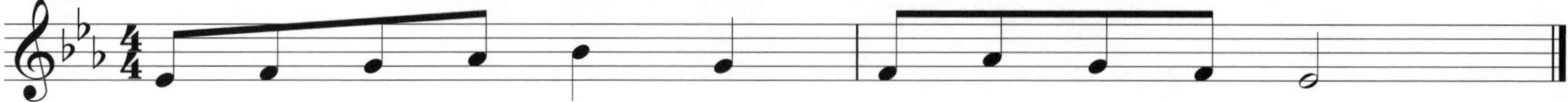

CHAPTER 1

Do, Re, Mi

MELODY

Syllables: Do, Re, Mi

To practice the Sol-Fa exercises, first choose a key to work with. You could change it every day or always use C. It does not matter, since the relationship between all the notes and the tonal center is always the same.

Play a low Do on your keyboard while you sing each solfege syllable in the exercises below. At first, you may need to check each note after you sing it, to confirm that you are singing the correct pitch. Later, this will not be necessary.

Do not play the note on the keyboard before you sing it. That's cheating! The goal is to internalize the note relationships and tonal center.

Inhale at each breath mark (/).

1. Do Re Mi / Mi Re Do / Re Mi Re / Mi Re Mi Do Re Mi /
2. Re Do Re Do Mi Re Mi / Do Mi Do Mi Do Re Mi Do /
3. Re Mi Do Re Mi Do Mi Re / Mi Do Re Mi Do Re Mi /
4. Do Mi Re Do Re Do Mi Re / Re Do Re Mi Re Do Re /
5. Mi Do Re Mi Do Re Do Re / Do Re Do Mi Re Do Mi /

After you go through the set, try improvising using those three syllables: Do, Re, Mi. Use a set rhythmic pattern or vary the rhythm. Experiment!

RHYTHM

The rhythms used in this chapter are:

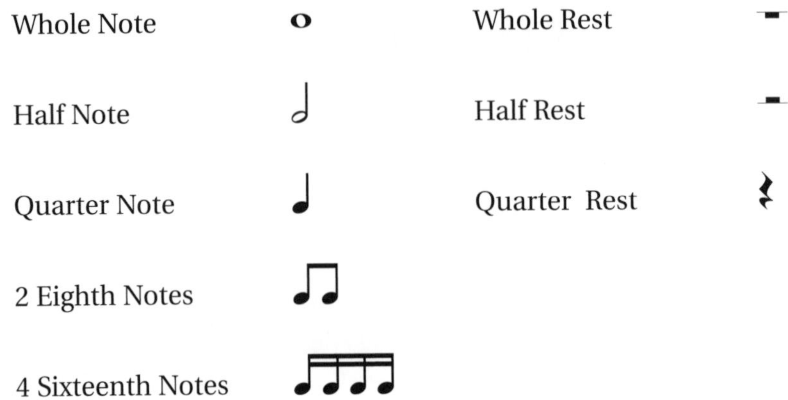

Sing each rhythm using the subdivision shown (1+2+3+4+, etc.). Use the subdivision syllables "1 + 2 + 3 + 4 +" (say "and" for +) for eighth notes.

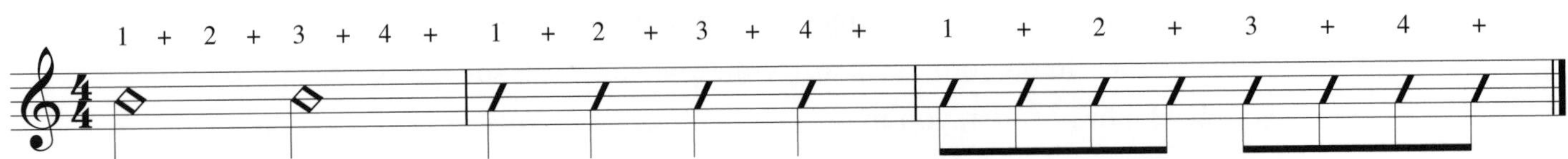

Use the subdivision syllables "1 e + a" (ee and uh) for sixteenth notes.

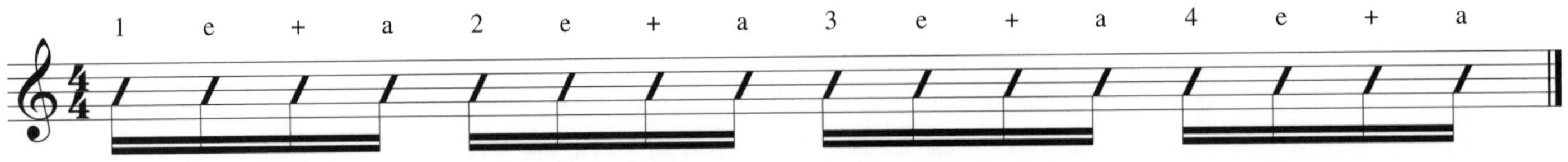

Practice the rhythms below. Use a three-step process:

1. Clap the rhythms as you count the beats and subdivisions aloud.
2. Count the beats and subdivisions silently, as you clap the rhythms.
3. Conduct and perform the rhythms.

TRACK 2

Check your singing against track 2.

1.

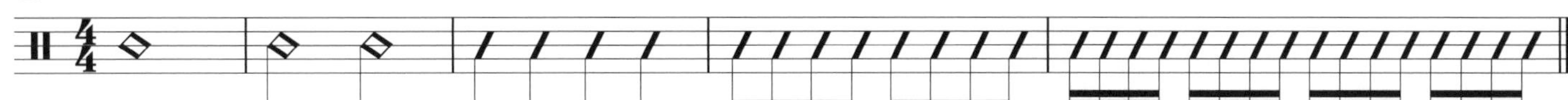

2.

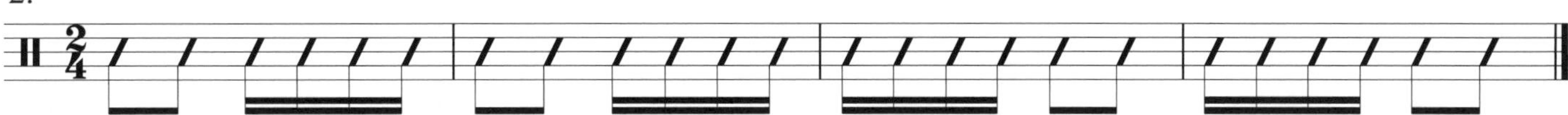

3.

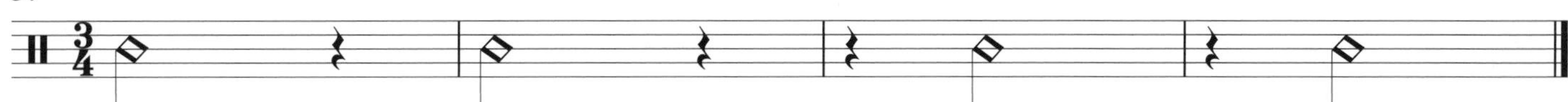

4.

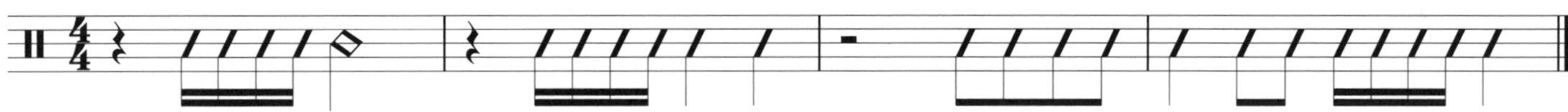

5.

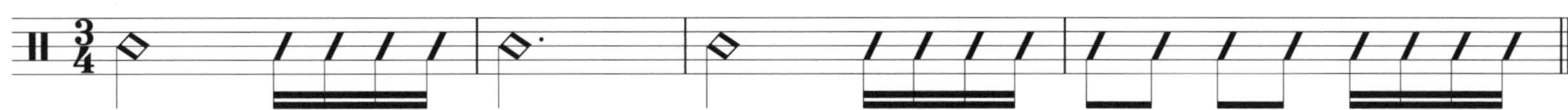

6.

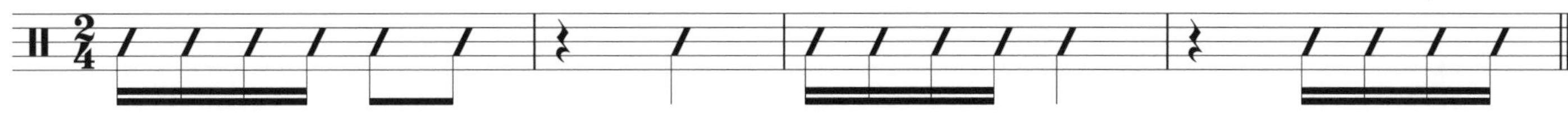

7.

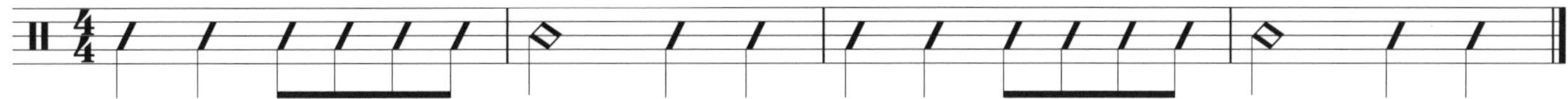

DICTATION

Transcribe each melody by following this procedure.

1. Listen to the CD track until you have memorized the melody.
2. Write the rhythms.
3. Write the solfege syllables.
4. Determine the correct octave, and then write out the notation.
5. Check your transcription against the answer key in appendix B.

Examples 1 to 6 are in C major.
Examples 7 to 12 are in F major.
Examples 13 to 18 are in B♭ major.

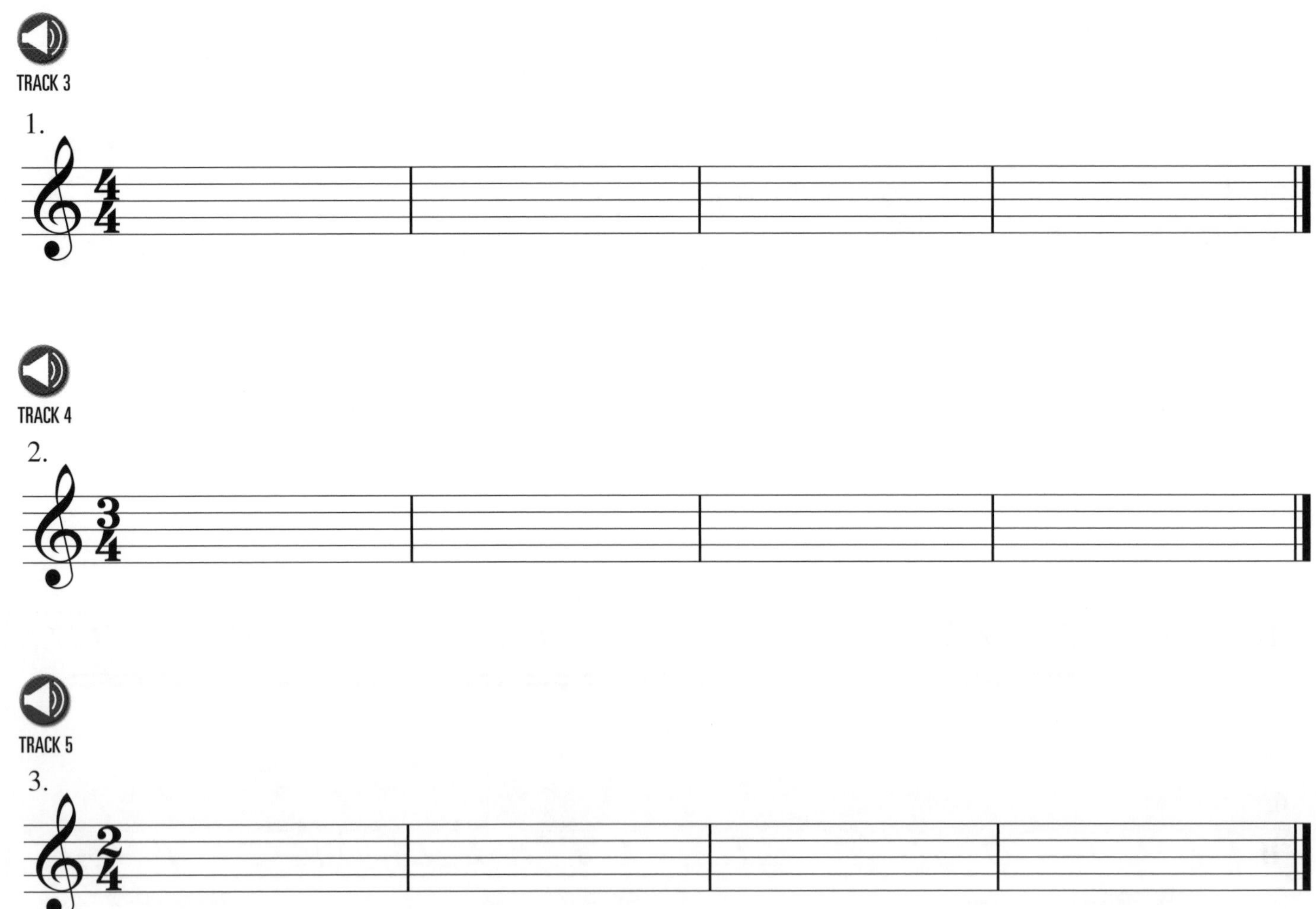

TRACK 6

4.

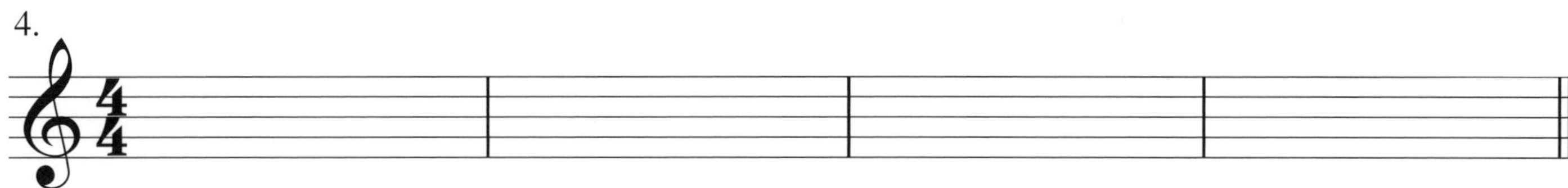

TRACK 7

5.

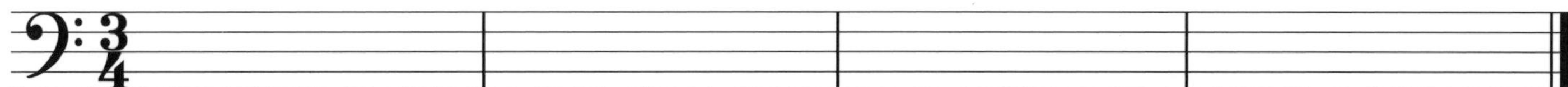

TRACK 8

6.

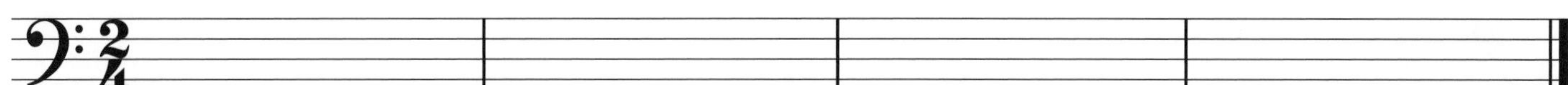

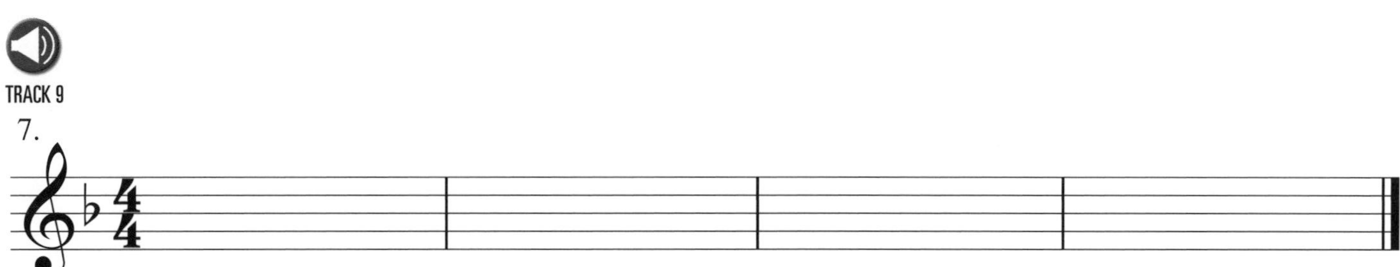

TRACK 9

7.

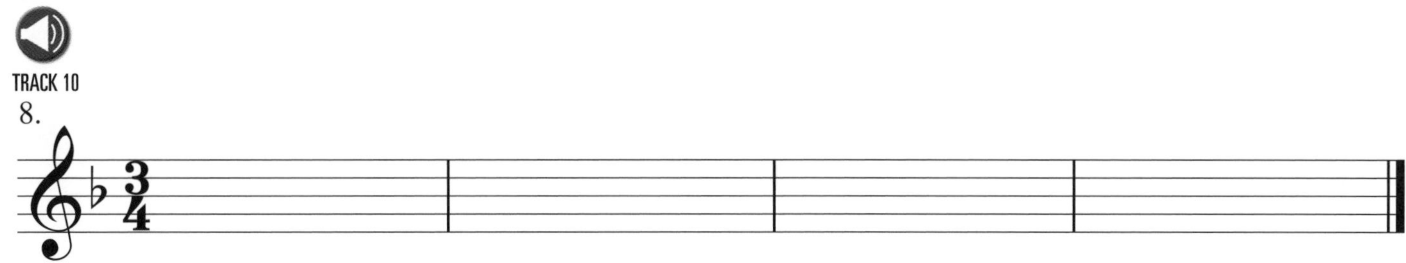

TRACK 10

8.

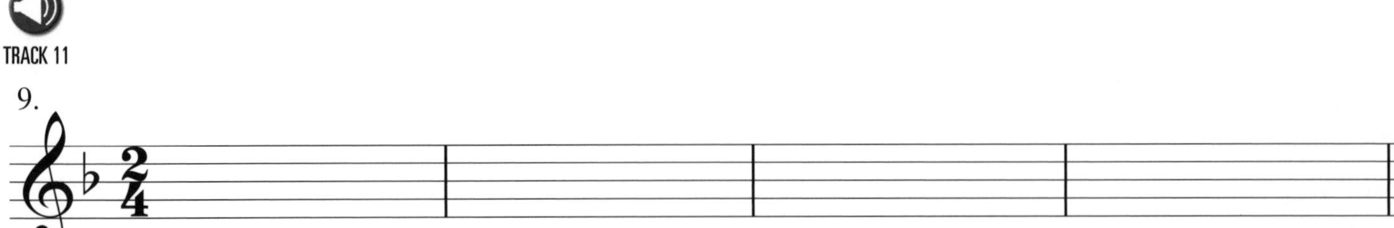

10.

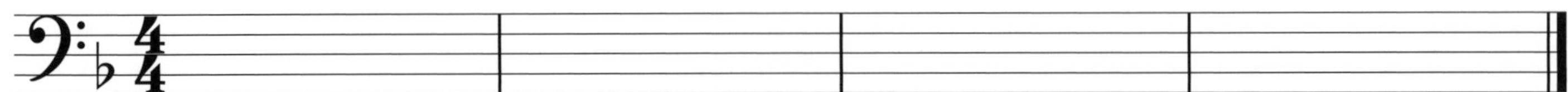

11.

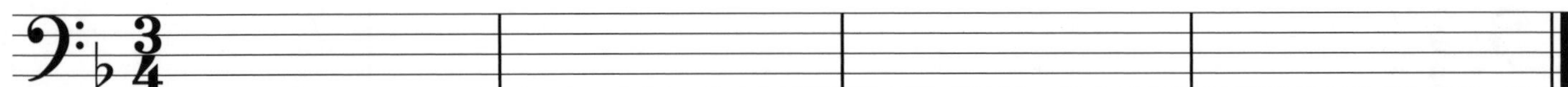

12.

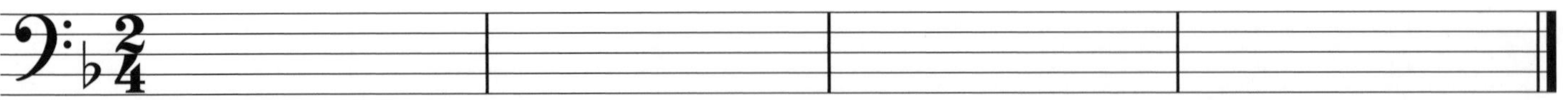

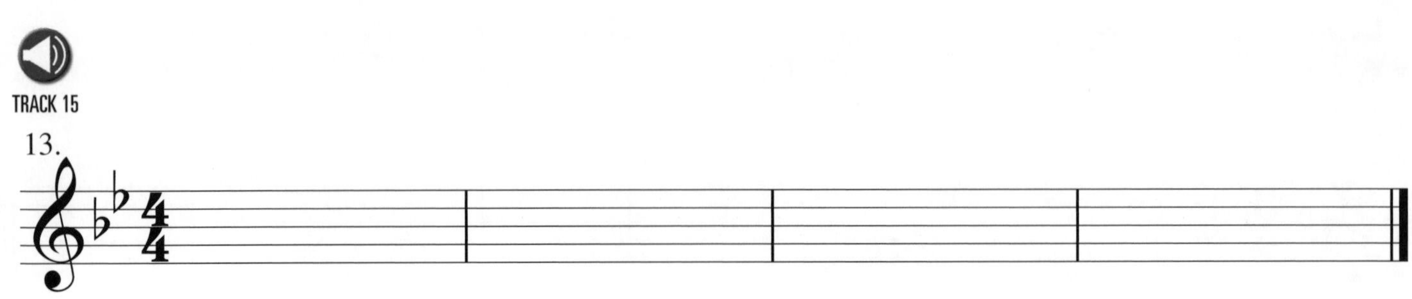

TRACK 16

14.

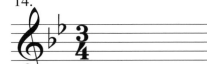

TRACK 17

15.

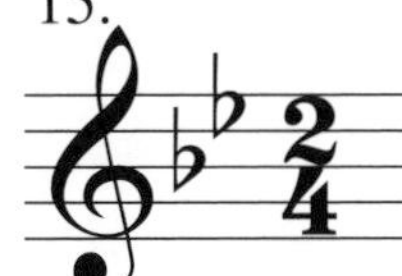

TRACK 18

16.

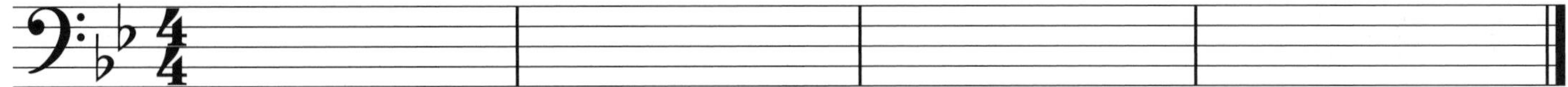

TRACK 19

17.

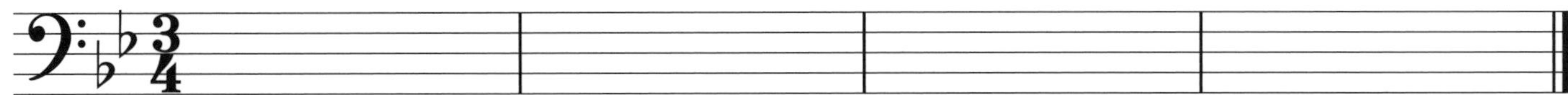

TRACK 20

18.

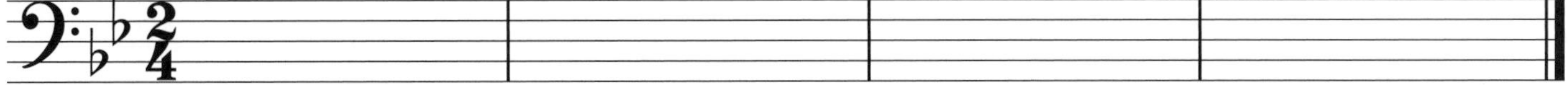

CHAPTER 2

Do, Re, Mi, Fa

MELODY

New Syllable: Fa

Tendency Tones: Re-Do, Fa-Mi

Practice the Sol-Fa exercises below following the same guidelines explained in chapter 1. Remember, speed is not the goal here. Strive for perfect accuracy of pitch.

1. Do Re Mi Fa / Fa Mi Re Do / Re Do Mi Fa Mi /
2. Re Fa Mi Do Mi Fa / Re Do Fa Mi Do Fa Re /
3. Mi Re Do Fa Mi Re Do / Mi Fa Re Mi Do Re Do /
4. Fa Do Mi Fa Mi Re Do / Fa Mi Fa Re Do Mi Re /
5. Fa Do Fa Do Mi Do Re Fa / Re Do Fa Re Mi Do Fa /
6. Do Re Mi Do Fa Mi Re Do / Re Fa Do Mi Fa Re Mi Do /
7. Mi Fa Do Mi Fa Re Fa Do Re Fa / Fa Mi Re Mi Fa Do Re /

Certain notes have the tendency to resolve to other notes. This is similar to physical gravity. Pairs of notes that tend to resolve to each other are called *tendency tones*. Two pairs of tendency tones are featured in the above exercises: Re resolving to Do and Fa resolving to Mi.

Practice these tendency tone pairs, focusing on how the more dissonant note resolves to the less dissonant note. They will be very useful later on for dictation and sight-singing purposes.

RHYTHM

New Rhythms:

Single Eighth Note: ♪

Eighth Rest: 𝄾

Tie: 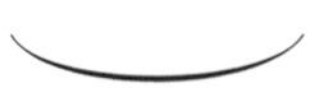

Pickup Notes: 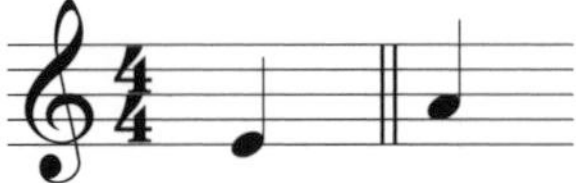

Eighth notes and rests last one half of a quarter-note beat. Ties combine the values of consecutive notes.

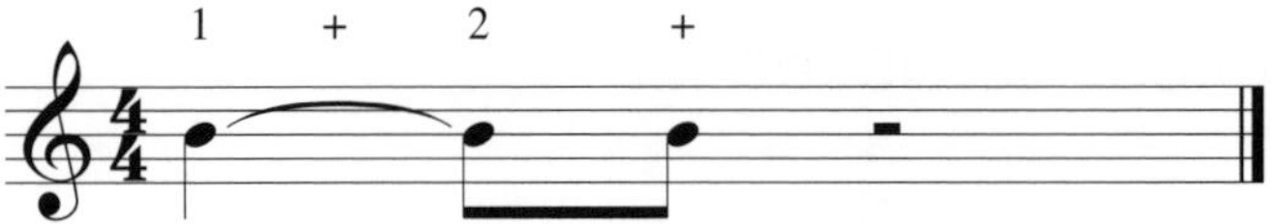

Ties sometimes lead to confusion, especially when they result in no attack on the downbeat. To help you keep your place in the measure, practice counting the beats and subdivisions and clapping the rhythms.

Pickup notes occur before beat 1 of a measure. A common example is the beginning of "Happy Birthday," where "Hap-py" comes before beat 1. In this lesson, we use two types of pickups: quarter- and eighth-note pickups. For a quarter-note pickup, count 1 + 2 + 3 +, and come in on 4.

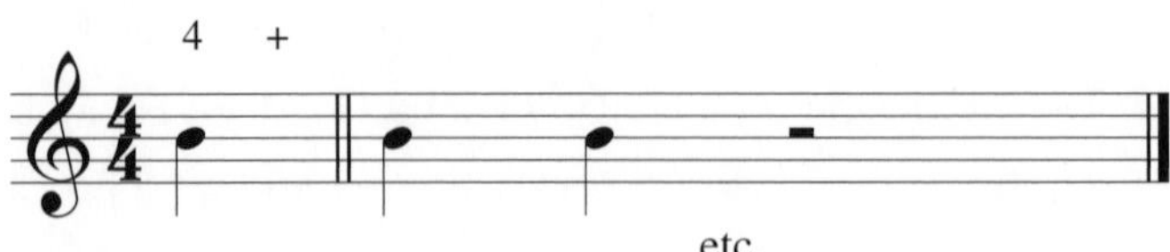

Eighth-note pickups occur off the beat. In 3/4 meter, you would count 1 + 2 + 3, and then come in on the + of beat 3.

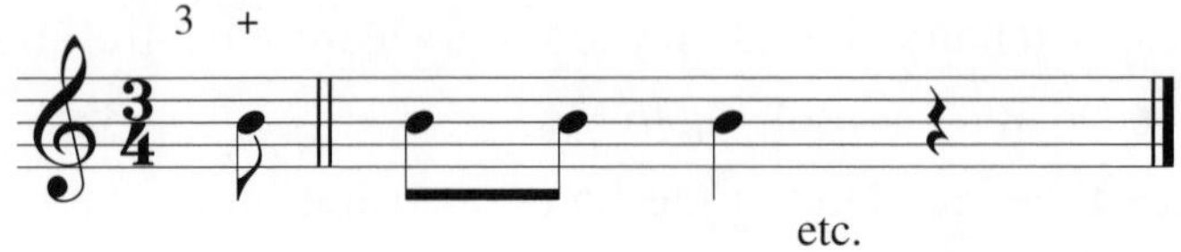

Practice the rhythms below. Use a three-step process:

1. Clap the rhythms as you count the beats and subdivisions aloud.
2. Count the beats and subdivisions silently, as you clap the rhythms.
3. Conduct and perform the rhythms.

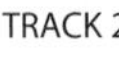

TRACK 21

Check your singing against track 21.

1.

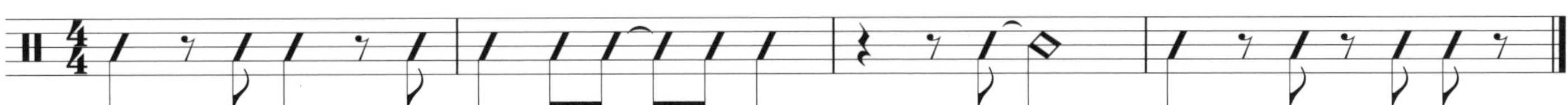

2.

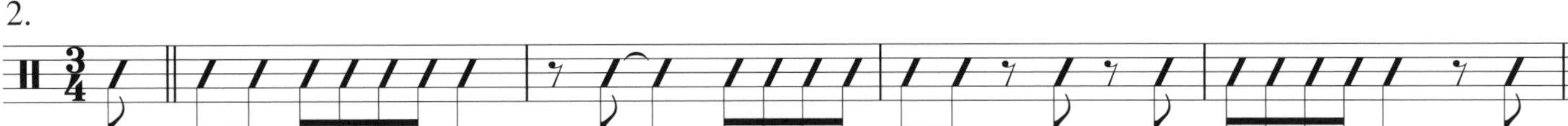

3.

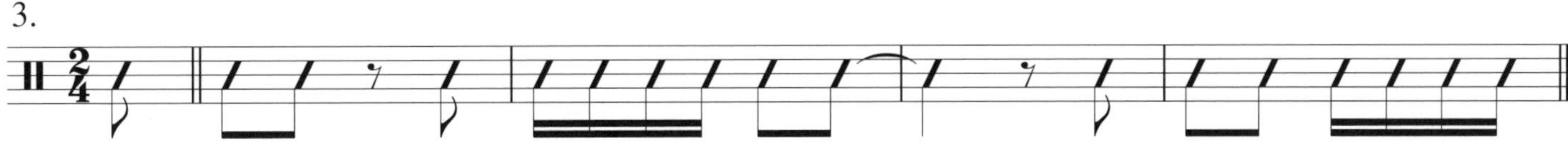

4.

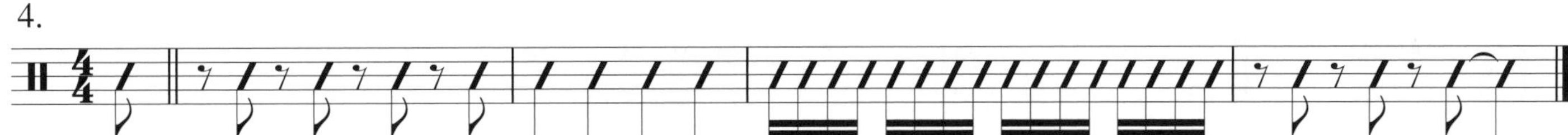

5.

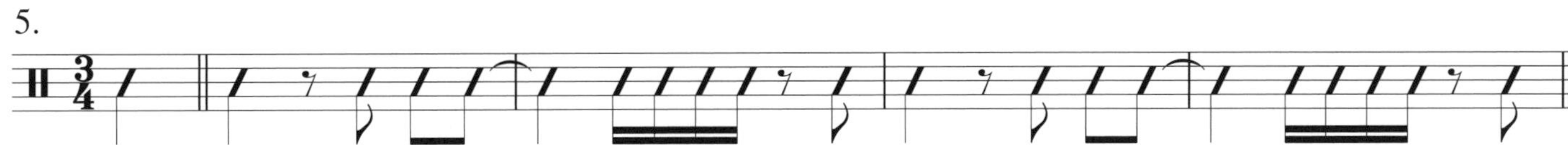

6.

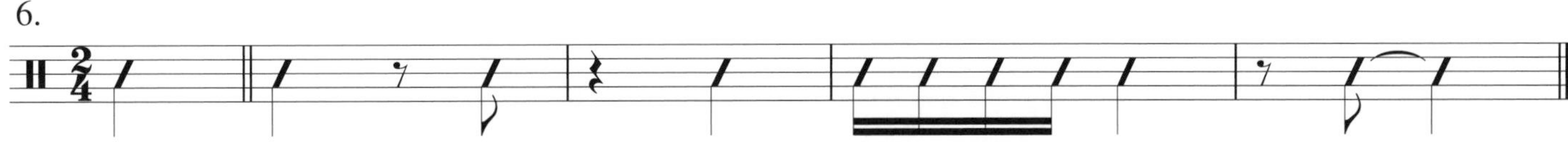

7.

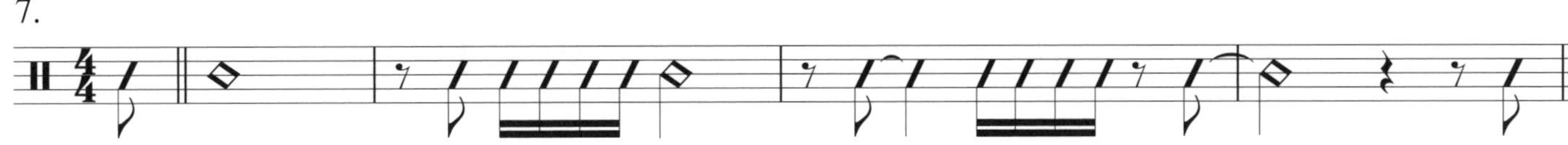

DICTATION

Transcribe each melody by following this procedure. A beginning double barline indicates that there is a pickup.

1. Listen to the CD track until you have memorized the melody.
2. Write the rhythms.
3. Write the solfege syllables.
4. Determine the correct octave, and then write out the notation.
5. Check your transcription against the answer key in appendix B.

Examples 1 to 6 are in E♭ major.
Examples 7 to 12 are in A♭ major.
Examples 13 to 18 are in D♭ major.

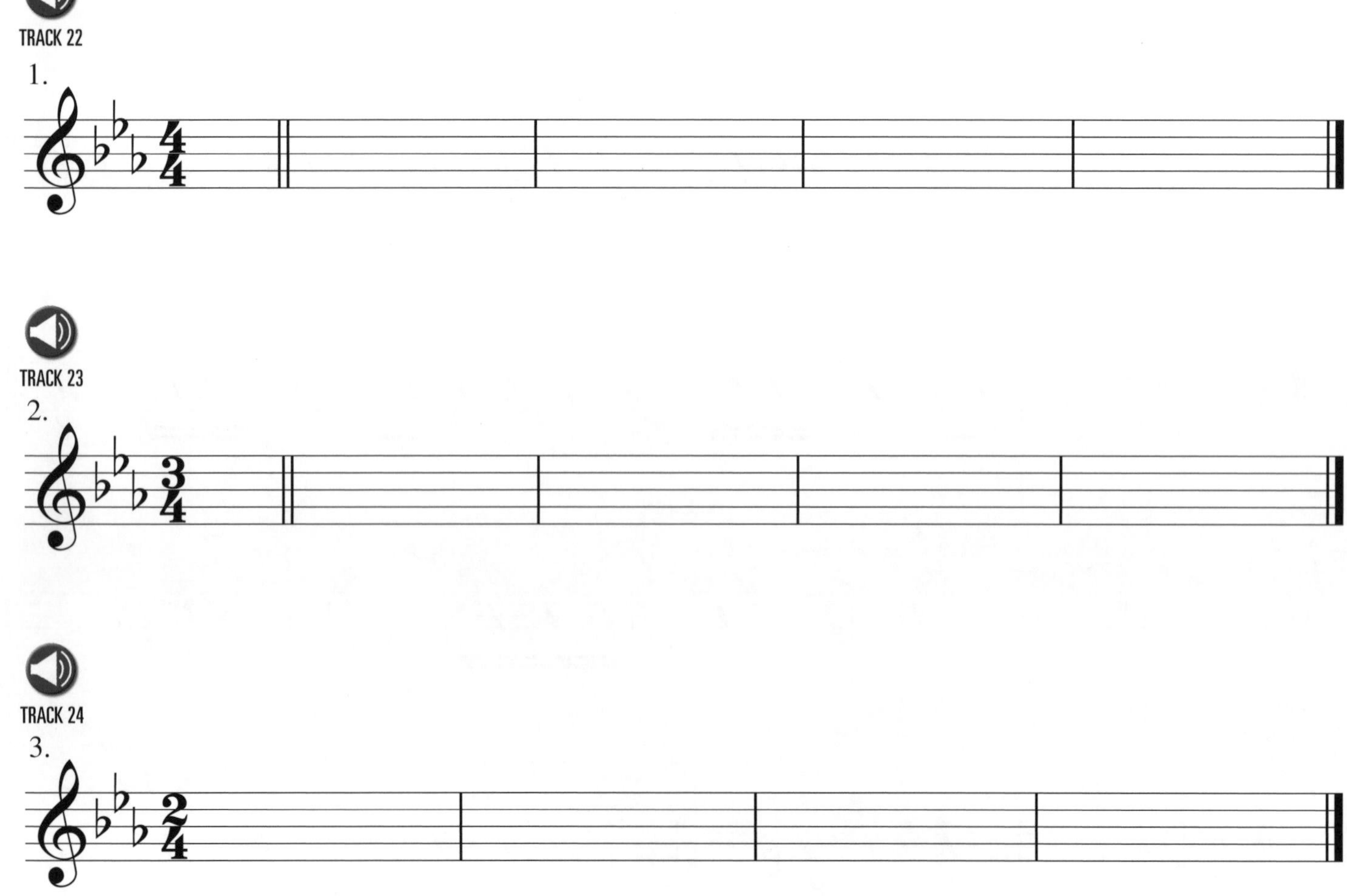

TRACK 25

4.

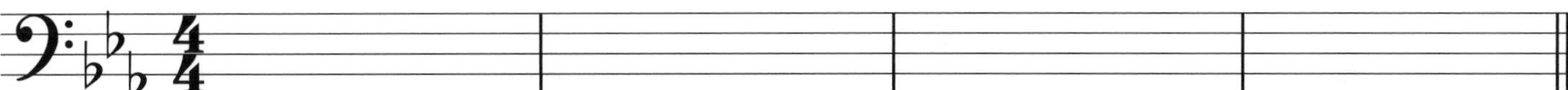

TRACK 26

5.

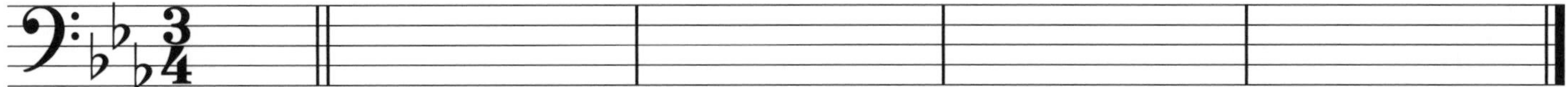

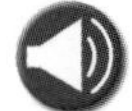

TRACK 27

6.

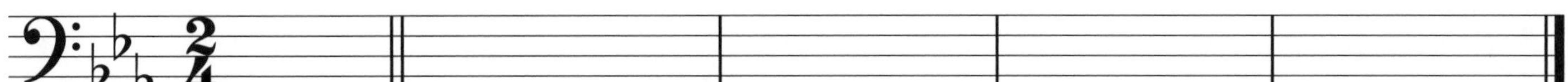

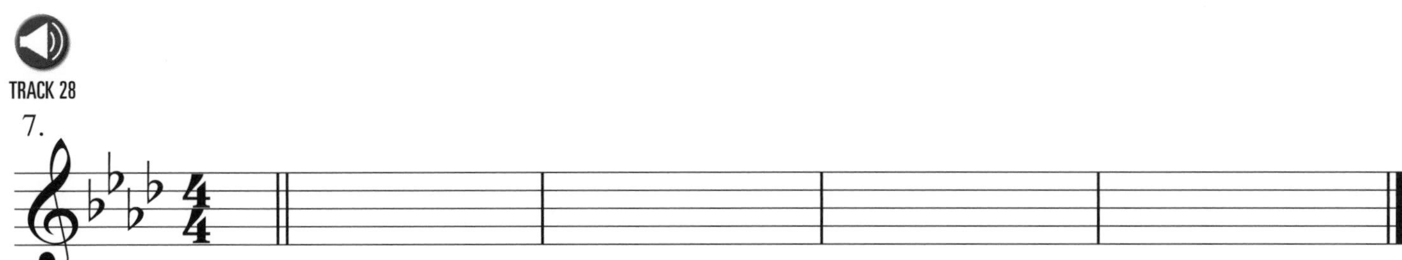

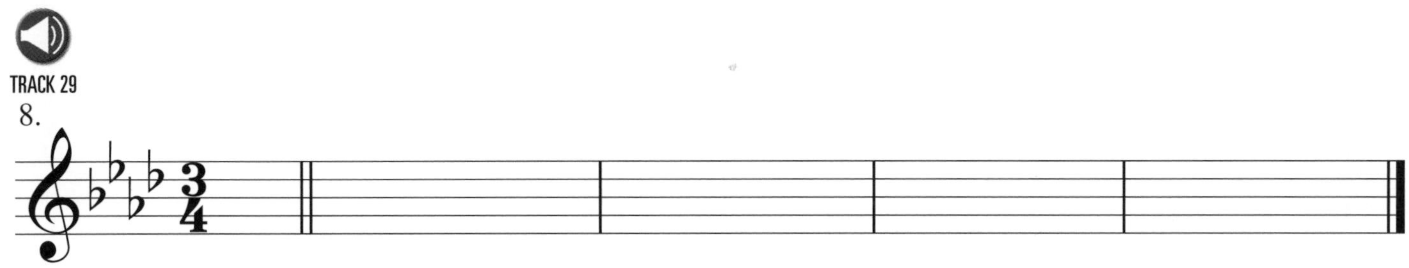

TRACK 30

9.

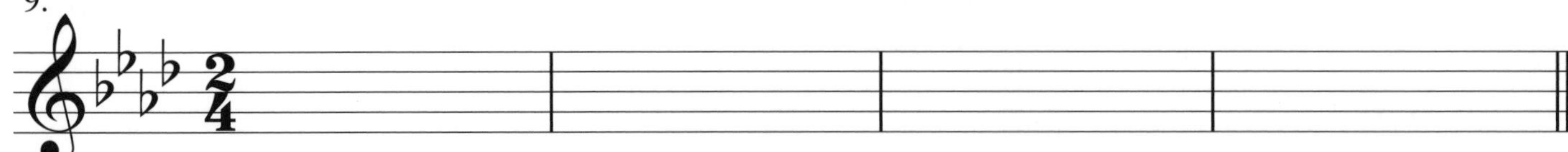

TRACK 31

10.

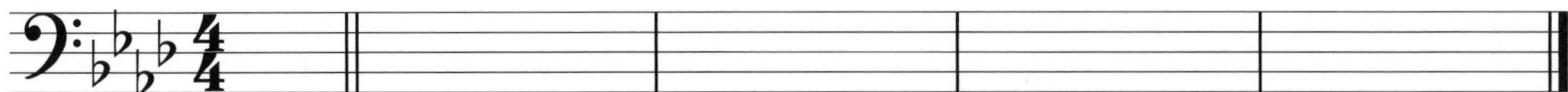

TRACK 32

11.

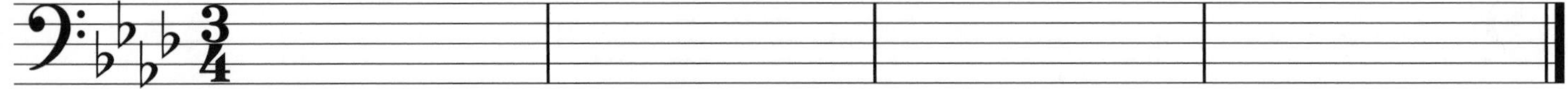

TRACK 33

12.

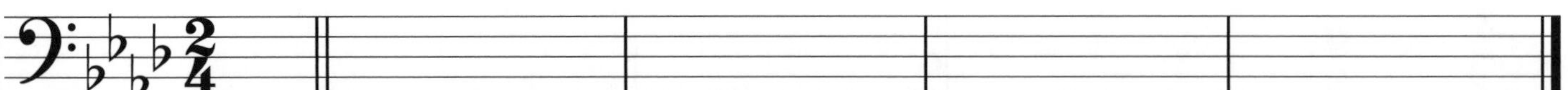

TRACK 34

13.

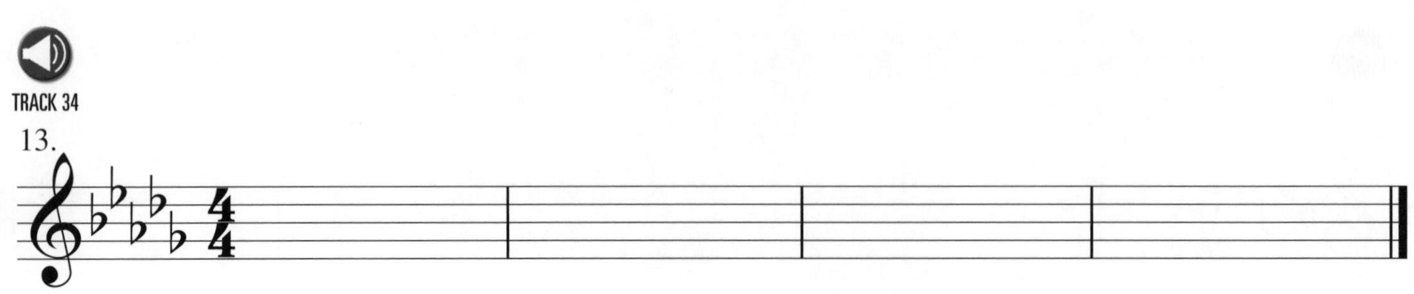

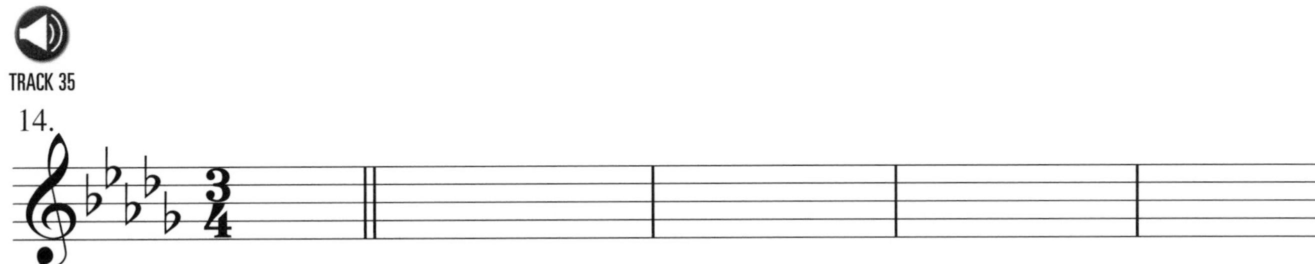

TRACK 35

14.

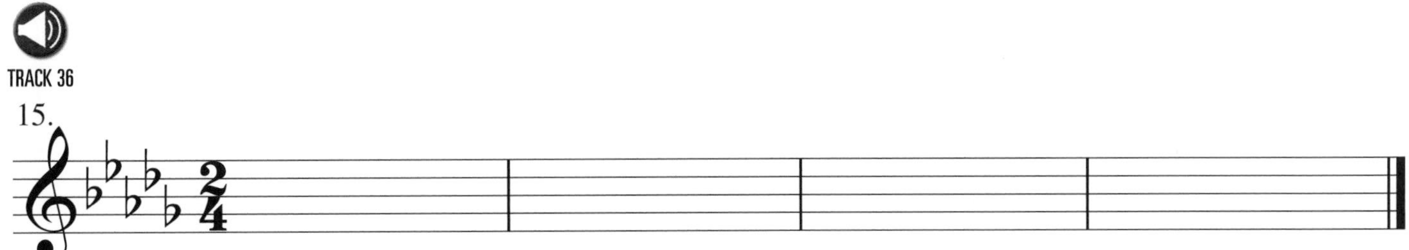

TRACK 36

15.

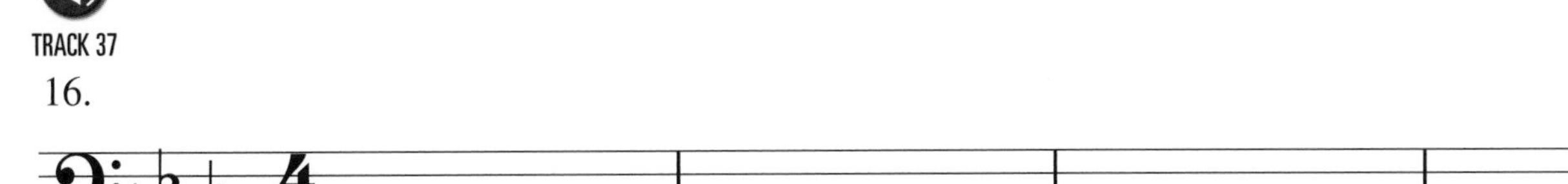

TRACK 37

16.

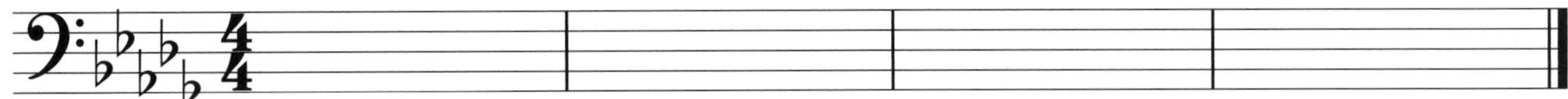

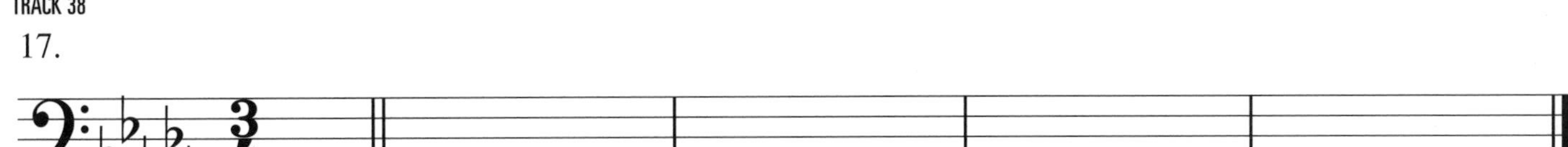

TRACK 38

17.

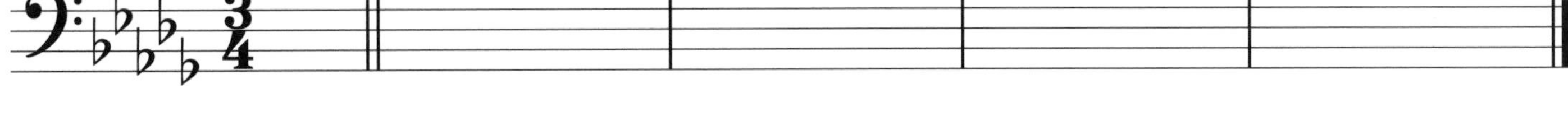

TRACK 39

18.

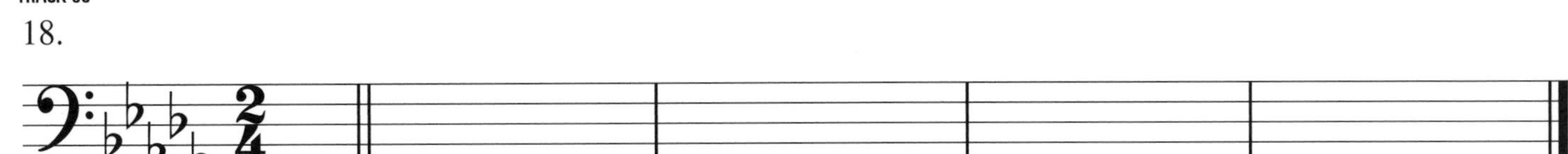

CHAPTER 3

Do, Re, Mi, Fa, Sol

MELODY

New Syllable: Sol

Tendency Tones: Sol-Fa

In the Sol-Fa exercises, you can go up or down, when singing the pitches.

With the addition of Sol, we get another tendency tone pair: Sol resolving to Do. Practice all three tendency tone pairs: Re-Do, Fa-Mi, and Sol-Do.

1. Do Re Mi Fa Sol / Sol Fa Mi Re Do /
2. Do Re Mi Sol Fa Mi Re / Do Mi Fa Re Mi /
3. Re Fa Mi Do Sol Fa Mi / Re Do Sol Fa Mi /
4. Mi Do Sol Fa Do Re / Mi Fa Sol Do Sol Mi /
5. Fa Do Sol Mi Fa Re Mi Do / Fa Do Re Sol Mi /
6. Sol Mi Fa Re Mi Do Sol Fa / Sol Re Sol Re Mi Fa /
7. Do Mi Re Fa Mi Do Re Sol / Re Fa Sol Mi Fa Re Sol /
8. Fa Sol Do Re Fa Sol Mi / Mi Do Fa Re Sol Mi Do Fa /
9. Mi Fa Re Sol Do Fa Re Sol / Mi Re Fa Sol Do Fa Re /
10. Fa Mi Do Re Fa Mi Do Sol / Re Sol Do Sol Re Fa Do /
11. Re Do Mi Fa Sol Do Mi Re / Mi Fa Do Sol Re Fa Mi Sol /

When you complete these exercises, write your own Sol-Fa sequence to a melody you create—without using an instrument. When you are finished, confirm that your syllables actually correspond to the pitches you had imagined.

RHYTHM

Eighth-Note Syncopation

A *syncopated* rhythm has an attack on the upbeat, rather than the downbeat. Try to find tunes you know that use syncopated rhythms (e.g., the guitar riff on "Cocaine" by Eric Clapton). Three syncopated rhythms are used in this lesson's rhythm exercises:

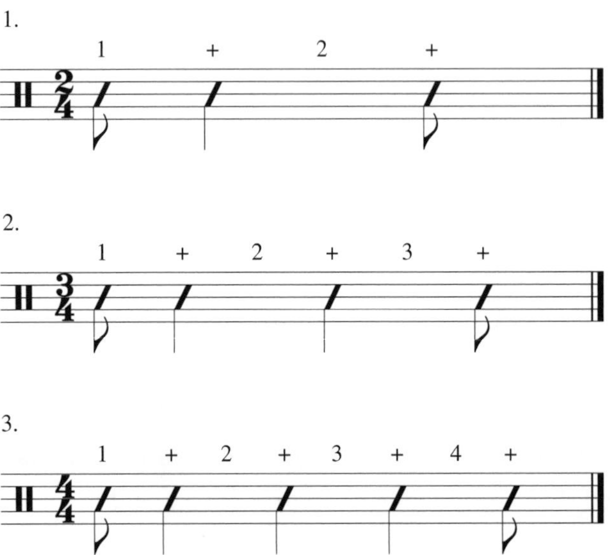

Practice syncopation by subdividing the beat aloud while you clap the rhythms: 1 + 2 + 3 + 4 +. Listen to the relationship between the notes and the downbeats.

The rhythm exercises also include these rhythmic cells:

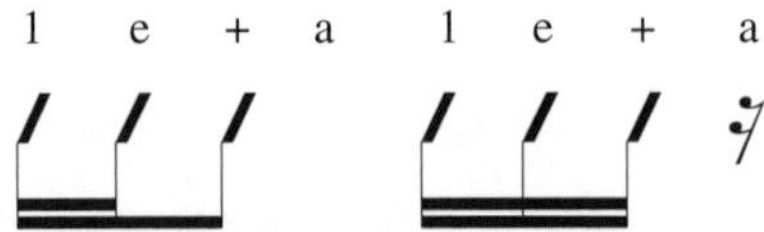

Practice each rhythmic cell:

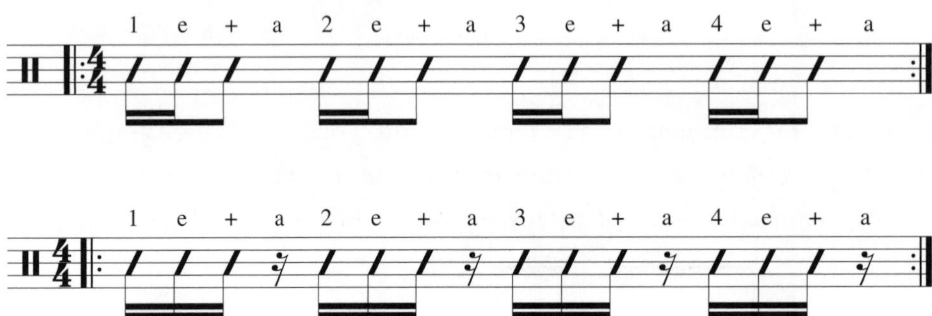

Practice the rhythms below. Use a three-step process:

1. Clap the rhythms as you count the beats and subdivisions aloud.
2. Count the beats and subdivisions silently, as you clap the rhythms.
3. Conduct and perform the rhythms.

TRACK 40

Check your singing against track 40.

1.

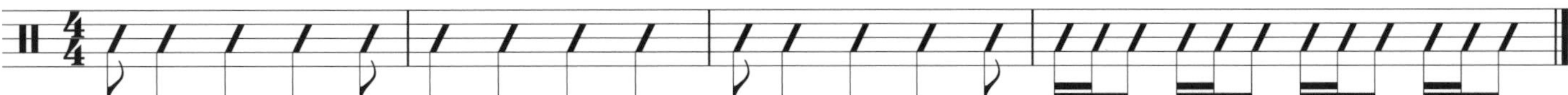

2.

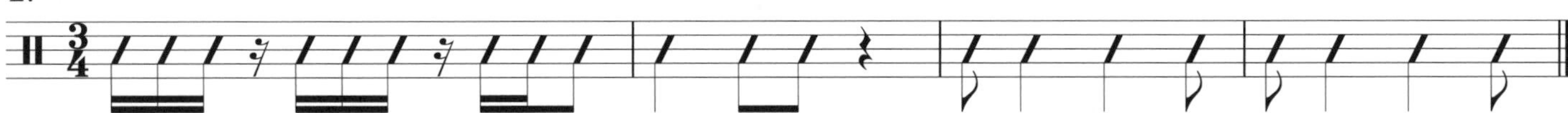

3.

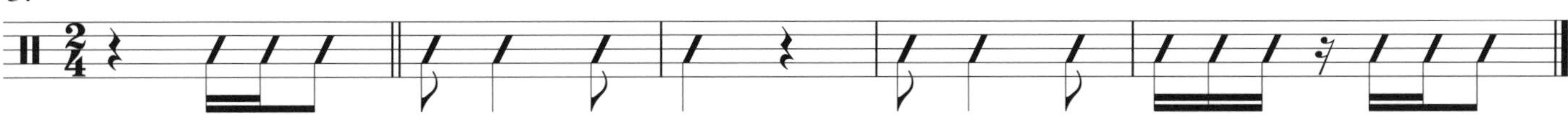

4.

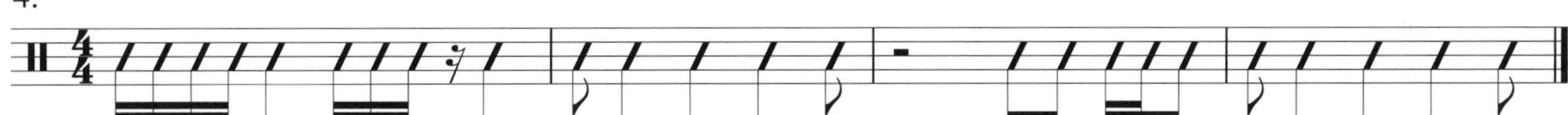

5.

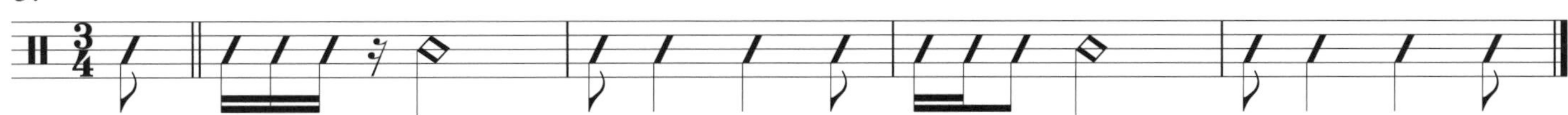

6.

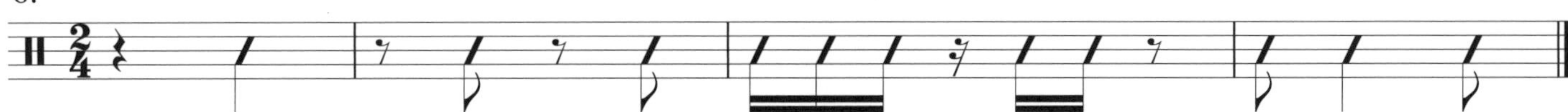

7.

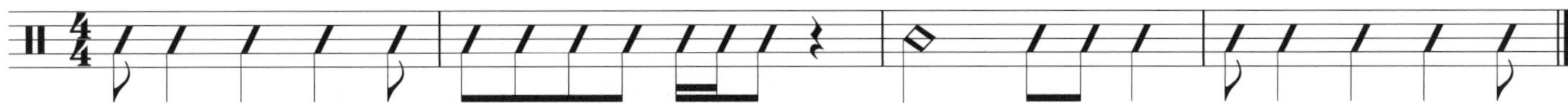

DICTATION

Transcribe each melody by following this procedure.

1. Listen to the CD track until you have memorized the melody.
2. Write the rhythms.
3. Write the solfege syllables.
4. Determine the correct octave, and then write out the notation.
5. Check your transcription against the answer key in appendix B.

Examples 1 to 6 are in G♭ major.
Examples 7 to 12 are in B major.
Examples 13 to 18 are in E major.

TIP

These keys might seem intimidating at first, but remember, the solfege syllables are the same: Do, Re, Mi, Fa, Sol.

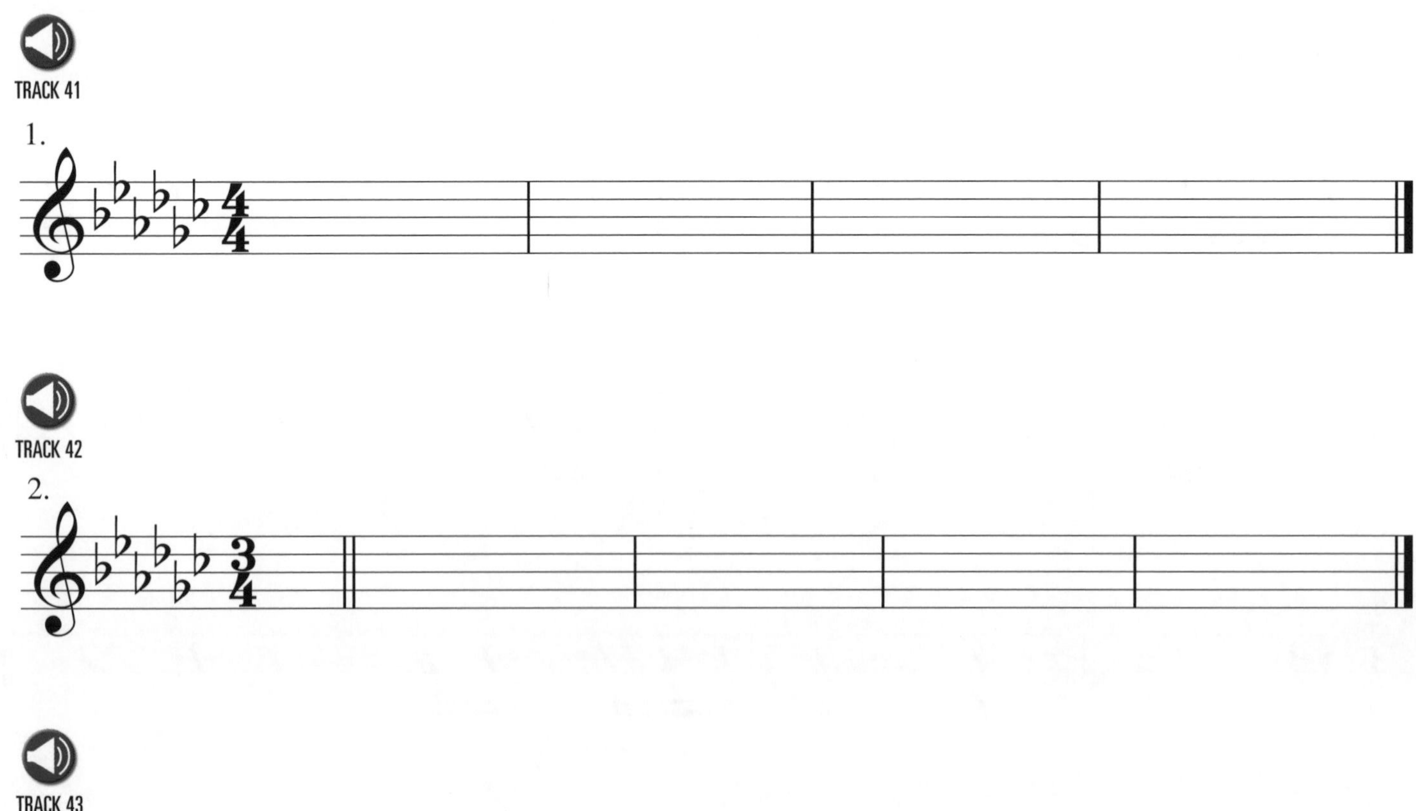

TRACK 44

4.

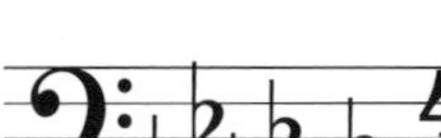

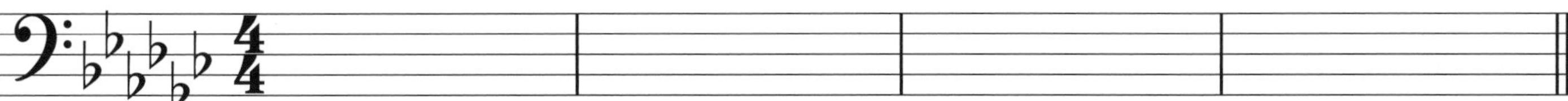

TRACK 45

5.

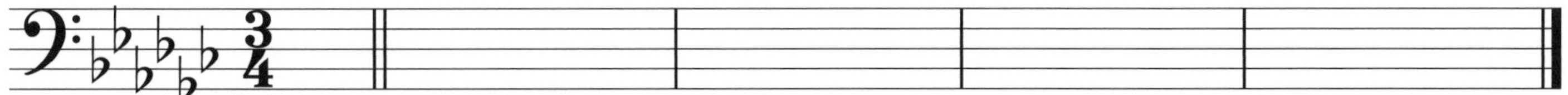

TRACK 46

6.

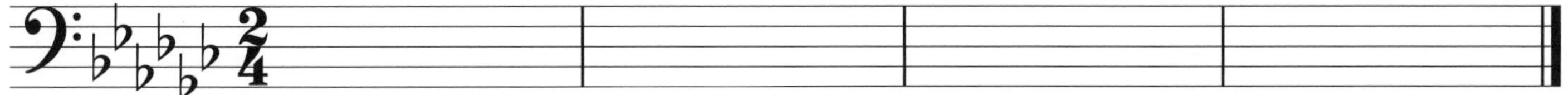

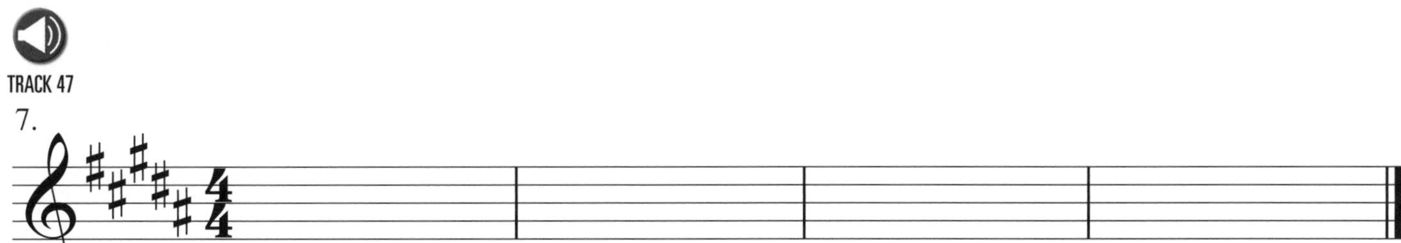

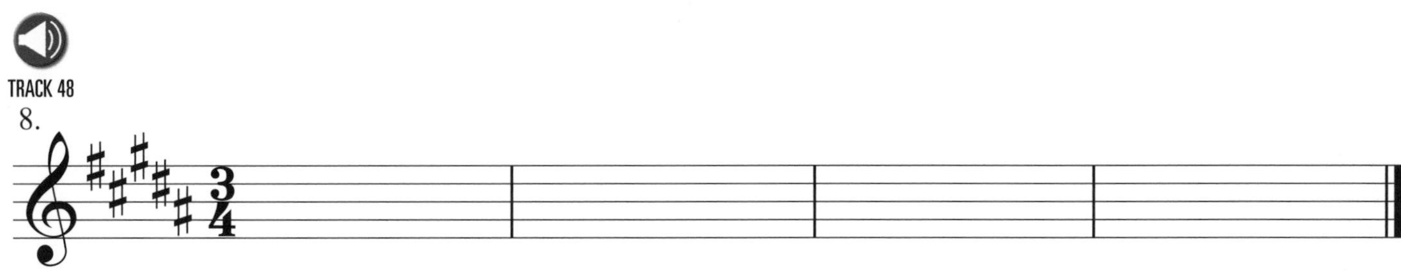

TRACK 49

9.

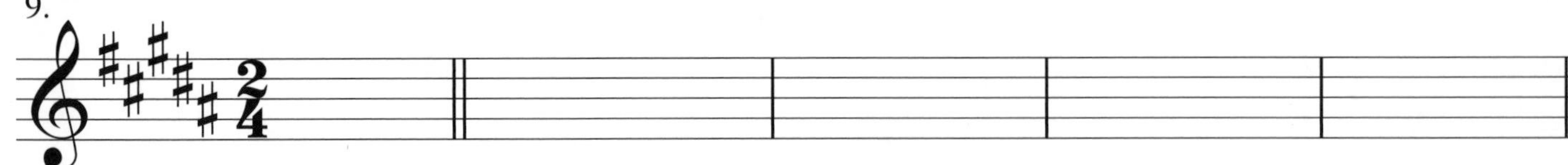

TRACK 50

10.

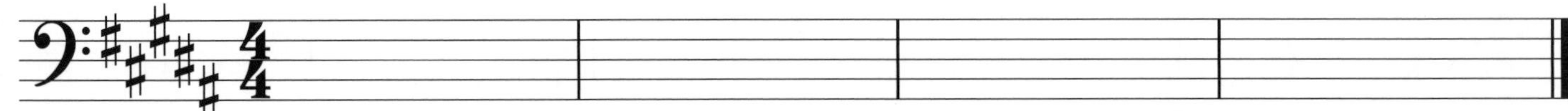

TRACK 51

11.

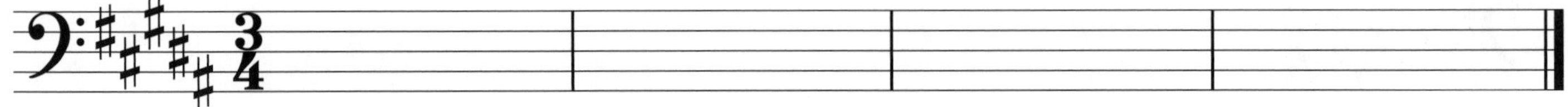

TRACK 52

12.

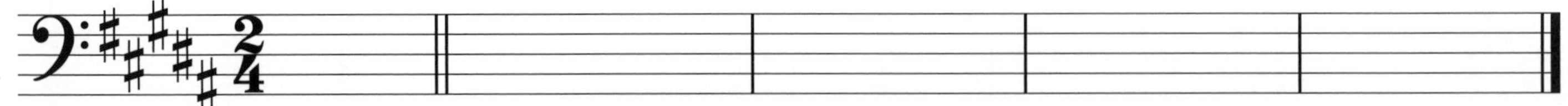

TRACK 53

13.

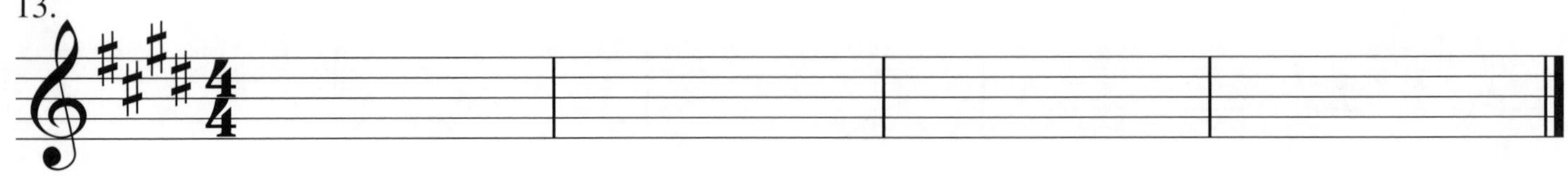

TRACK 54

14.

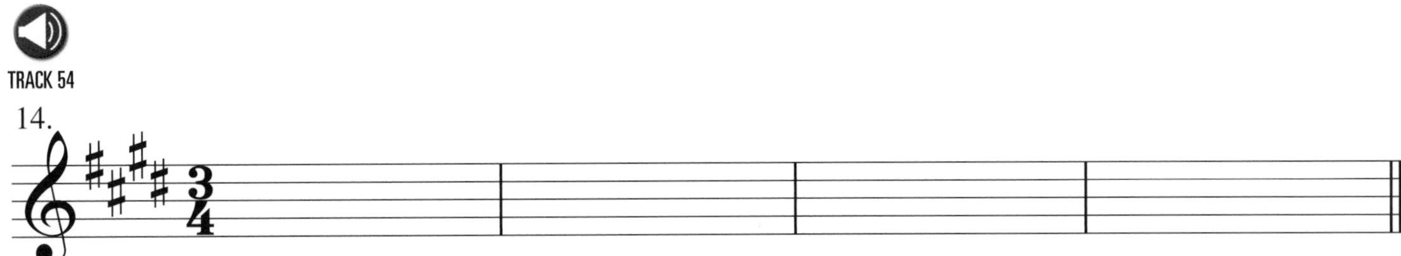

TRACK 55

15.

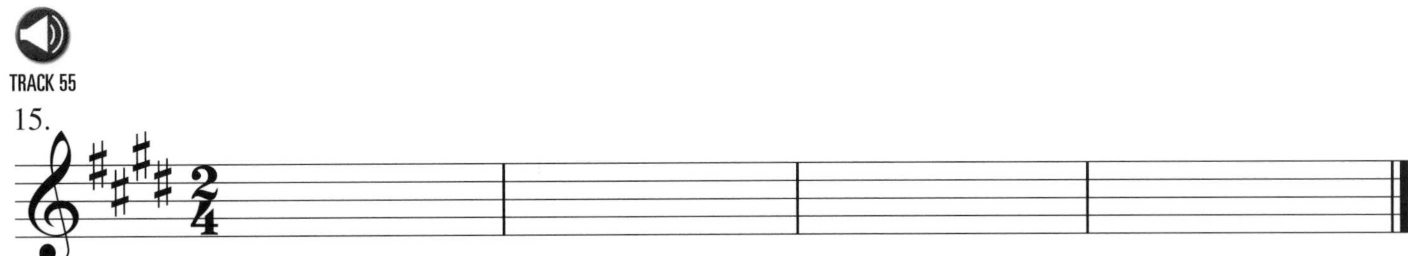

TRACK 56

16.

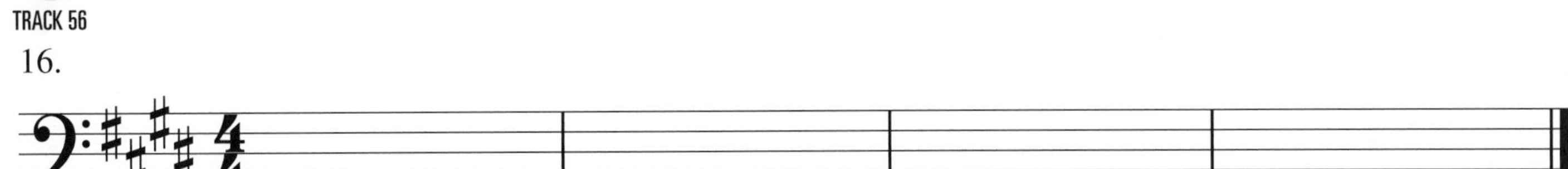

TRACK 57

17.

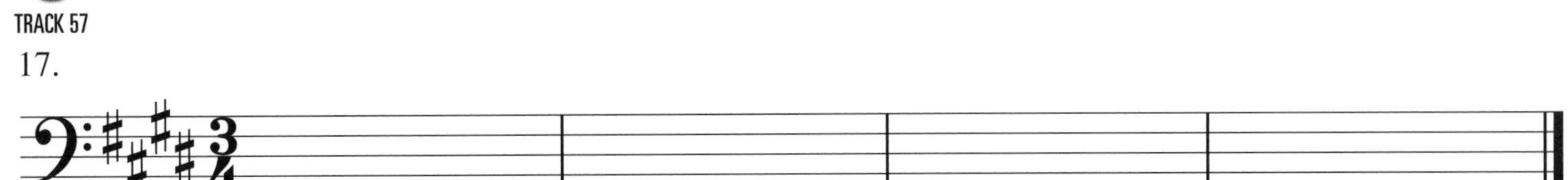

TRACK 58

18.

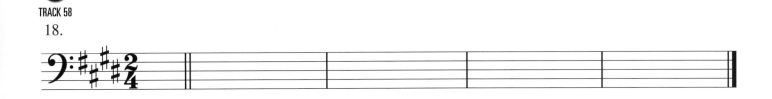

CHAPTER 4

Do, Re, Mi, Fa, Sol, La

MELODY

New Syllable: La

Tendency Tones: La-Sol

Practice four sets of tendency tones: Re-Do, Fa-Mi, Sol-Do, and La-Sol.

Focus on the natural tendency of the tones that are less consonant—and therefore, unstable—to resolve to more consonant and stable tones. Tension and resolution is the basis of all music.

1. Do Re Mi Fa Sol La / La Sol Fa Mi Re Do /
2. Do Mi Re Fa La Sol Fa Mi / Do Fa Re Sol La Sol Re /
3. Re Fa La Sol La Fa Mi / Re Mi Do Mi Fa La Sol Fa /
4. Mi Sol Fa La Sol Mi Re Do / Mi Re Mi Sol La Fa Mi /
5. Fa Do Fa Do La Sol La Fa Re / Fa Re Sol Do Fa La /
6. Sol La Mi Fa Sol Mi Do / Re Mi Fa La Sol Fa Do Sol /
   La Mi Sol La Fa La Sol / Re Sol Do Fa La Mi /
7. Mi Do La Re Fa Sol Mi Do / Do Sol Re La Mi Sol /
8. La Re Fa Do Sol Mi Fa Mi / Do La Sol Fa Re Mi La /
9. Fa Mi Do Re Sol Fa La / La Do La Re La Mi La Fa /
10. Fa Re Mi La Do Re Sol / Re La Do Fa La Mi Sol Re /

Remember to improvise after you complete the Sol-Fa exercises.

RHYTHM

New Rhythms:

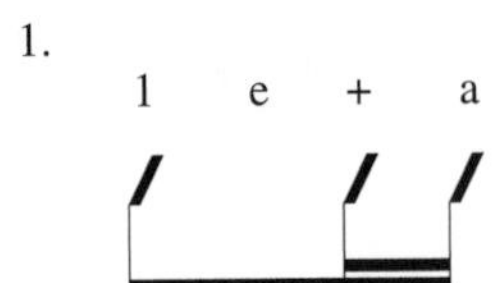

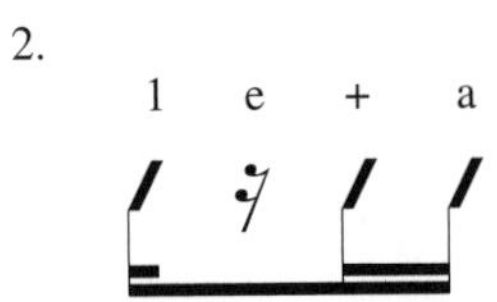

First, practice these rhythmic cells separately:

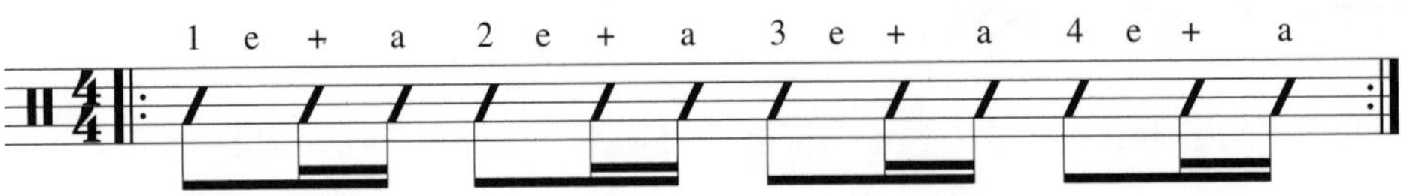

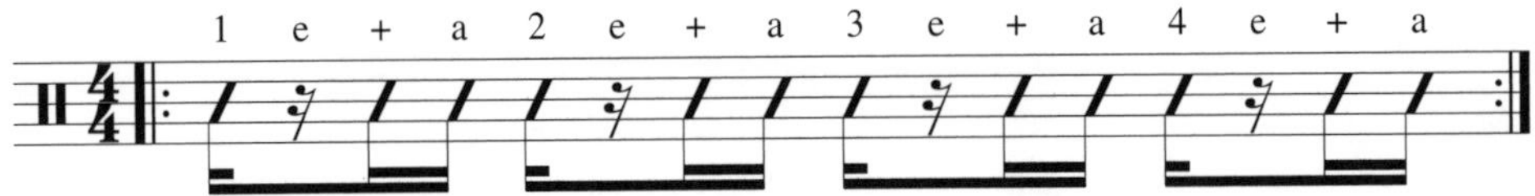

Then, practice the rhythms below. Use a three-step process:

1. Clap the rhythms as you count the beats and subdivisions aloud.
2. Count the beats and subdivisions silently, as you clap the rhythms.
3. Conduct and perform the rhythms.

Check your singing against track 59.

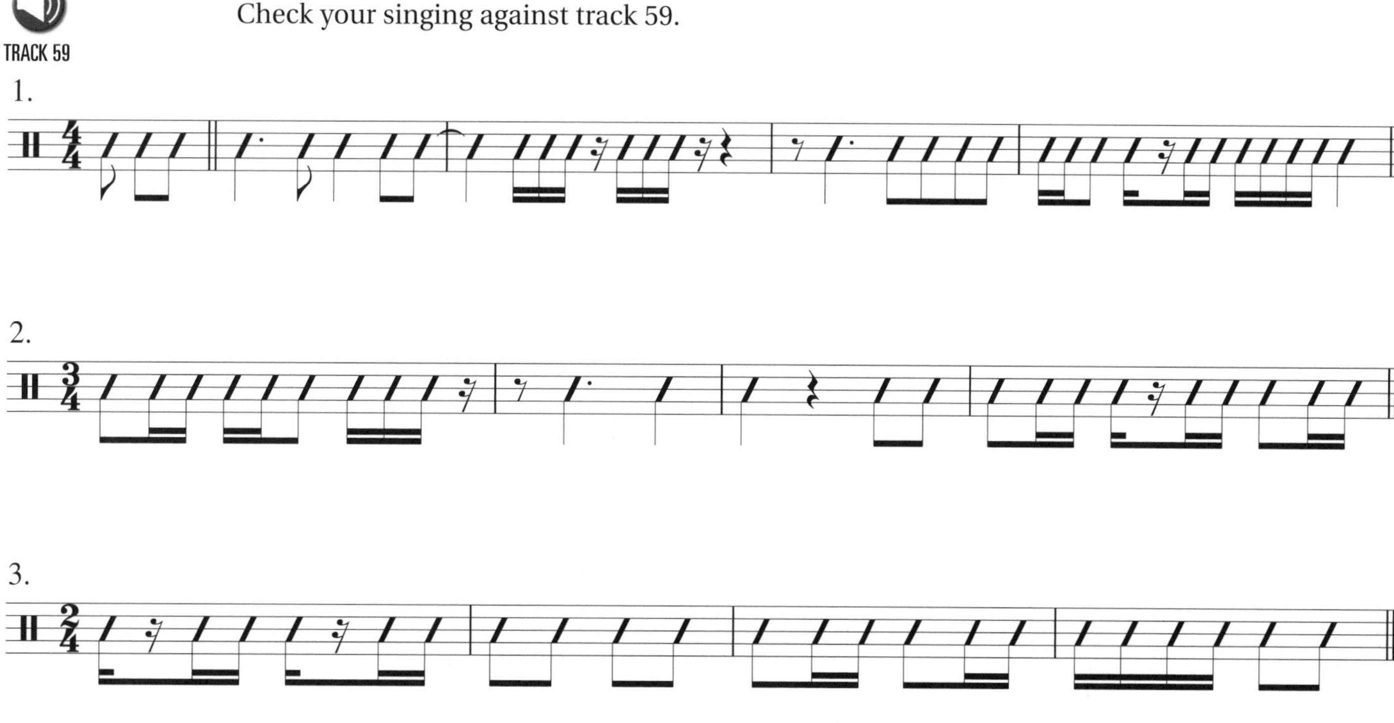

4.

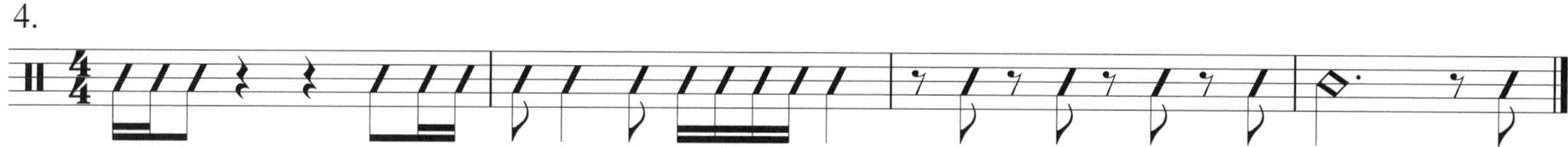

5.

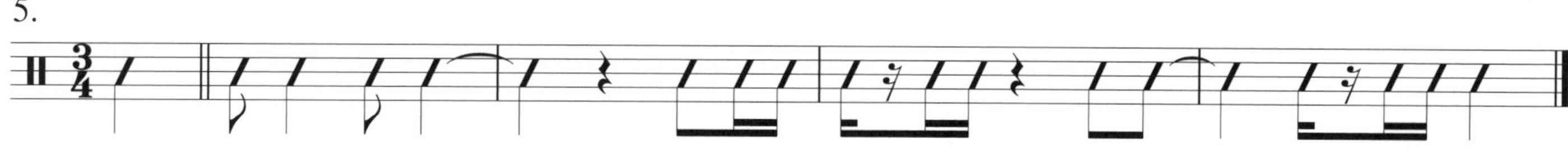

6.

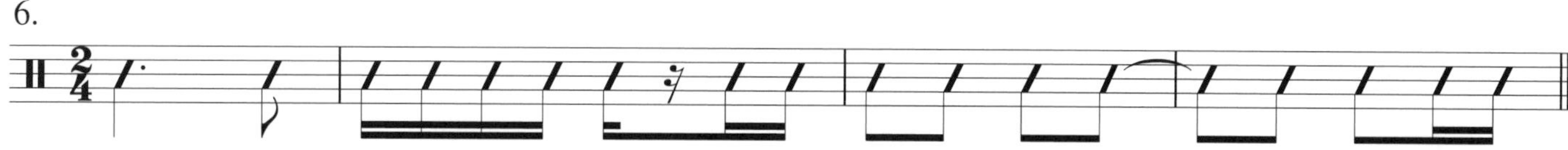

7.

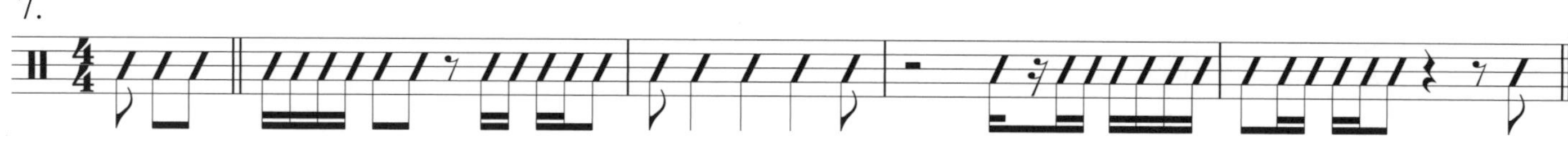

DICTATION

Transcribe each melody by following this procedure.

1. Listen to the CD track until you have memorized the melody.
2. Write the rhythms.
3. Write the solfege syllables.
4. Determine the correct octave, and then write out the notation.
5. Check your transcription against the answer key in appendix B.

Examples 1 to 6 are in A major.
Examples 7 to 12 are in D major.
Examples 13 to 18 are in G major.

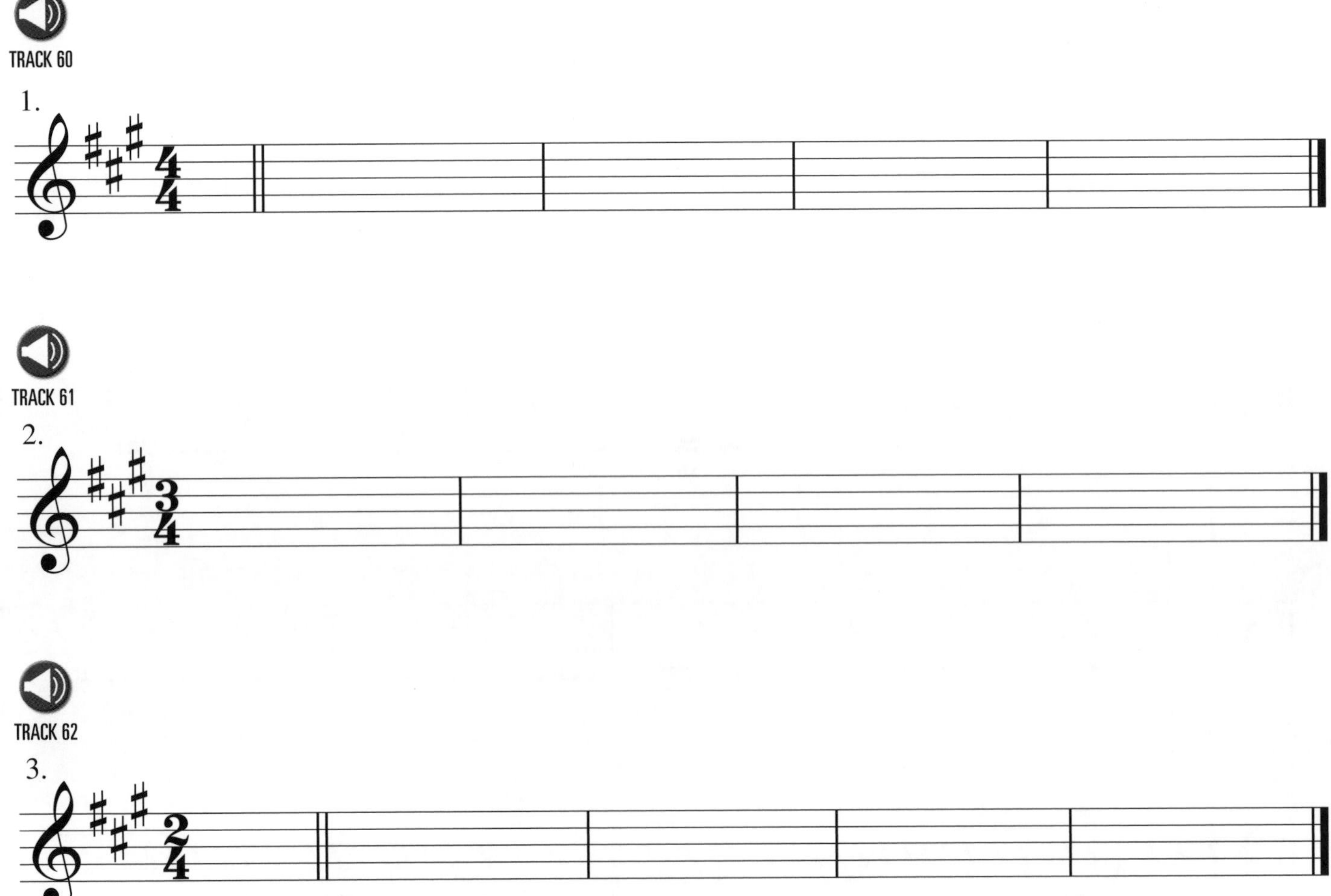

TRACK 63

4.

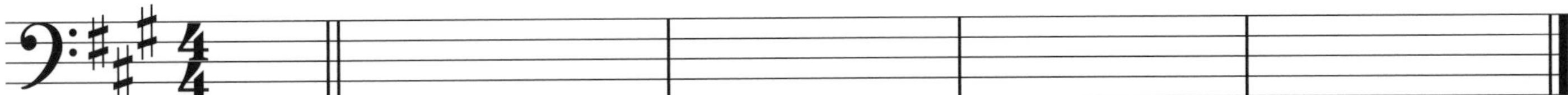

TRACK 64

5.

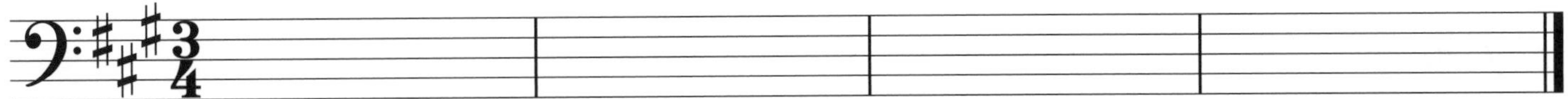

TRACK 65

6.

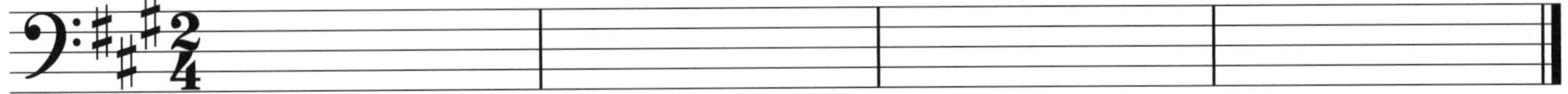

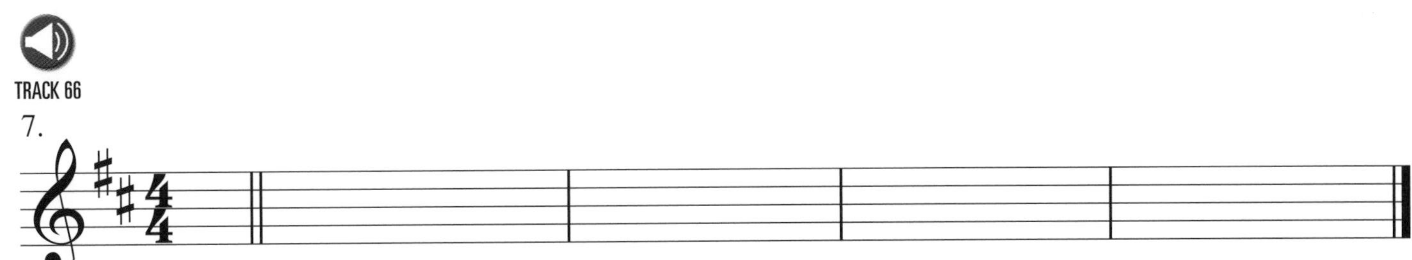

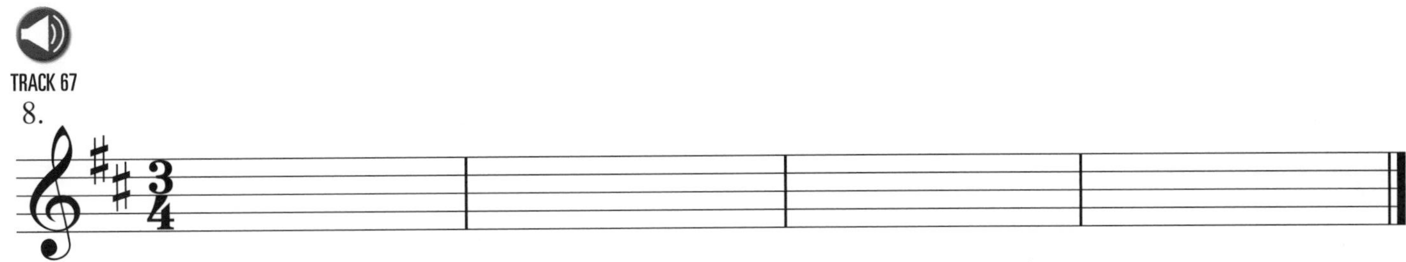

TRACK 68

9.

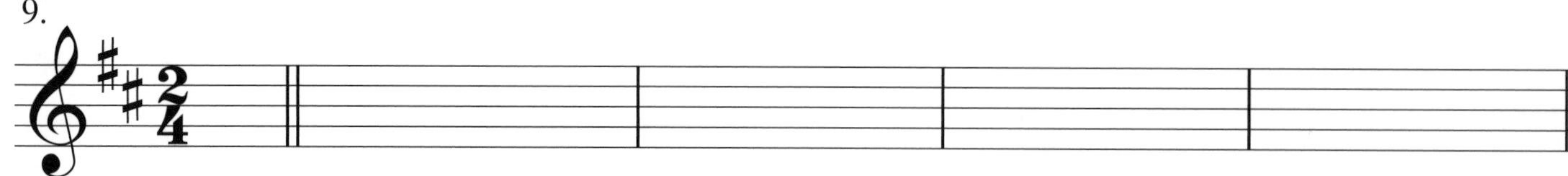

TRACK 69

10.

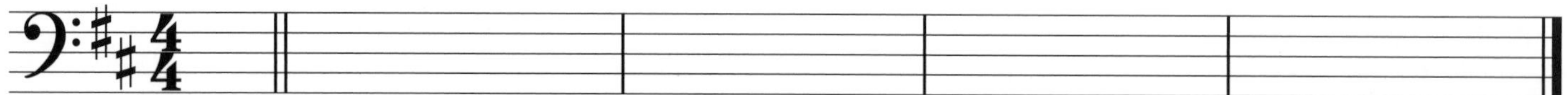

TRACK 70

11.

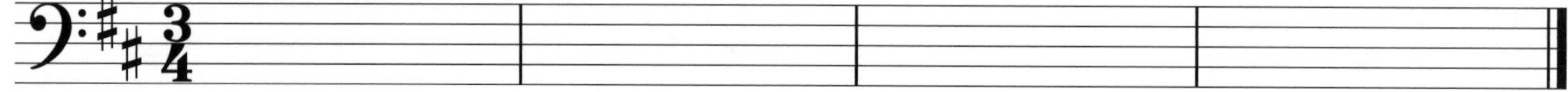

TRACK 71

12.

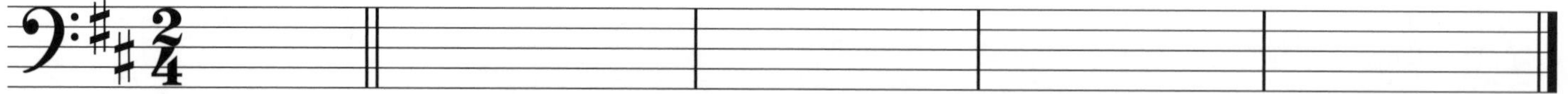

TRACK 72

13.

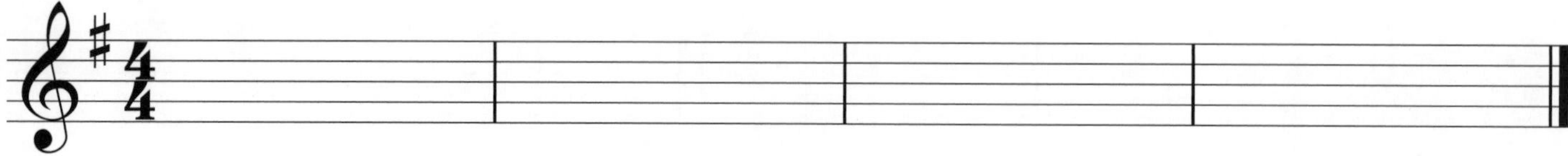

TRACK 73

14.

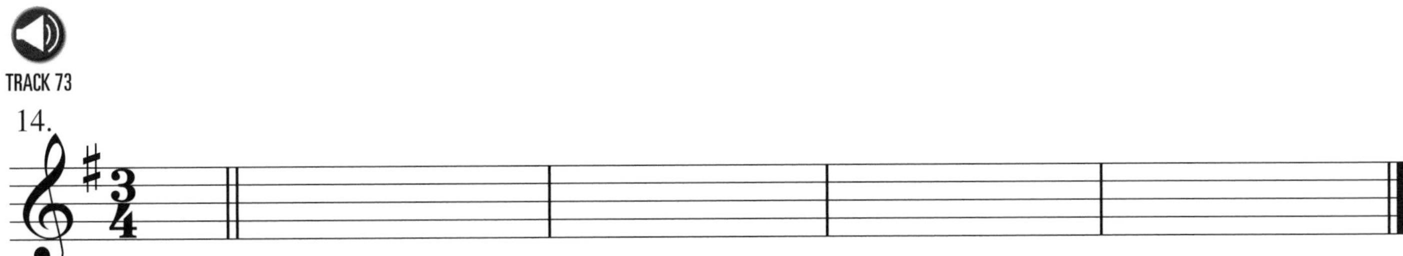

TRACK 74

15.

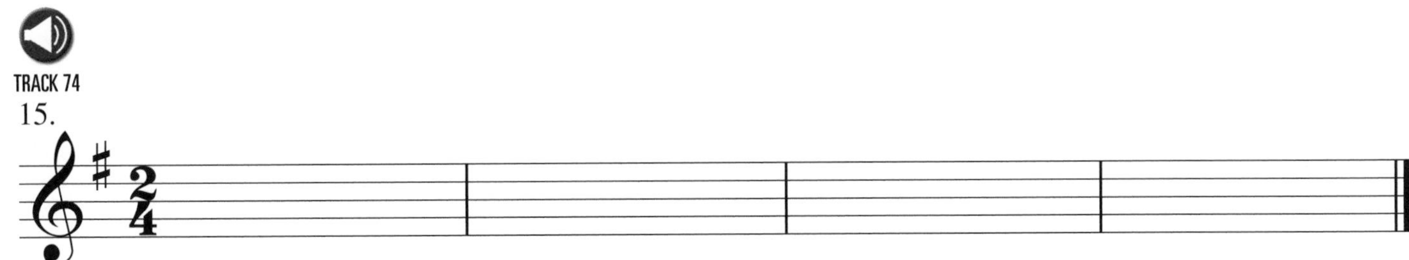

TRACK 75

16.

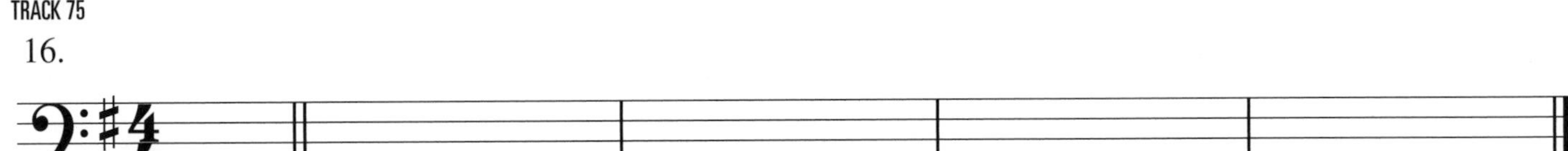

TRACK 76

17.

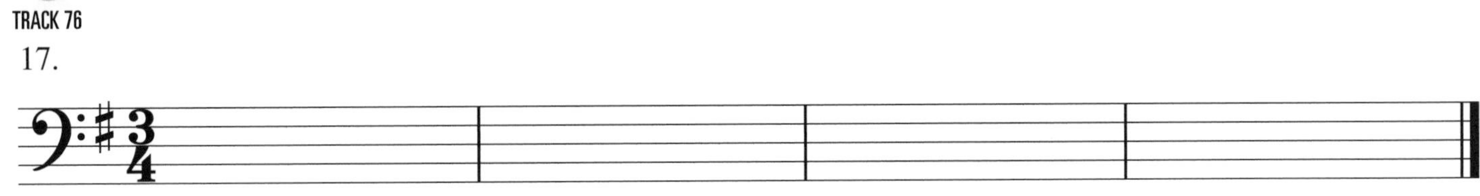

TRACK 77

18.

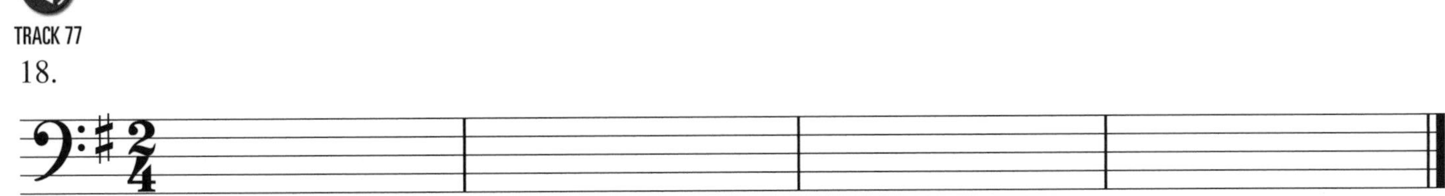

CHAPTER 5

Do, Re, Mi, Fa, Sol, La, Ti

MELODY

New Syllable: Ti

Tendency Tones: Ti-Do

Sing the tendency tones in the order we have studied them: Ti-Do, Re-Do, Fa-Mi, Sol-Do, La-Sol, and Ti-Do. Notice that there is low Ti-Do and high Ti-Do. Gradually, vary the order until you can sing any pair of tendency tones randomly.

1. Do Re Mi Fa Sol La Ti Do / Do Ti La Sol Fa Mi Re Do / Do Re La Mi Re Fa La Sol Fa Mi /
2. Re Fa La Sol Ti Do / Re Fa Mi Sol La Sol Fa / Mi Sol Ti Re Do Fa Re Mi Fa / Mi La Ti Sol Do Ti La Sol Re /
3. Mi La Ti Do Sol Mi Do Mi / Fa La Ti La Fa Ti La Sol / Fa Mi Do Ti Re Sol La / Sol Mi Re Mi Do Ti Re Fa /
4. Sol Ti Re Ti Do La Sol Fa / Sol Ti Re Ti Do Mi Sol / La Fa Re Ti Mi Re Sol Mi Sol / La Ti Re Ti Do Mi Fa Do Ti /
5. Do Fa Do Ti Do Fa Do Ti / Do Fa Ti Do Fa Ti Re Do / Ti Re Do Ti Do Mi Fa Mi Ti / Do Ti Fa Mi Sol La Sol /
6. La Ti Fa Mi Re Ti Sol Fa Re / Mi La Re Do Sol Fa / Mi La Re Sol Do Fa / Do Fa Ti Mi La Re Sol /

Now, the real music-making starts. Get a pencil and paper, and start singing your own Sol-Fa exercises. As you sing a note, write it down. When you're done, check on your instrument that what you wrote corresponds to the correct pitch.

RHYTHM

New Rhythms:

4-beat pattern:

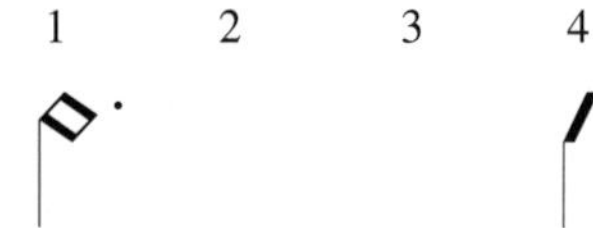

2-beat pattern:

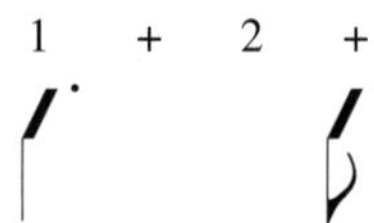

1-beat pattern:

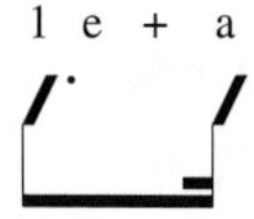

and

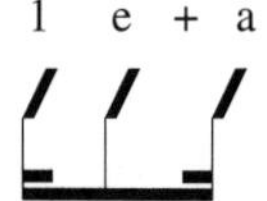

TIP

Review the rhythm exercises in previous lessons. This will help you to build a solid foundation, by constantly reinforcing your learned vocabulary. Look beyond this book at other notation examples, and try reading and transcribing every rhythm you can find.

Practice the rhythms below. Use a three-step process:

1. Clap the rhythms as you count the beats and subdivisions aloud.
2. Count the beats and subdivisions silently, as you clap the rhythms.
3. Conduct and perform the rhythms.

TRACK 78

Check your singing against track 78.

1.

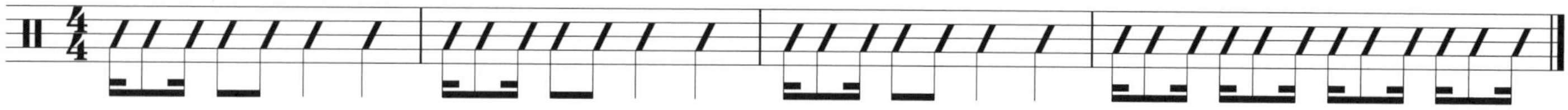

2.

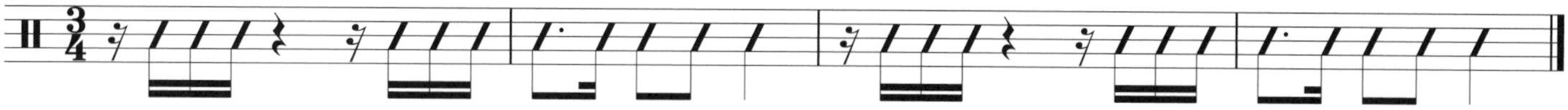

3.

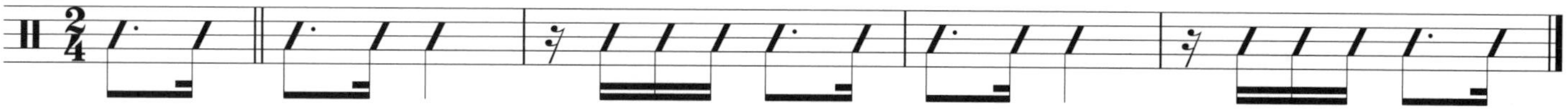

4.

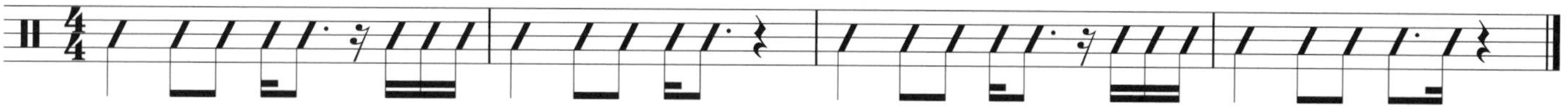

5.

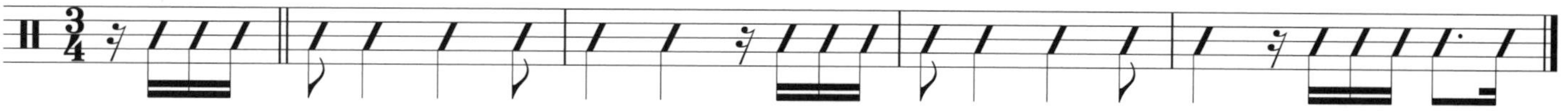

6.

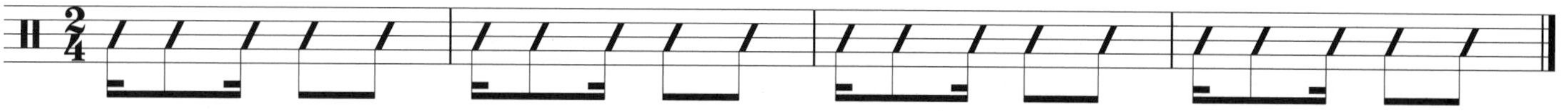

7.

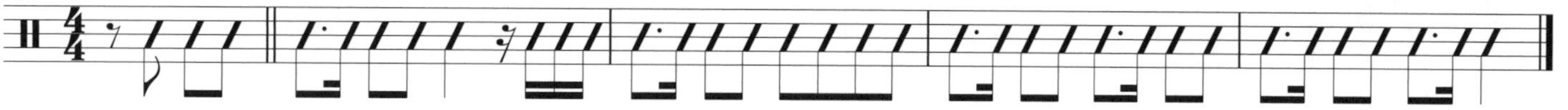

DICTATION

Transcribe each melody by following this procedure.

1. Listen to the CD track until you have memorized the melody.
2. Write the rhythms.
3. Write the solfege syllables.
4. Determine the correct octave, and then write out the notation.
5. Check your transcription against the answer key in appendix B.

Example 1 is in C major.
Example 2 is in D major.
Example 3 is in E major.
Example 4 is in G♭ major.
Example 5 is in A♭ major.
Example 6 is in B♭ major.
Example 7 is in B major.
Example 8 is in D♭ major.
Example 9 is in E♭ major.
Example 10 is in F major.
Example 11 is in G major.
Example 12 is in A major.
Example 13 is in B major.
Example 14 is in C♯ major.
Example 15 is in E♭ major.
Example 16 is in C major.
Example 17 is in G major.
Example 18 is in D♭ major.

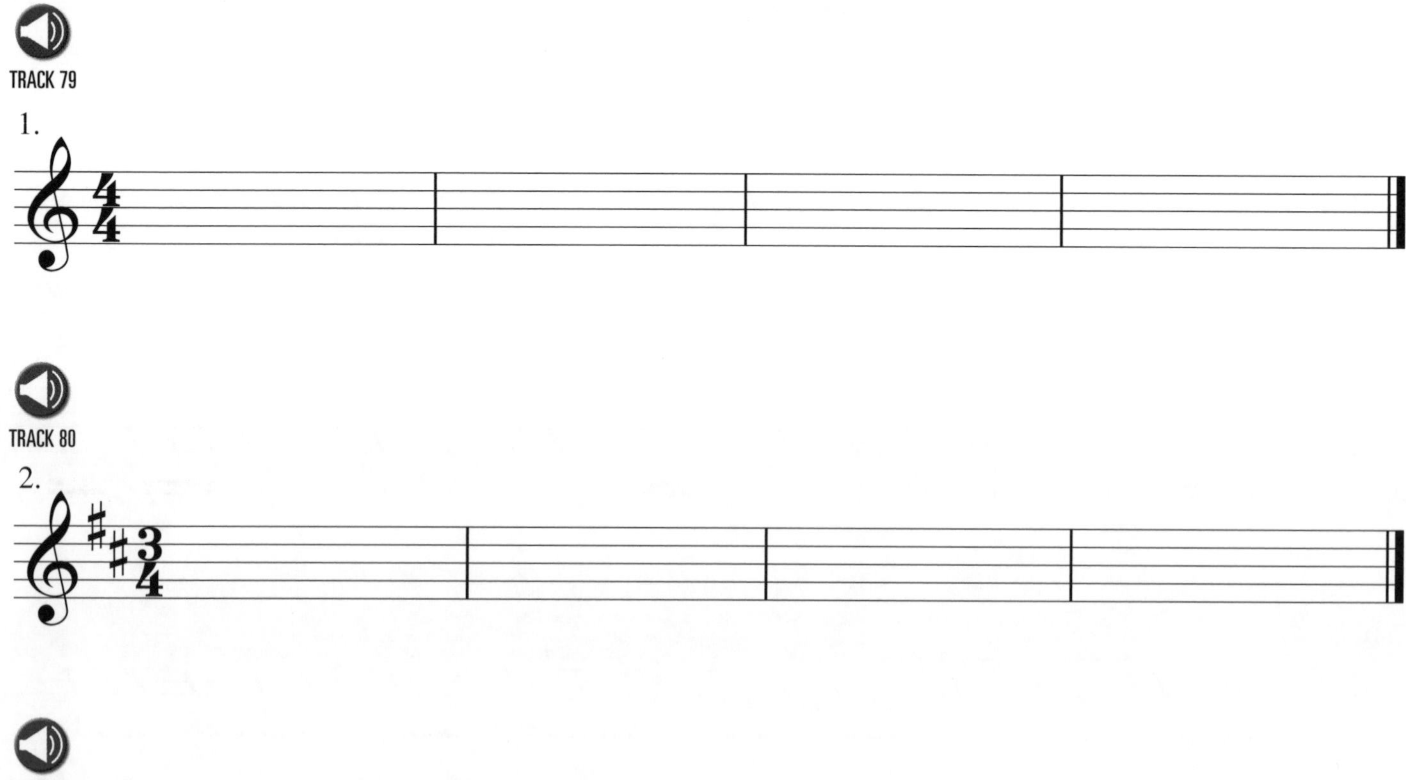

TRACK 82

4.

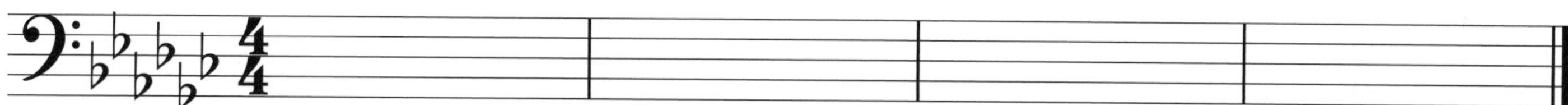

TRACK 83

5.

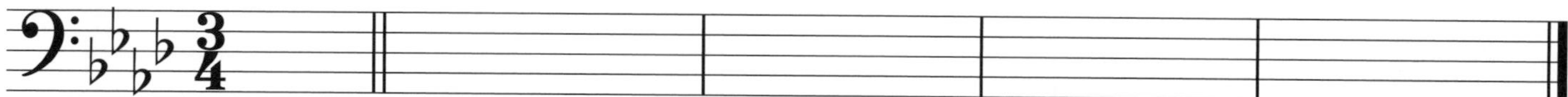

TRACK 84

6.

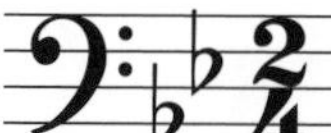

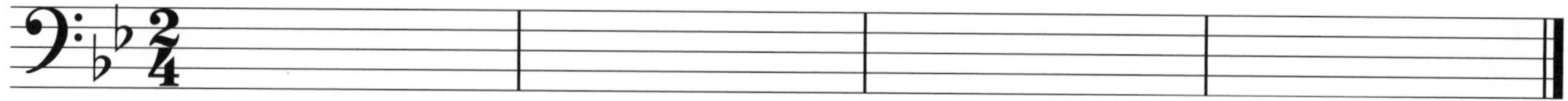

TRACK 85

7.

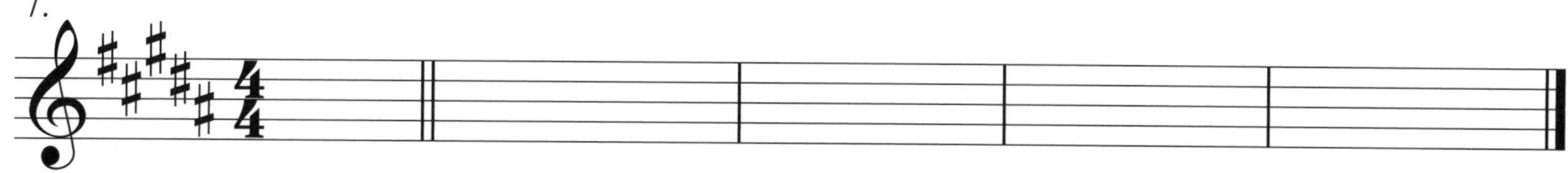

TRACK 86

8.

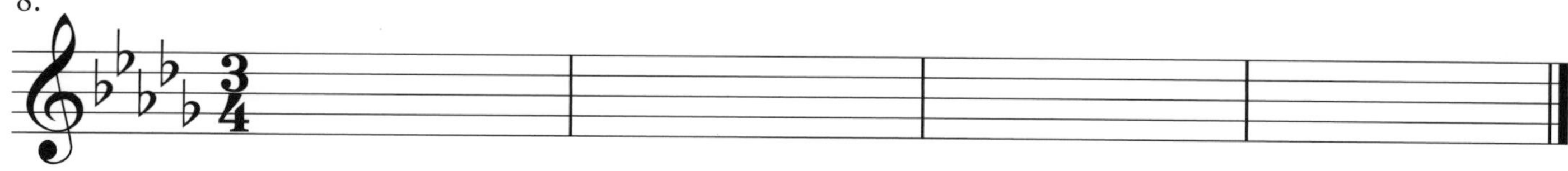

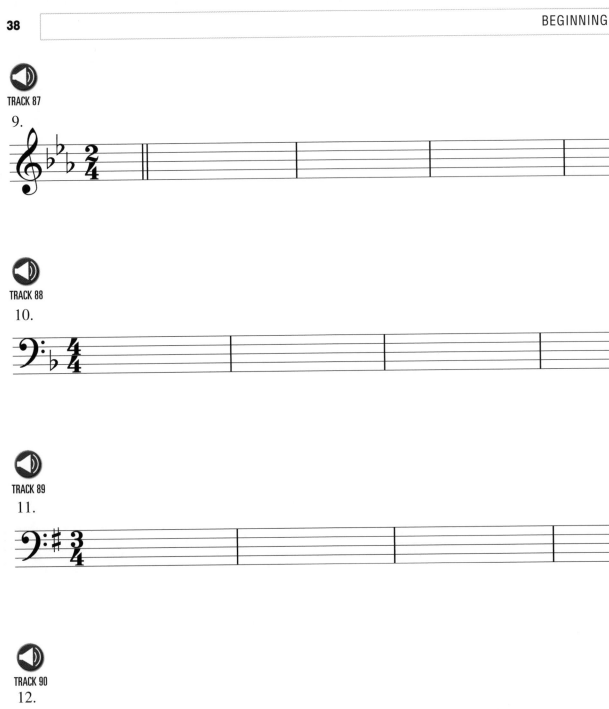

TRACK 87

9.

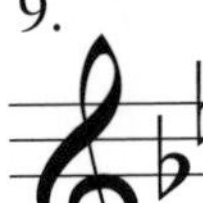

TRACK 88

10.

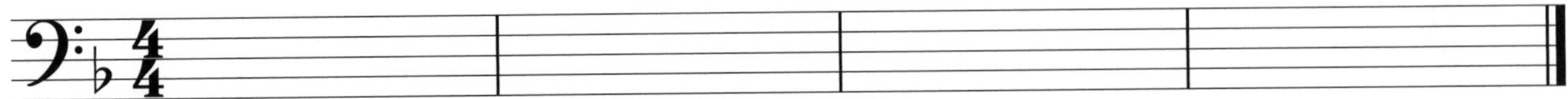

TRACK 89

11.

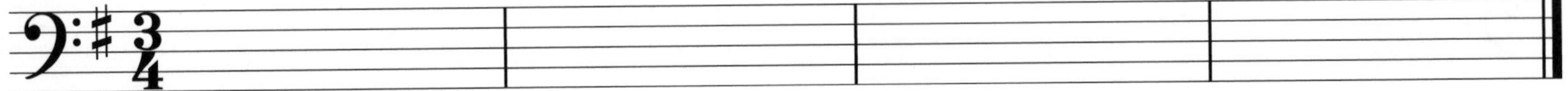

TRACK 90

12.

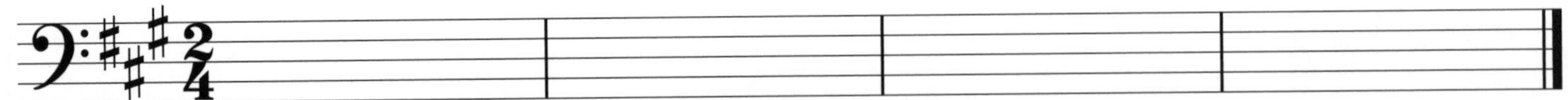

TRACK 91

13.

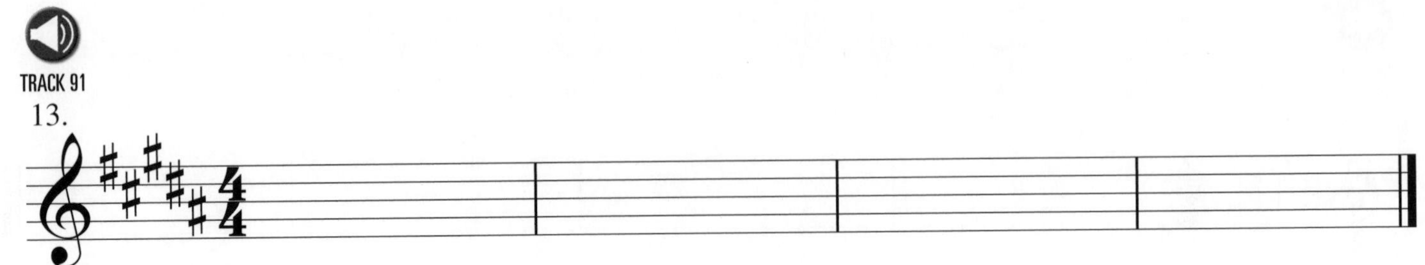

TRACK 92

14.

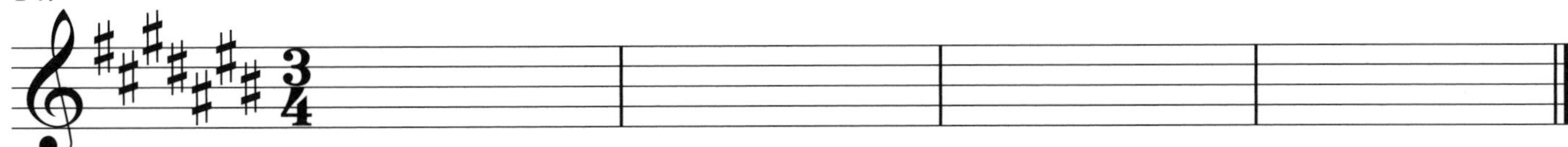

TRACK 93

15.

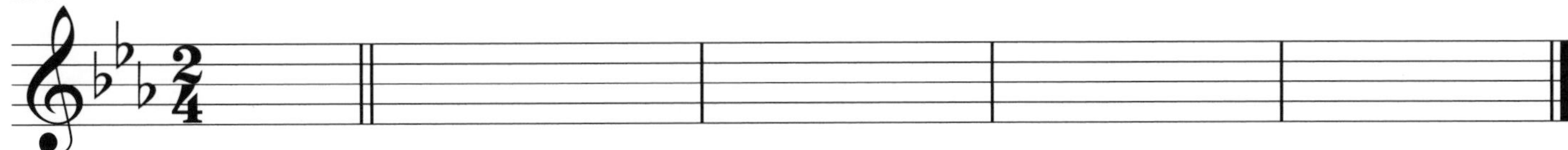

TRACK 94

16.

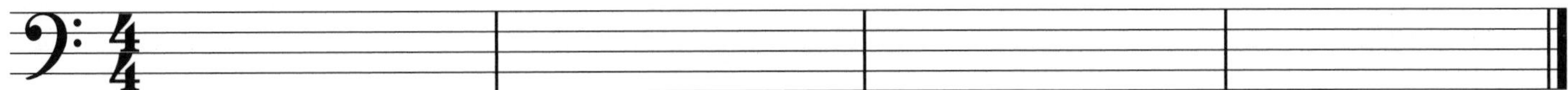

TRACK 95

17.

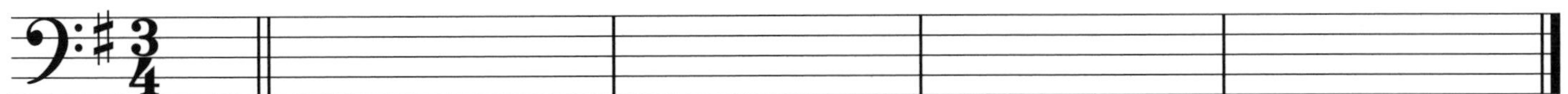

TRACK 96

18.

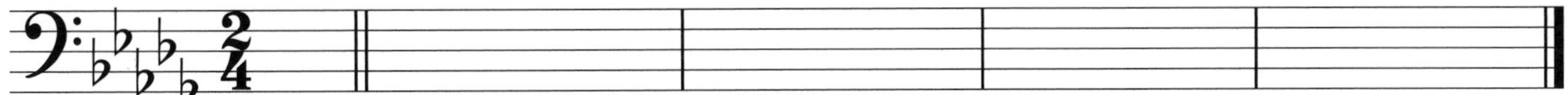

CONCLUSION

"A great way to develop the ability to hear melodies, harmonies, and rhythms is to copy things from recordings. This way of learning is actually the most standard, and the most traditional, way of learning that exists in the world."

—Chick Corea (*Contemporary Keyboard Magazine,* 1976)

Congratulations on completing the exercises in this book. Being able to sing them all perfectly is a significant accomplishment—by no means, a small feat.

Now, you are ready to use these skills on other types of music. Start transcribing everything that sparks your interest: an Eric Clapton guitar solo, Eddie Palmieri's montunos, your favorite television show themes—whatever music interests you.

Make a commitment with yourself to try to learn music by ear, instead of just from lead sheets or published transcriptions. Only by ear will you learn to capture the articulation, personality, and spirit of the music.

—Gilson Schachnik

APPENDIX A

Scales

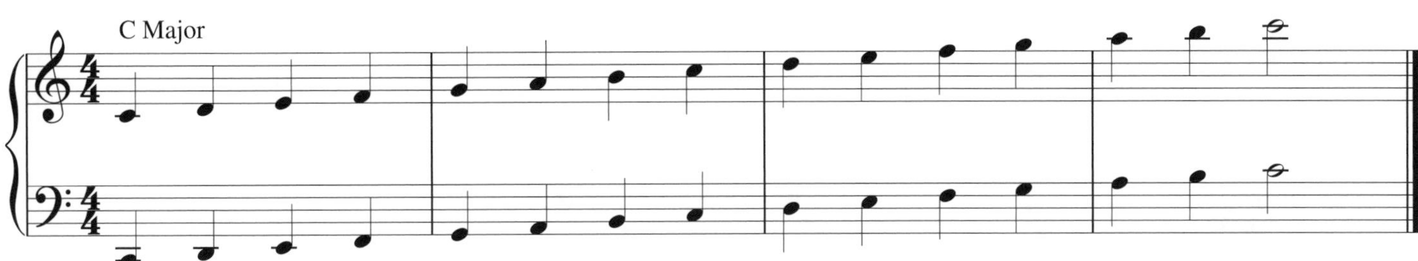

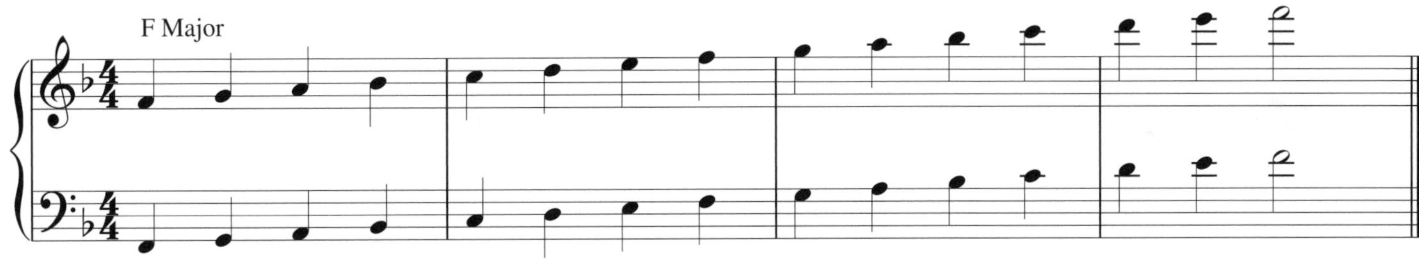

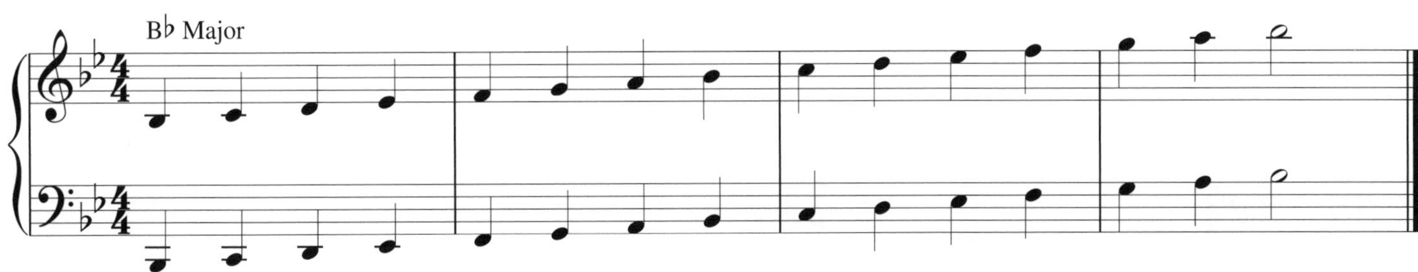

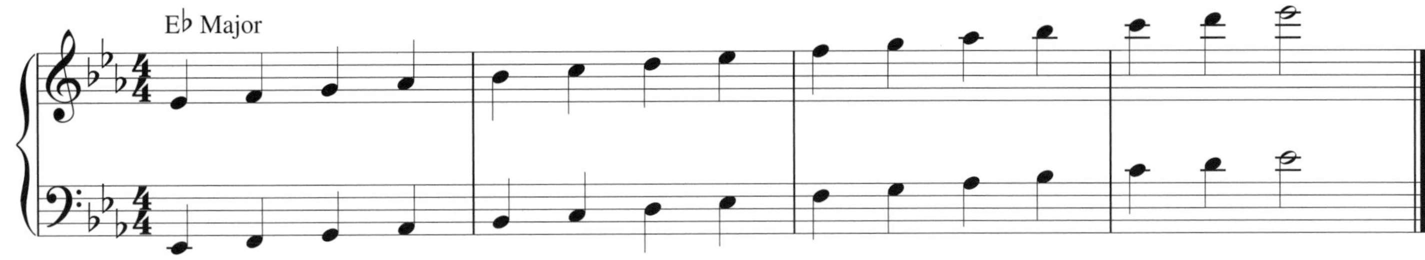

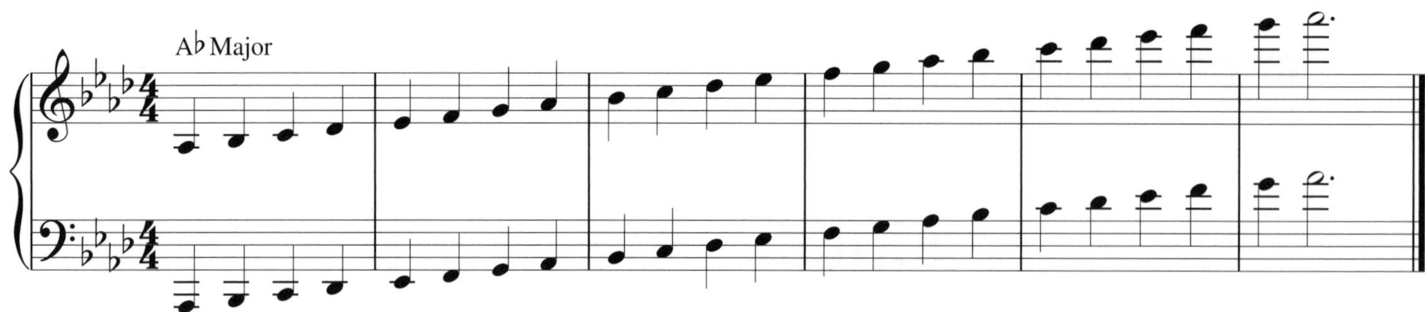
A♭ Major

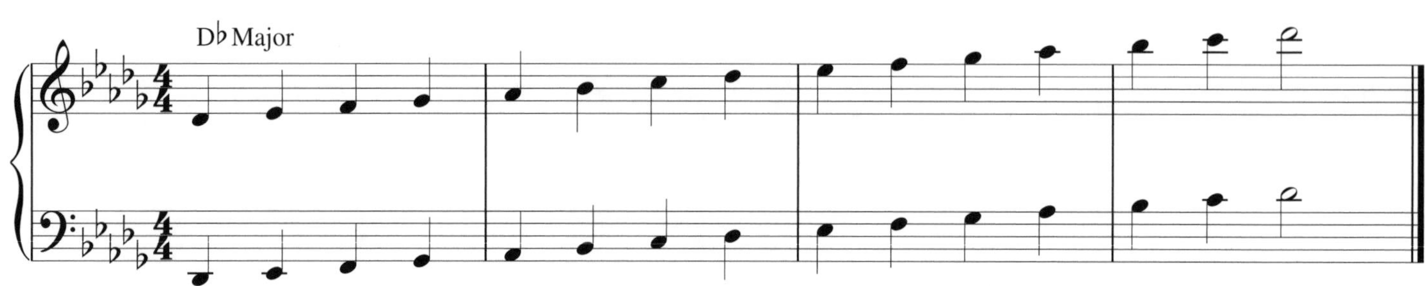
D♭ Major

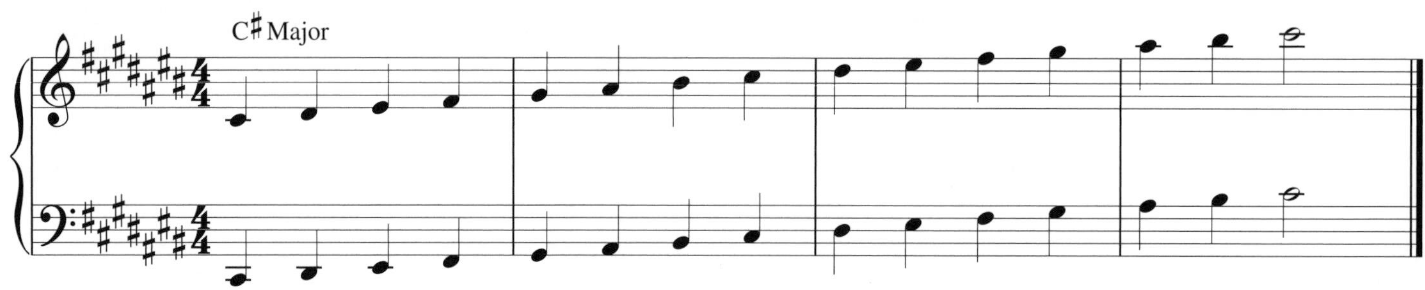
C♯ Major

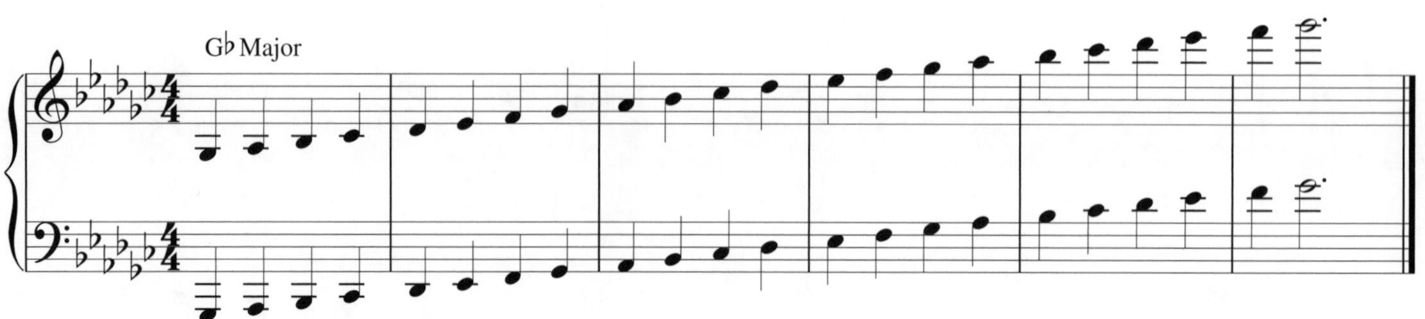
G♭ Major

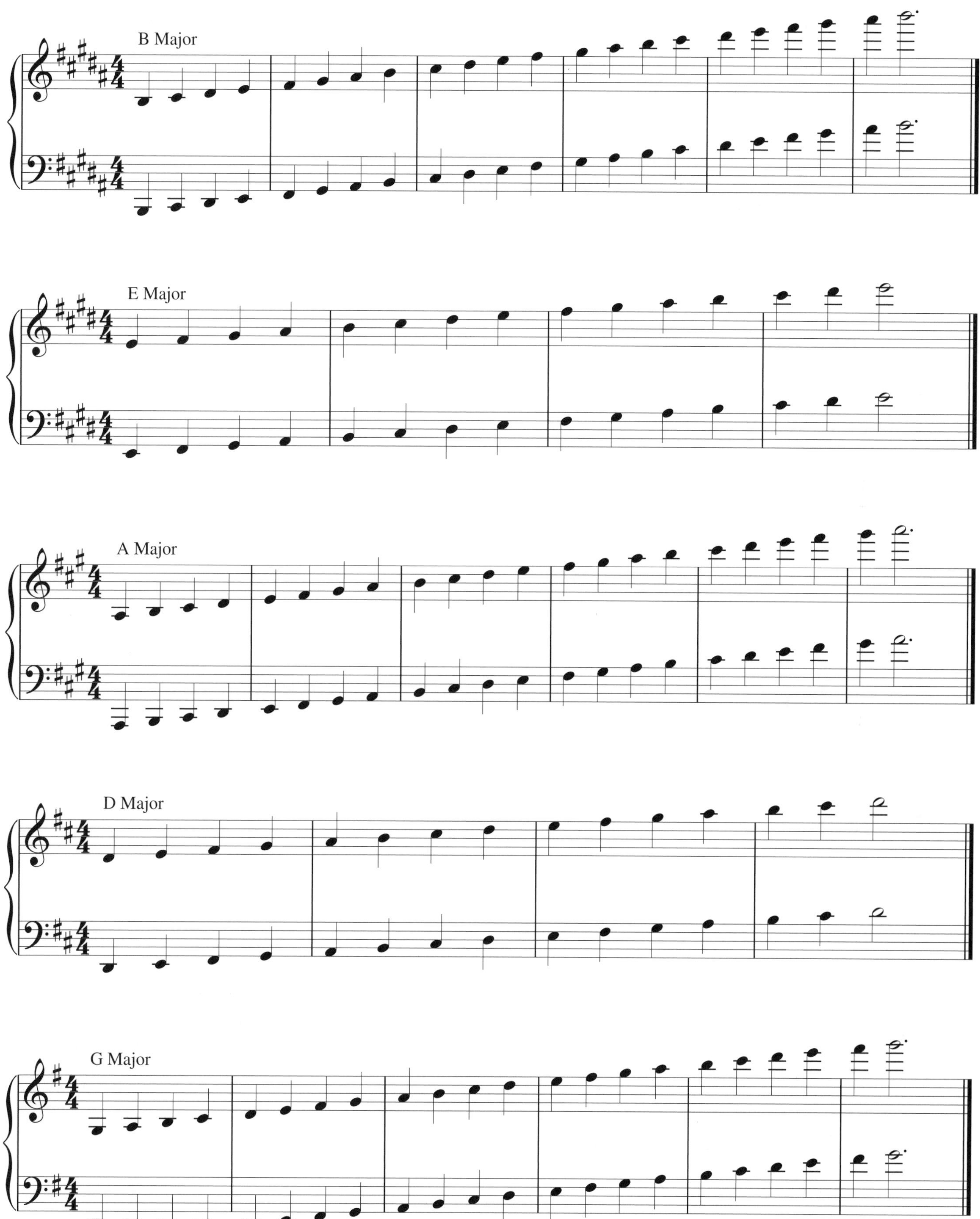
B Major
E Major
A Major
D Major
G Major

APPENDIX B

Dictation Answers

Chapter 1

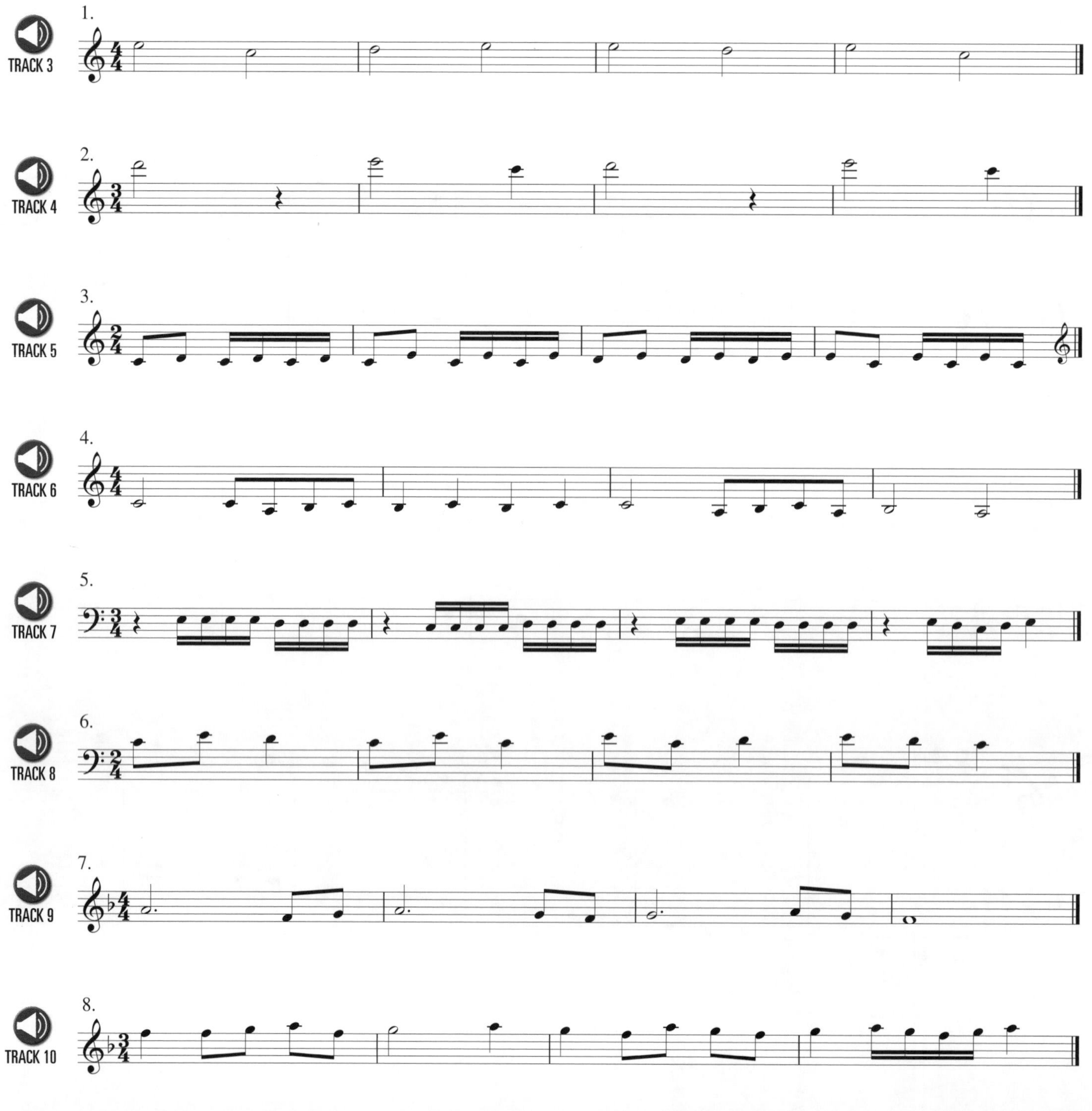

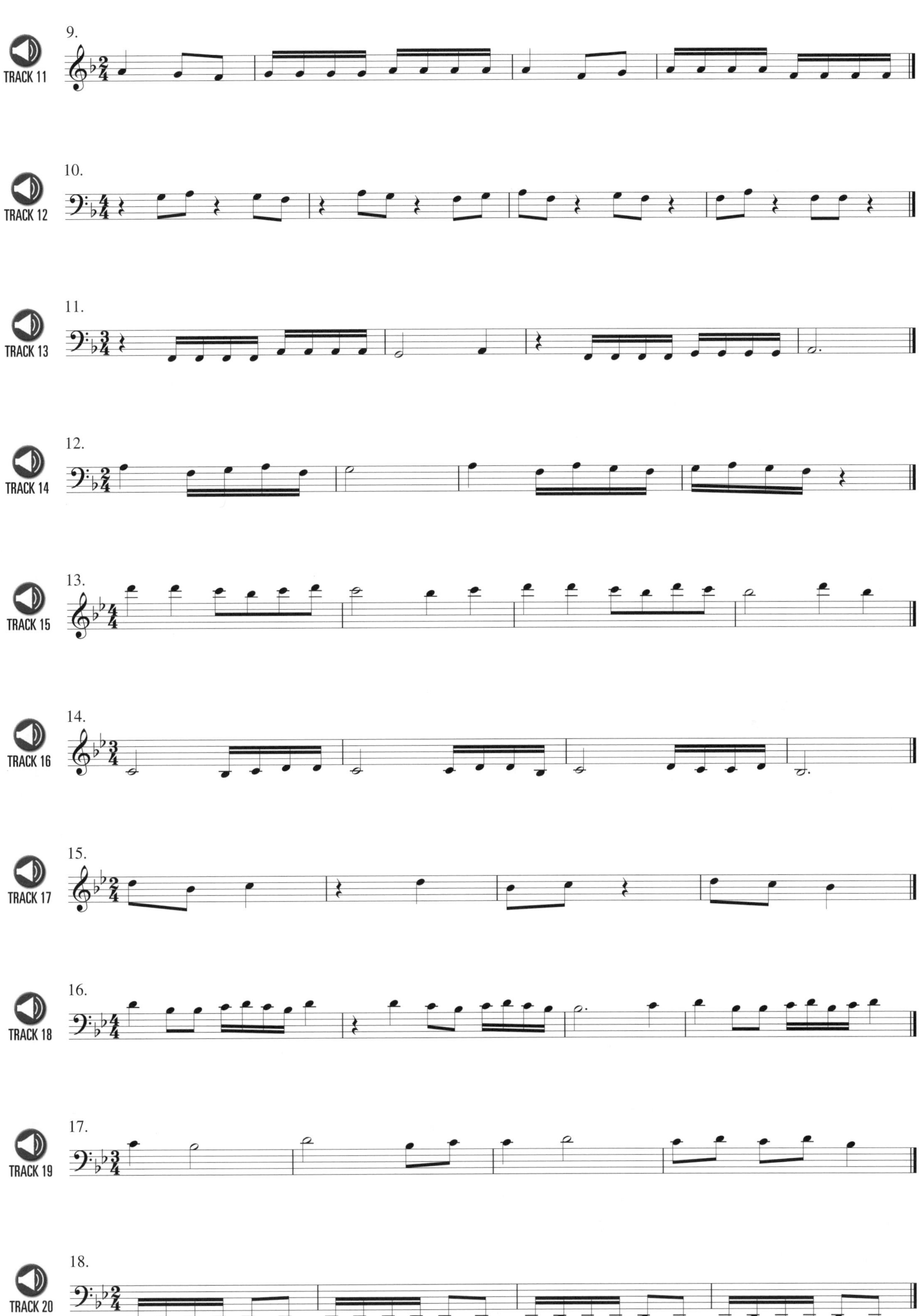
9.
TRACK 11
10.
TRACK 12
11.
TRACK 13
12.
TRACK 14
13.
TRACK 15
14.
TRACK 16
15.
TRACK 17
16.
TRACK 18
17.
TRACK 19
18.
TRACK 20

Chapter 2

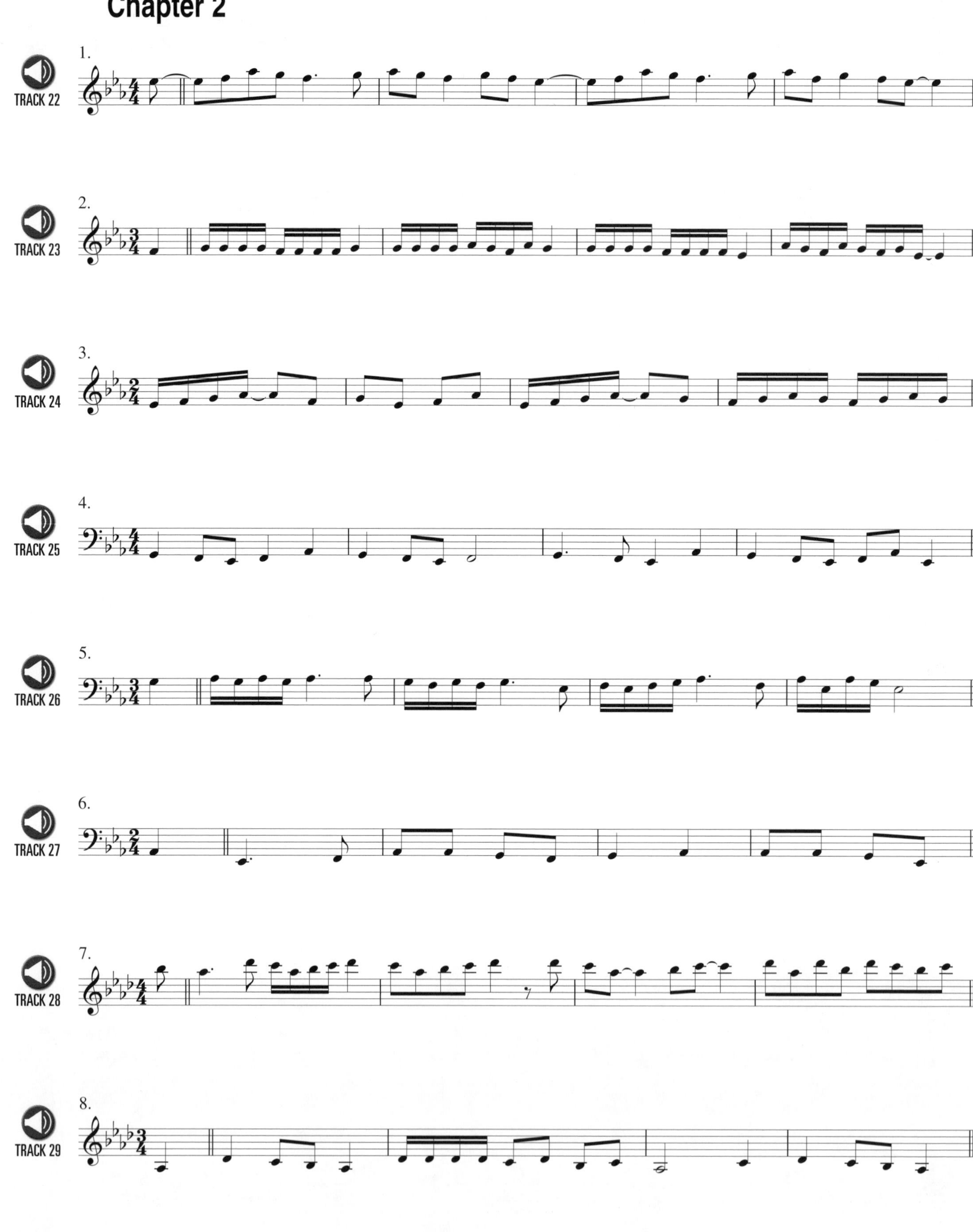
1.
TRACK 22
2.
TRACK 23
3.
TRACK 24
4.
TRACK 25
5.
TRACK 26
6.
TRACK 27
7.
TRACK 28
8.
TRACK 29
9.
TRACK 30

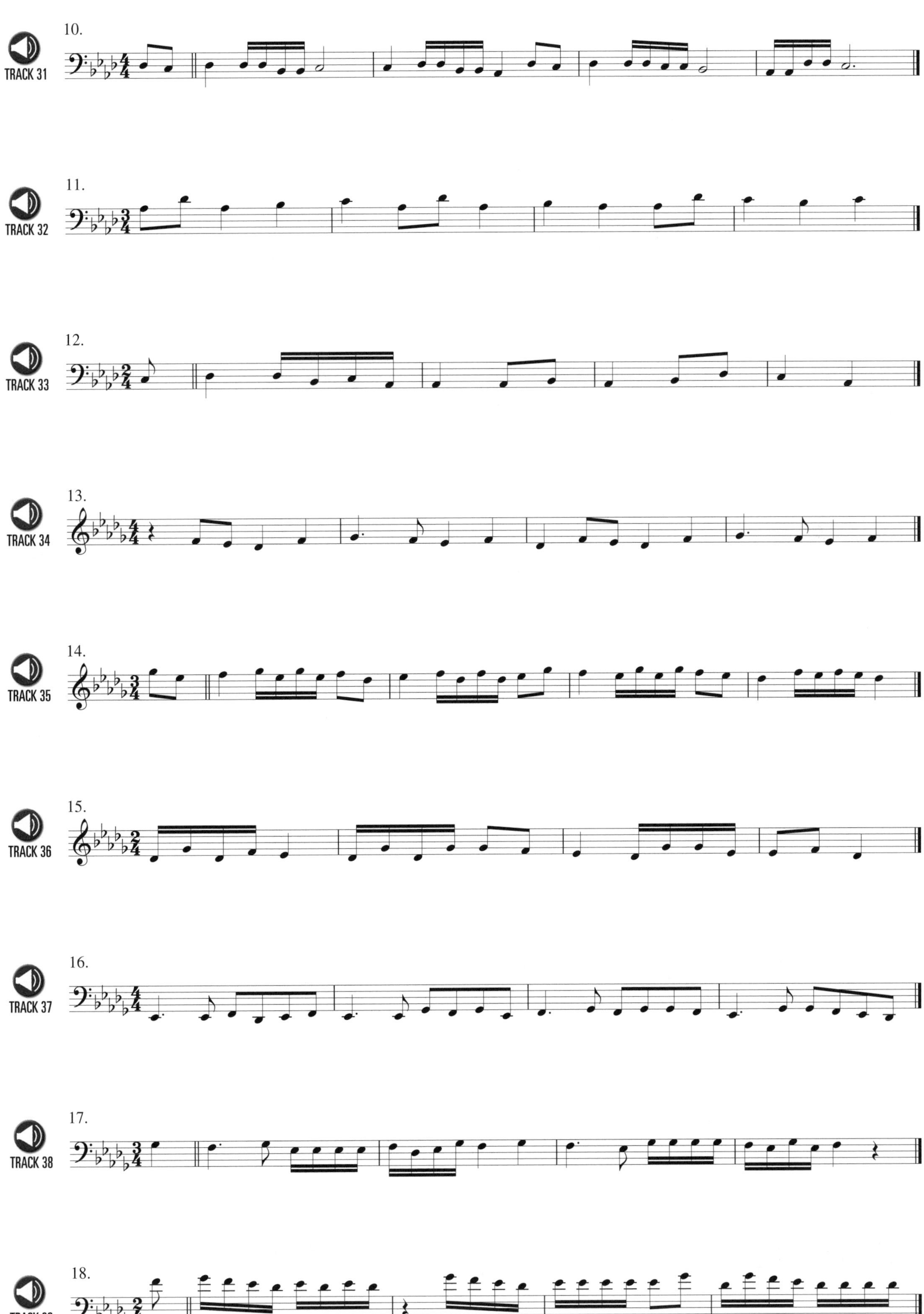
10.
TRACK 31
11.
TRACK 32
12.
TRACK 33
13.
TRACK 34
14.
TRACK 35
15.
TRACK 36
16.
TRACK 37
17.
TRACK 38
18.
TRACK 39

Chapter 3

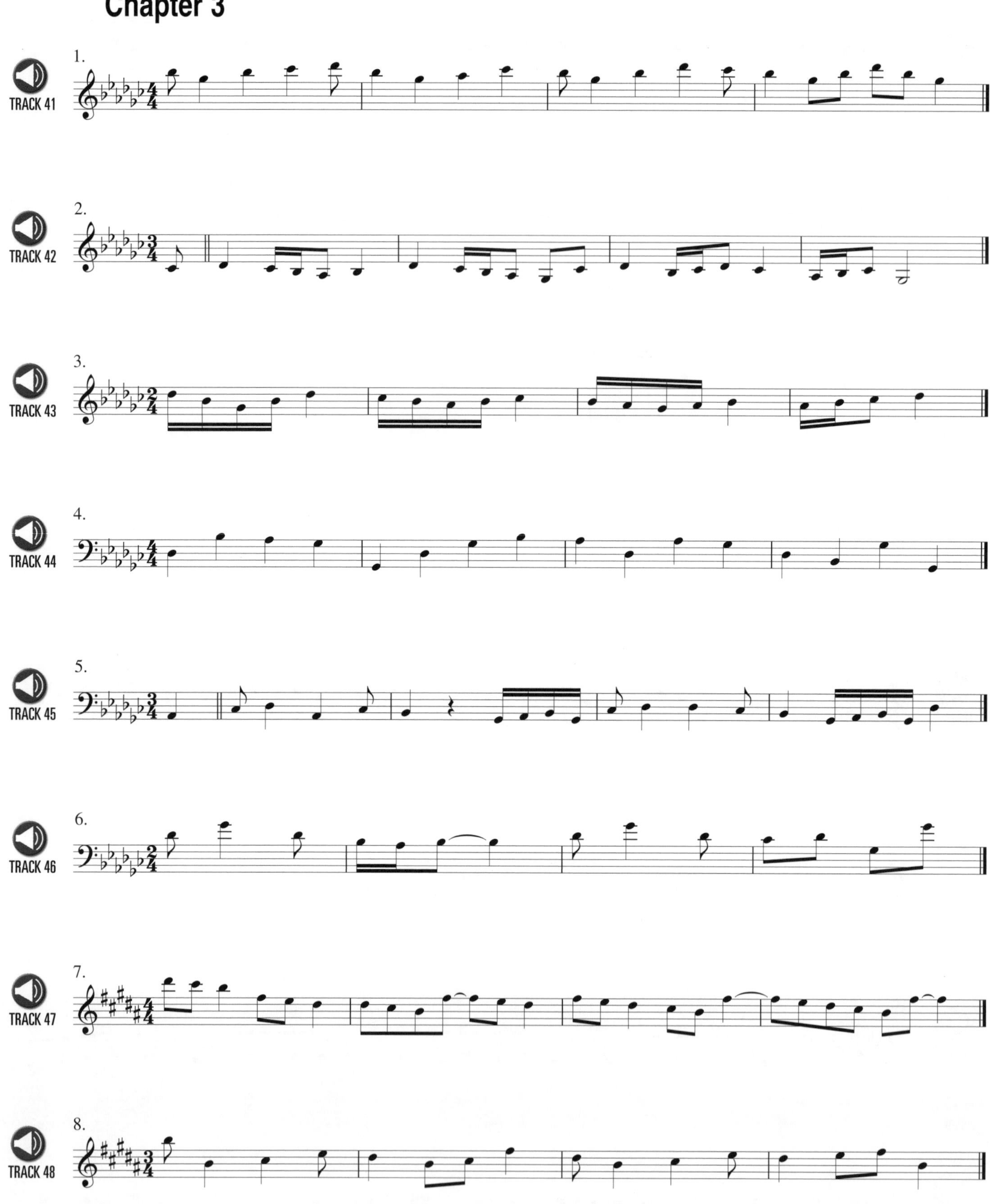
1.
TRACK 41
2.
TRACK 42
3.
TRACK 43
4.
TRACK 44
5.
TRACK 45
6.
TRACK 46
7.
TRACK 47
8.
TRACK 48
9.
TRACK 49

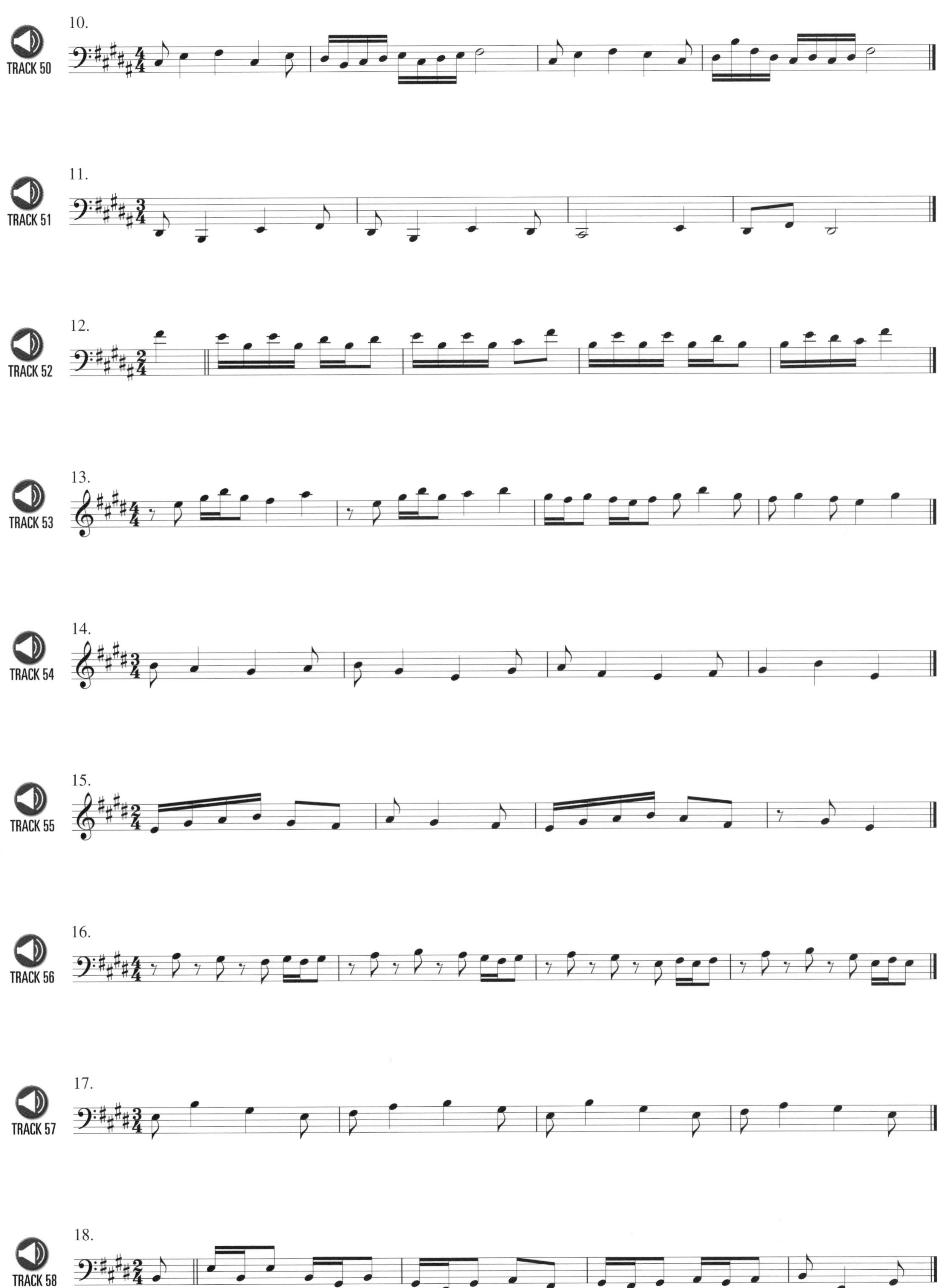
10.
TRACK 50
11.
TRACK 51
12.
TRACK 52
13.
TRACK 53
14.
TRACK 54
15.
TRACK 55
16.
TRACK 56
17.
TRACK 57
18.
TRACK 58

Chapter 4

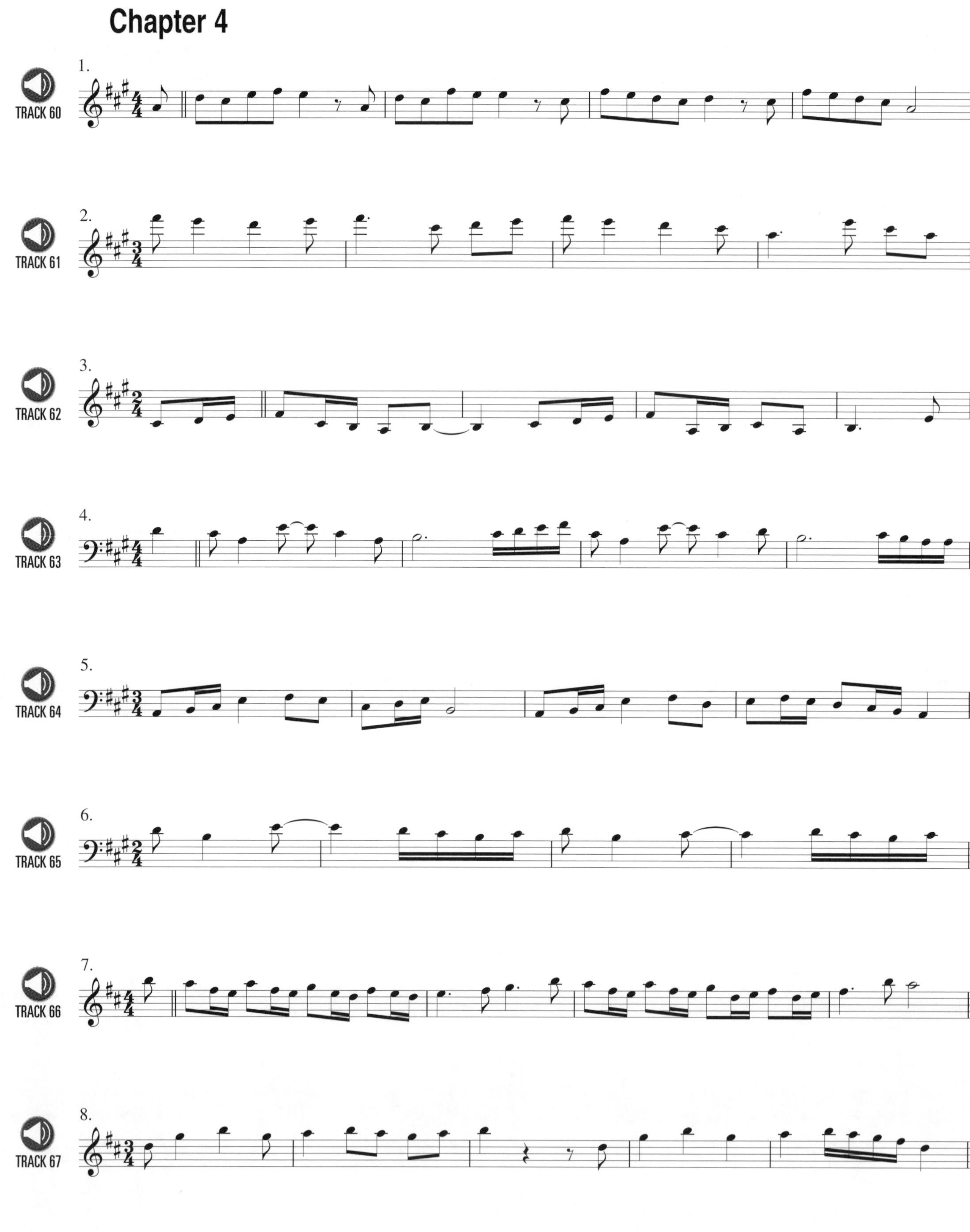
1.
TRACK 60
2.
TRACK 61
3.
TRACK 62
4.
TRACK 63
5.
TRACK 64
6.
TRACK 65
7.
TRACK 66
8.
TRACK 67
9.
TRACK 68

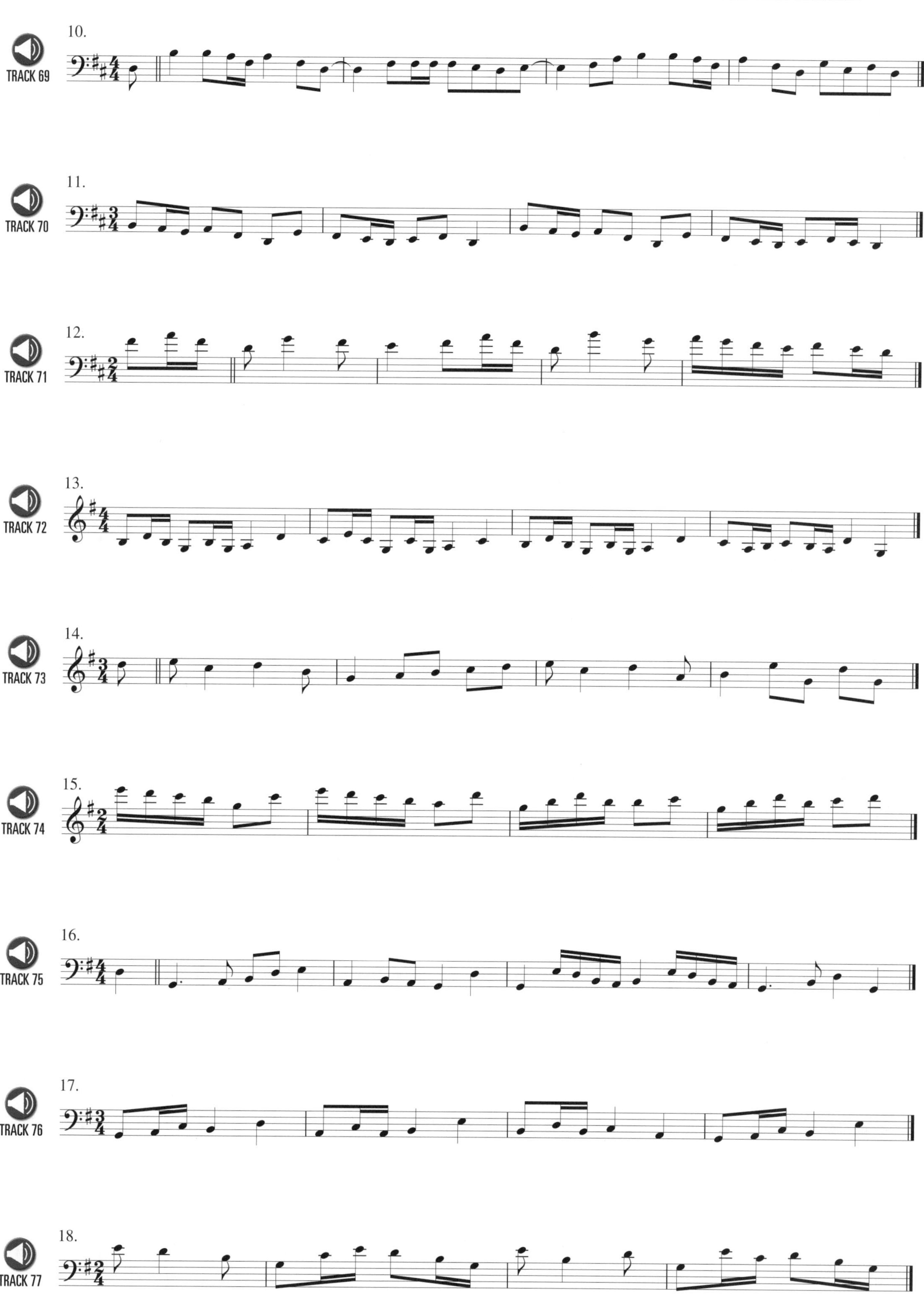
10.
TRACK 69
11.
TRACK 70
12.
TRACK 71
13.
TRACK 72
14.
TRACK 73
15.
TRACK 74
16.
TRACK 75
17.
TRACK 76
18.
TRACK 77

Chapter 5

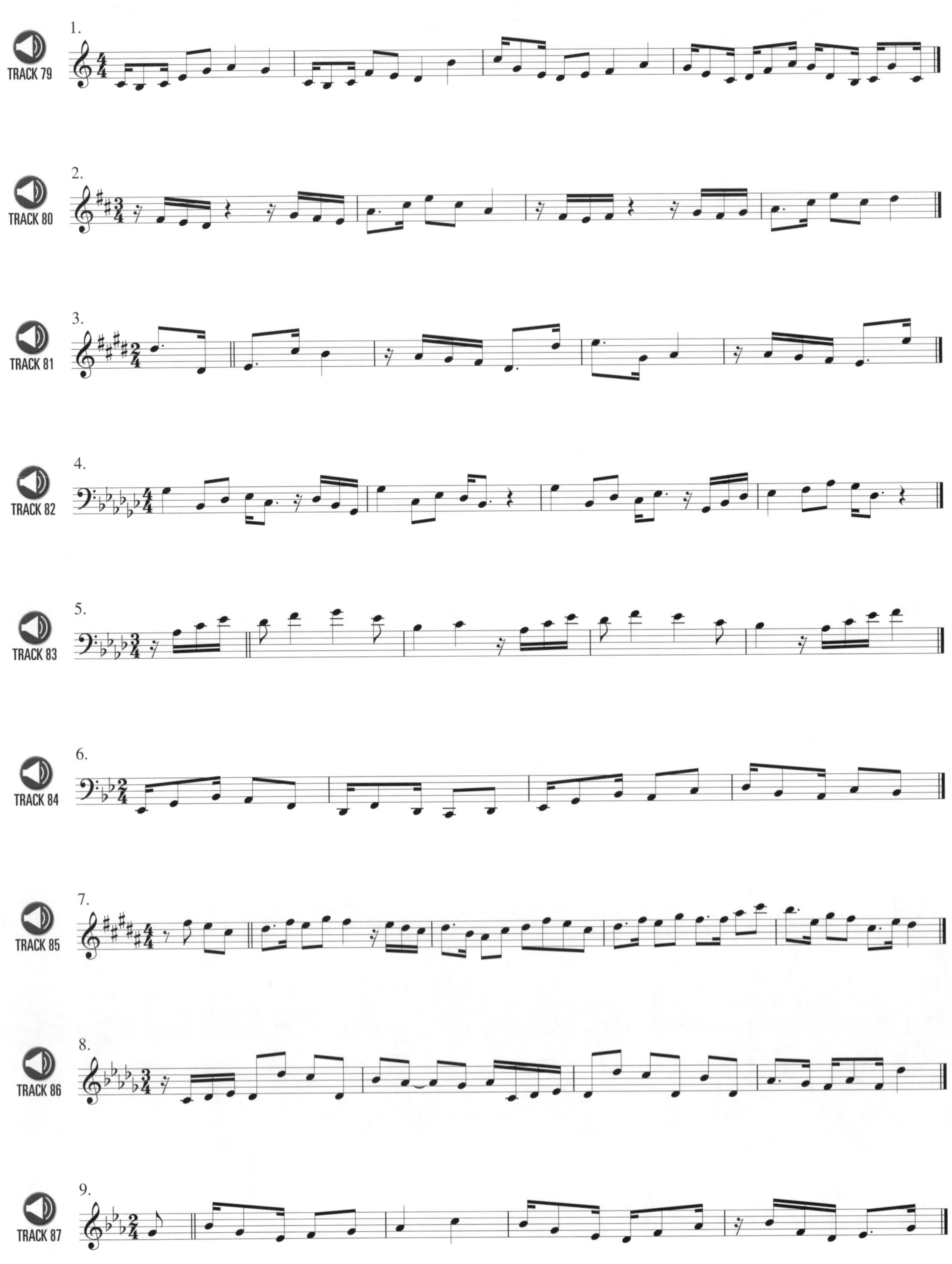
1.
TRACK 79
2.
TRACK 80
3.
TRACK 81
4.
TRACK 82
5.
TRACK 83
6.
TRACK 84
7.
TRACK 85
8.
TRACK 86
9.
TRACK 87

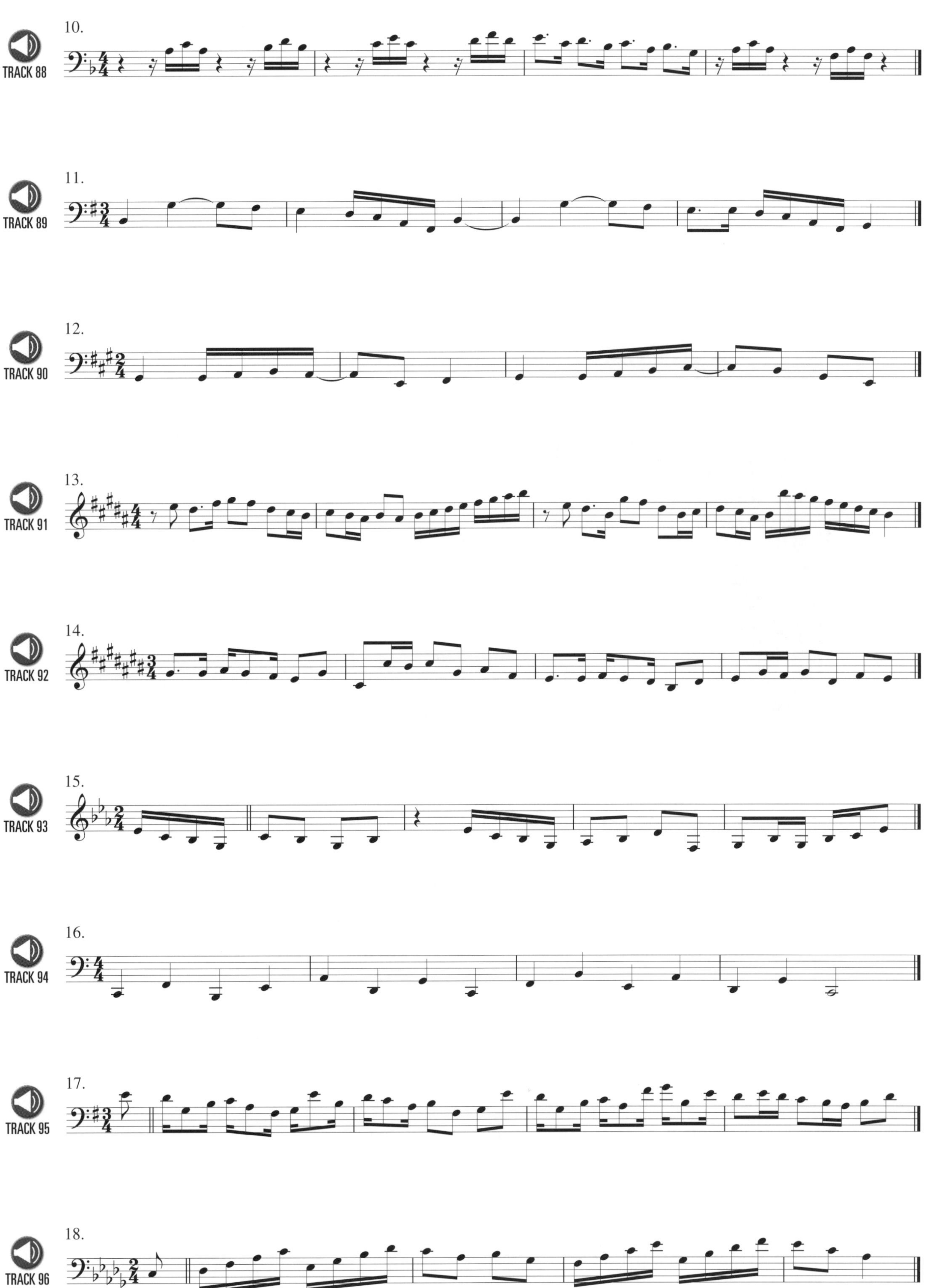
10.
TRACK 88
11.
TRACK 89
12.
TRACK 90
13.
TRACK 91
14.
TRACK 92
15.
TRACK 93
16.
TRACK 94
17.
TRACK 95
18.
TRACK 96

About the Author

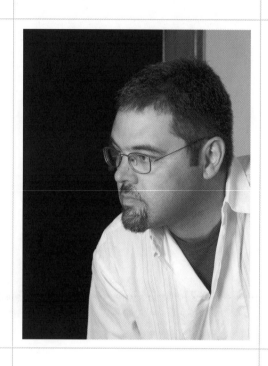

Photo by Liz Linder

Born in Sao Paulo, Brazil, 1963, Gilson Schachnik is an active keyboardist, composer, and arranger. He has played keyboards alongside some of the most important names in the jazz and Brazilian music scenes, including Claudio Roditti, Bill Pierce, Romero Lubambo, Yoron Israel, Jerry Bergonzi, Luciana Souza, Mick Goodrick, John Lockwood, Paulo Braga, Peri Ribeiro, Antonio Sanchez, Miguel Zenon, and Cafe. His mentors include Danilo Perez, Charlie Banacos, and Bob Durso.

As a composer, Gilson's credits include jingles (BASF cassette tapes, *Playboy* magazine, and others), and soundtracks for the acclaimed children's television program *Ratimbum* (awarded Best TV Show by the New York Film Festival) and the feature film *Fogo e Paixao*.

Gilson's debut CD, *Raw* (Brownstone: 1998) received rave reviews. Bob Young, of the *Boston Herald* and *Jazziz* magazine, wrote, "Gilson Schachnik creates the kind of all-encompassing jazz mix that fans of the music's new world order now demand: entertaining, unclichéd, and flavored with tastes from around the globe." *Raw* was nominated for the 1999 Boston Music Awards.

Gilson's CD *Lampiao* (Candid Records: 2005) features an all-star Latin jazz ensemble: drummer Antonio Sanchez, saxophonist Miguel Zenon, bassist Fernando Huergo, guitarist Guilherme Monteiro, and percussionist Sula da Silva.

Gilson is an assistant professor of ear training at Berklee College of Music.

Contact Gilson with any questions or comments via his Web site at www.gilsonmusic.com.

Berklee to Go.

Take your music career further. Learn about the future of the music industry. Discover how to set up a recording studio for that perfect sound. Strengthen your performance chops. You'll find all the tools you need with books and DVDs from Berklee Press.

DVDs

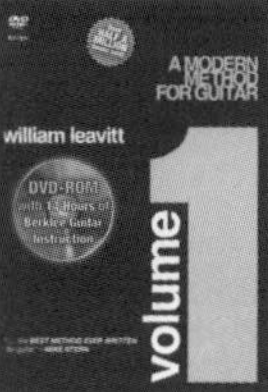

A Modern Method for Guitar Volume 1
Featuring Larry Baione and William Leavitt
14 hours of instruction! A year's worth of guitar lessons at Berklee College of Music.

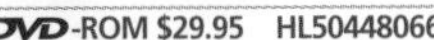

DVD-ROM $29.95 HL50448066

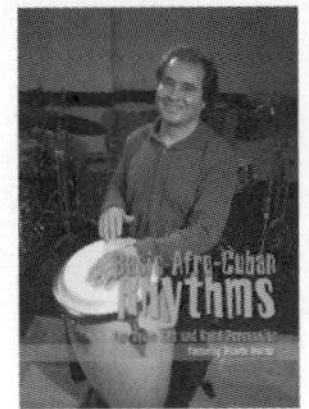

Basic Afro-Cuban Rhythms
Featuring Ricardo Monzón
Learn the classic rhythms of Afro-Cuban music as master percussionist Monzón demonstrates the patterns and instruments that form its beating heart.

DVD $19.95 HL50448012

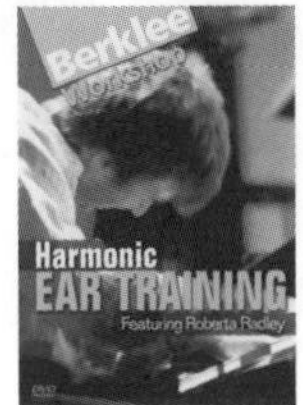

Harmonic Ear Training
Featuring Roberta Radley
A vital introduction to ear training for songwriters and performers looking to improve their listening skills and become better musicians.

DVD $19.95 HL50448039

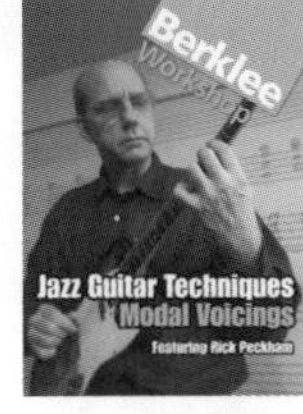

Jazz Guitar Techniques: Modal Voicings
Featuring Rick Peckham
Extend your capabilities by integrating a variety of new voicings and articulations into your playing.

DVD $19.95 HL50448016

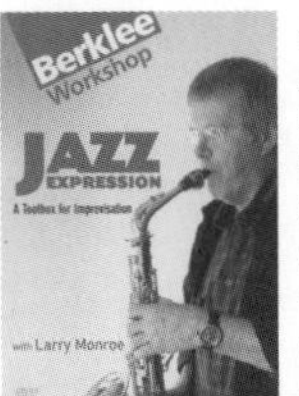

Jazz Expression: A Toolbox for Improvisation
Featuring Larry Monroe
Learn to develop your own style as you work with the building blocks of expression and articulation to craft your personal musical interpretation of a song.

DVD $19.95 HL50448036

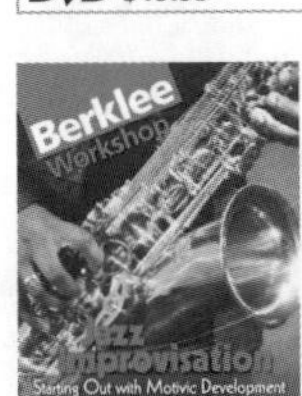

Jazz Improvisations: Starting out with Motivic Development
Learn techniques for creating graceful solos from a two-, three- or four-note riff or motive. Add depth and variety by stringing several motives together.

DVD $29.95 HL50448014

Kenwood Dennard: The Studio/ Touring Drummer
Find the right groove for any session or performance with one of the industry's most in-demand drummers.

DVD $19.95 HL50448034

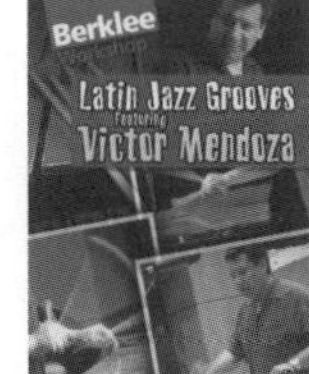

Latin Jazz Grooves
Featuring Victor Mendoza
Learn to apply your musical vocabulary and knowledge of rhythm, scales and chord progressions to explore this rich musical style. Includes practice and play-along tracks.

DVD $19.95 HL50448003

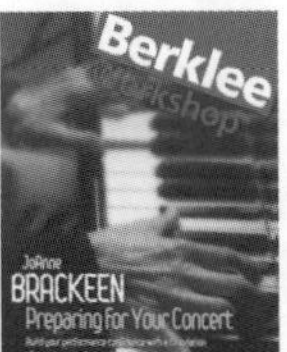

Preparing for Your Concert
Featuring JoAnne Brackeen
Learn routines and exercises to get you physically and mentally primed to walk out on stage and deliver an amazing performance.

DVD $19.95 HL50448018

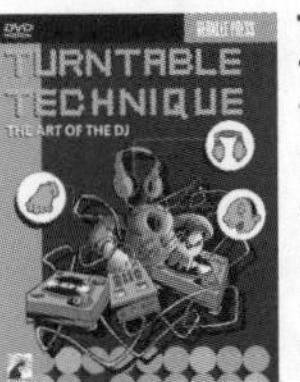

Turntable Technique: The Art of the DJ
Featuring Stephen Webber
Learn about basic equipment set-up, beat matching, creative mixing skills, and scratching techniques like cutting, stabs, crabs and flares.

DVD $29.95 HL50448025
VIDEO $19.95 HL50448026

The Ultimate Practice Guide for Vocalists
Featuring Donna McElroy
Learn to use the whole body to become the best singer you can be. Includes simple everyday exercises to increase vocal strength and endurance.

DVD $19.95 HL50448017

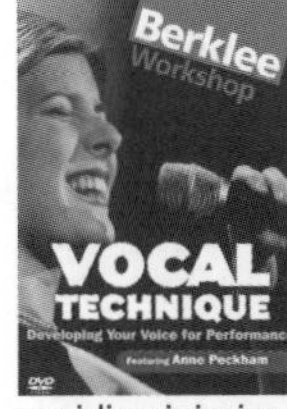

Vocal Technique: Developing Your Voice for Performance
Featuring Anne Peckham
Gain technical and expressive command of your voice while avoiding injuries and maximizing your vocal potential.

DVD $19.95 HL50448038

BOOKS

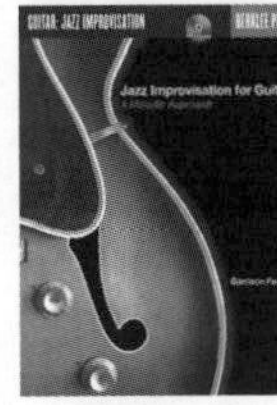

Jazz Improvisation for Guitar A Melodic Approach
By Garrison Fewell
Build solos from chord tones and melodic extensions, using guide tones to connect melodic ideas and "play the changes."

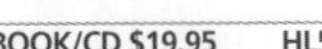

BOOK/CD $19.95 HL50449503

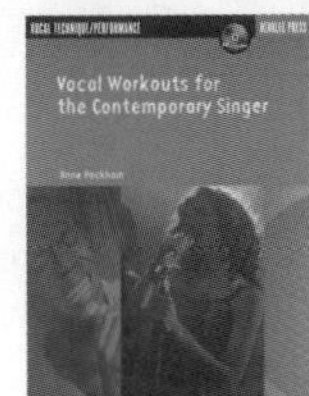

Vocal Workouts for the Contemporary Singer
By Anne Peckham
Warm up before you sing and continually develop the range, power, and expressive scope of your voice with this essential workout book and CD.

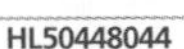

BOOK/CD $19.95 HL50448044

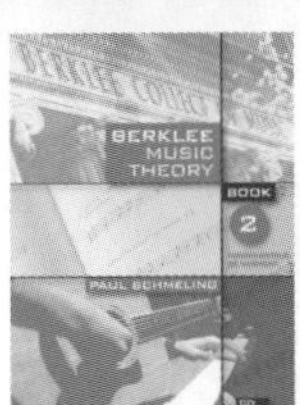

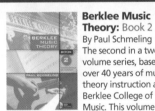

Berklee Music Theory: Book 2
By Paul Schmeling
The second in a two-volume series, based on over 40 years of music theory instruction at Berklee College of Music. This volume focuses on harmony and voice leading.

BOOK/CD $19.95 HL50448062

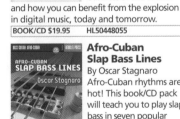

The Future of Music Manifesto for the Digital Music Revolution
By David Kusek and Gerd Leonhard
Discover the top 10 truths about the music business of the future and how you can benefit from the explosion in digital music, today and tomorrow.

BOOK/CD $19.95 HL50448055

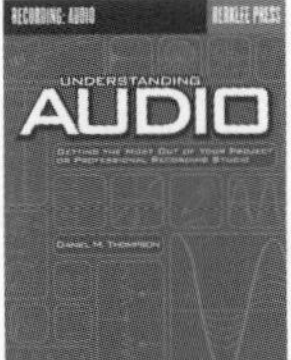

Understanding Audio Getting the Most out of Your Project or Professional Recording Studio
By Daniel M. Thompson
Develop a thorough understanding of the underlying principles of sound. Learn how equipment setup affects the quality of your recordings.

BOOK $24.95 HL50449456

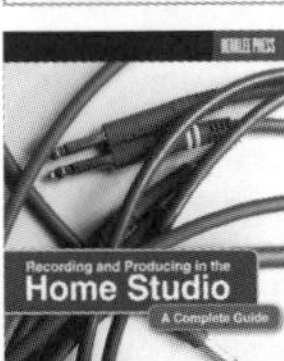

Recording and Producing in the Home Studio A Complete Guide
By David Franz
This comprehensive guide will show you how to create the highest quality recordings by teaching fundamental production skills and engineering techniques.

BOOK $24.95 HL50449498

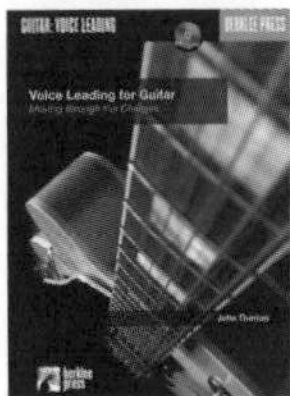

Voice Leading for Guitar Moving Through the Changes
By John Thomas
Berklee Associate Professor of Guitar John Thomas shows you how to voice lead both chord tones and tensions, and will help you add a new level of sophistication to your music.

BOOK/CD $24.95 HL50449498

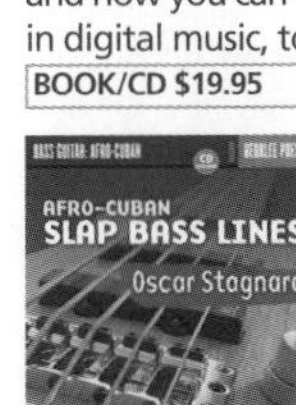

Afro-Cuban Slap Bass Lines
By Oscar Stagnaro
Afro-Cuban rhythms are hot! This book/CD pack will teach you to play slap bass in seven popular Afro-Cuban styles.

BOOK/CD-ROM $19.95 HL50449512

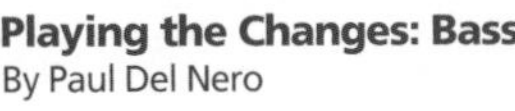

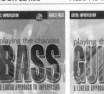

Playing the Changes: Bass
By Paul Del Nero

Playing the Changes: Guitar
By Mitch Seidman and Paul Del Nero

Each book/CD pack presents a unique improvisation strategy based on ear training and a linear interpretation of note/chord relationships.

HL50449510 HL50449509 EACH BOOK/CD $19.95

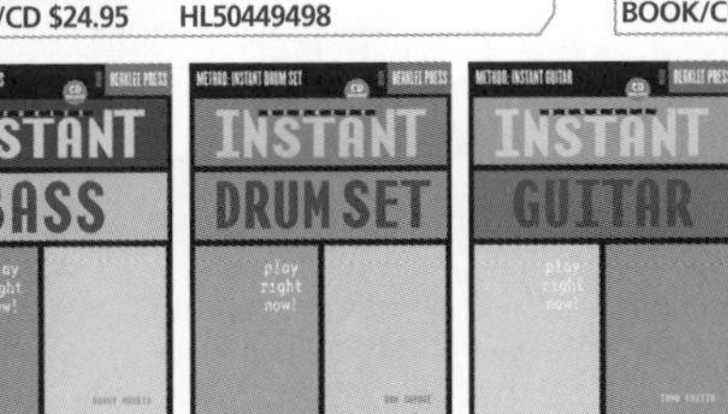

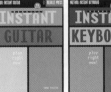

BERKLEE INSTANT SERIES
Absolute beginners can learn to play instantly with this revolutionary method! Each book/CD pack includes a wealth of playing tips, a jam-along CD and much more.

HL50449502 HL50449513 HL50449522 HL50449525 EACH BOOK/CD $14.95

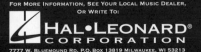

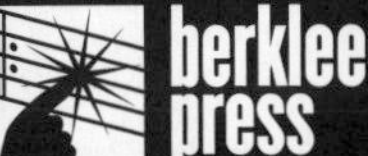

as serious about music as you are.
866-berklee (237-5533) berkleepress.com

For More Information, See Your Local Music Dealer, Or Write To:

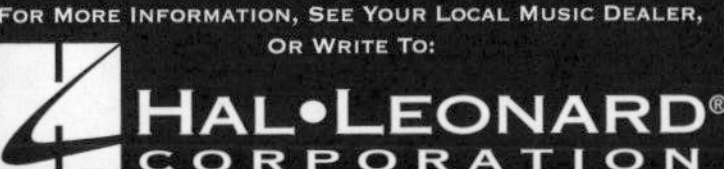

7777 W. Bluemound Rd. P.O. Box 13819 Milwaukee, WI 53213